Dr. Susan Love's Menopause and Hormone Book

ALSO BY SUSAN M. LOVE, M.D., WITH KAREN LINDSEY

Dr. Susan Love's Breast Book

DR. SUSAN LOVE'S MENOPAUSE AND HORMONE BOOK

MAKING INFORMED CHOICES

Previously published as *Dr. Susan Love's Hormone Book*

SUSAN M. LOVE, M.D., WITH KAREN LINDSEY

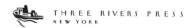
THREE RIVERS PRESS
NEW YORK

Grateful acknowledgement is made to the following for permission to use specified material:

John Boik: Table 10.1: "Natural Agents That Affect Hormone Bioavailability" from *Cancer and Natural Medicine* by John Boik. Reprinted by permission.

Key Porter Books, Dutton Signet, a division of Penquin Books USA Inc., and Janine O'Leary Cobb: Table 3.1: "Menopausal Ailments" from *Understanding Menopause* by Janine O'Leary Cobb. Copyright © 1988 by Key Porter Books. Copyright © 1993 by Janine O'Leary Cobb. Rights throughout the United States are controlled by Dutton Signet, a division of Penquin Books USA Inc. Reprinted by permission of Key Porter Books, Dutton Signet, a division of Penquin Books USA Inc., and Janine O'Leary Cobb.

Rodale Press, Inc.: Table from article entitled "Get Your Isoflavones Here" by Holly McCord, R.D., with Teresa Yeykal from *Prevention* magazine (August 1996). Copyright © 1996 by Rodale Press, Inc. Reprinted by periimission of Rodale Press, Inc. For subscription information, please call 1-800-666-2503.

Marcia Williams: Illustrations by Marcia Williams. Reprinted by permission of the illustrator.

Published by Three Rivers Press, New York, New York. Member of the Crown Publishing Group, a division of Random House, Inc.

www.randomhouse.com

THREE RIVERS PRESS is a registered trademark and the Three Rivers Press colophon is a trademark of Random House, Inc.

Originally published in hardcover in slightly different form as *Dr. Susan Love's Hormone Book* by Random House, Inc., New York, in 1997. A revised edition was subsequently published in paperback by Times Books, a division of Random House, Inc., New York, in 1998.

Printed in the United States of America

DESIGN BY ELINA D. NUDELMAN

Library of Congress Cataloging-in-Publication Data
Love, Susan M.
    Dr. Susan Love's menopause and hormone book: making informed choices / Susan M. Love with Karen Lindsey.
Includes index.
1. Menopause—Popular works. 2. Menopause—Hormone therapy—Popular works. I. Title: Doctor Susan Love's menopause and hormone book. II. Title: Menopause and hormone book. III. Lindsey, Karen, 1944-   IV. Title. [DNLM: 1. Menopause—Popular Works. 2. Estrogen Replacement Therapy—Popular Works. WP 120 L897d 2002]
RG186 .L683 2002
618.1'75061—dc21   2002015811

ISBN 0-609-80996-2

10 9 8 7 6 5 4 3 2 1

Revised Paperback Edition

This revised edition is dedicated to the courageous women who participated in the Women's Health Initiative and all of the other randomized controlled studies of menopause and its treatments. Your generous spirits will help countless women with the scientific data they need to make decisions about their lives.

CONTENTS

Acknowledgments

This second edition took almost as much work as the first. Karen Lindsey, my coauthor, has always cleaned up my writing and made sure that everything was understandable to the "science phobic" reader. I am thankful as always to my agent, Jill Kneerim, a constant source of support, wisdom, and encouragement. I also appreciate the work of Emily Loose, my editor.

Connie Long, my assistant, is the diligent detail person who makes sure that the references match. I thank her for her cheerful and willing spirit that keeps my life well managed and on an even keel. Ewa Witt is the wonderful person who gets me that one article I need when I need it. Her contribution is vital.

On top of the wonderful professionals who helped me with the first edition, I need to add Bruce Ettinger, Steve Cummings, Deborah Grady, Elizabeth Barrett-Connor, and Marcie Richardson. As always, the errors in fact or interpretation are mine but the wonderful insights are probably theirs.

I need in this edition to also thank all the women and men who stood by me when my position was criticized. They were willing to listen to the data and make up their own minds. It is their support that keeps me going.

The Susan Love MD Breast Cancer Research Foundation and the staff of www.SusanLoveMD.org are my work family now. Liz Thompson, Ada Lauren, Michelle Woodhouse, and all the members of the board of the foundation deserve thanks for their support for this work and their unflagging loyalty. Sue Rochman always keeps me abreast and challenged. Deborah Jenkins and John Carpenter keep the website working, and Judy Hirshfield-Bartek, Barbara Kalinowski, Sherry Goldman, and

Ellen Mahoney help me reach women all over the world with the answers to their most pressing questions.

Finally, I need to thank my family—especially my life partner of more than twenty years, Helen Sperry Cooksey, and our daughter, Katie Love-Cooksey. Their love and support are my foundation.

INTRODUCTION

We have entered a new age in women's health. As I write the update to this book I cannot help reflecting on all that has happened since the first edition. In 1997 I was cautioning women about hormone replacement therapy (HRT). I explained how we had not proven that hormones taken after menopause could decrease heart disease, Alzheimer's, or even the fractures that occur with osteoporosis. I pointed out the fears many of us had that long-term use of hormones might increase breast cancer. I felt like the kid in the story, yelling that the emperor might really be naked.

I was not alone in my position, but I certainly was a lightning rod for much of the criticism from doctors, the public, and the press. *The New Yorker* in June 1997 printed an article entitled "How Wrong Is Susan Love?" The American College of Obstetrics and Gynecology invited me to their annual meeting in New Orleans in May 1998 to debate the use of postmenopausal hormones and then attacked me personally and professionally rather than discuss the issues. I was accused of being anti-estrogen and having "oncovision"—that is, of being blinded to the benefits of hormones by my many years of taking care of women with breast cancer. As *Slate* magazine put it, "Love had been treated by much of the medical establishment as a dangerous New Age nut who'd forgotten to get out of the menstrual hut in time to take her own estrogen."[1]

Why did I go out on that limb? I had carefully researched the subject and found that estrogen and progestins, commonly and casually prescribed to women in the second half of their lives, needed a lot more studying. We really were not sure of the safety of these drugs nor of their benefits. I was optimistic about the Women's Health Initiative Study, begun in 1993 and scheduled to go on until 2006; the largest-ever study of its kind, it randomized 161,809 postmenopausal women from ages fifty to seventy-nine. It was set up to study estrogen alone, estrogen and progestin, as well as diet and calcium supplements. This study had been launched as a result of pressure from congresswomen, Bernadine Healy (then head of the National Institutes of Health), and women's health activists and would provide solid data on which we could make our decisions.

Well, my hopes were well founded. One of the parts of the Women's Health Initiative (WHI) was halted prematurely and abruptly in July 2002, creating a rush of headlines. The participants who were taking estrogen and progestin demonstrated more risks than benefits, and researchers did not want to risk harming any more women.

At least six million women in this country were aghast. "What happened?" they asked. Over the last several years they had read books and magazines, listened to TV pundits, and talked to doctors and friends, all of whom assured them that taking hormone replacement therapy for the rest of their lives would keep them healthy. Suddenly their world shifted. Their daily little wonder pill offered less health benefit than they'd been told—and worse, it brought with it the risk of a very scary disease. How could this be?

What happened is that medical practice, as it so often does, got ahead of the science. Researchers made observations and developed hypotheses . . . and then forgot to prove them. A combination of media hype and great marketing led the public and much of the medical profession to believe that the data were more solid than they were said to be. Hormone replacement therapy became the standard of care without the scientific underpinnings usually required before exposing so many people for so long to preventative drugs.

The research had, quite properly, begun with observational studies, in which groups of people are observed to see if there are any clues about a given disease. All that this kind of study can do is find associations: it can't prove cause and effect. As a first step, it's invaluable, pointing the way to future research. But it should never be taken as conclusive.

With HRT there were many observational studies. They all found that women on HRT had a lower incidence of heart disease, stroke, colon cancer, and fracture. It sounded wonderful. But it was treated by doctors and the media as though it was the answer, rather than a step toward the answer. No one had bothered to look at other possible causes for the women's good health, and yet those causes were there. These women were also more likely to see a doctor regularly (which is how they were put on HRT and got their prescriptions renewed), to exercise, and to eat a healthful diet than the women who were not taking HRT. Did hormones make women healthy, or did healthy women take hormones? To answer this question, we needed a randomized controlled study. One of the studies of the Women's Health Initiative (WHI) enrolled 16,608 healthy women from ages fifty to seventy-nine and randomly assigned them to take estrogen and progestin (Prempro) or placebo. Much to everyone's surprise, after 5.2 years this study showed that the risks of estrogen and progestins outweighed the benefits in preventing disease. (A separate study looking at estrogen alone in women who had undergone hysterectomies is still ongoing as planned and will be completed in 2006.)

Many are already arguing that the study was poorly designed, or that its results are limited to one type of HRT, or that "natural" or "bioidentical" hormones will be safe. The first argument is ridiculous: this is the most thorough kind of study medicine can do (as we discuss in Chapter 4). It is true that only Prempro was studied, but, as I hope we have learned, the fact that other formulations have not been studied does not mean that they are safe. We should assume that they are all dangerous until we have evidence otherwise. Any woman taking them long term outside of a study is being used as an unwitting guinea pig.

For me, the underlying question the study raises is the whole idea that we need to "replace" hormones long term. Menopause is normal. Women need high levels of hormones to reproduce; then we shift down to lower levels for the second half of life. Hot flashes and all the other symptoms of menopause are really symptoms not of low estrogen but of hormonal change: puberty in reverse. As with puberty, the symptoms are transient, usually lasting between three and four years. They vary enormously. Ten percent of women have no symptoms at all, and only 50 percent of women complain of hot flashes. For them, it is perfectly reasonable to take HRT for up to four years. At that point, a woman can either stop cold turkey (50 percent of women will do fine) or taper off gradually over several months. In only rare cases will a woman continue to have menopausal symptoms after her body has settled into its new rhythm.

Unfortunately, HRT has been marketed as a lifetime need for all women. Underlying all the controversy about HRT is the pernicious idea that menopause is a disease. We have been told that we were estrogen deficient and that nature didn't intend for us to live beyond our reproductive years. The ovaries were seen as expendable organs once reproduction was done. Diseases of aging, like heart disease and osteoporosis, were reclassified as diseases caused by menopause. And the standard of care was to give all women who had stopped menstruating the "replacement" that they needed to "be normal."

The studies of the last couple of years have punctured that bubble as well. It is amazing to me to hear former proponents of HRT now talking about individualized therapy, as opposed to the one-size-fits-all approach they had pushed for years. They are criticizing the WHI because it studied only one drug, ignoring the fact that this was the most common drug used to treat menopause in America. They talk about bioidentical hormones, or hormones more like the ones our own bodies make, contrasting them with the Premarin they have been prescribing for decades. They can't seem to give up the dream of a fountain of youth—a cure for the "disease" of being women who grow old. I don't think it will turn out to be any more real than the last panacea. In fact, most of the plant-based bioidentical hormones are "bioidentical" to the hormones our bodies make pre-menopausally—not what is natural postmenopausally. There are no data showing these are any safer than the nonbioidentical ones. We hear about "low doses" of hormones, but the data we have tell us only that lower doses work, not that they are safe in long-term use. The former proponents of HRT criticize the study because the women who were randomized were in their sixties and their risks of chronic diseases were really low. These are the same experts who accepted without criticism the observational data suggesting that *all* women without a contraindication should be on HRT for the rest of their lives. Finally, there are some menopause experts who are blaming the progestin. This is based on the fact that the estrogen–alone study is still ongoing. This means only that it has not yet reached a point where risk is higher than benefit. It does not mean that estrogen alone will prove to be safe or beneficial. The studies of women with heart disease have shown the same risk in women on estrogen alone as on estrogen and progestin. In addition, the observational studies have shown that estrogen alone increases breast cancer as well, just at a lower rate. It is very likely that when the estrogen–alone study is completed, it will show a risk-benefit ratio similar to that of estrogen and progestin.

Most researchers are now agreeing with my statements of 1997 that the only value of HRT is for women with severe symptoms and then only for a few years. Chronic diseases of aging, such as heart disease and osteoporosis, are better prevented with lifestyle changes and drugs that have been proven to work in randomized controlled studies such as statins and bisphosphonates. What a sea change!

In the wake of the newer studies, many women feel betrayed and confused, and they are right. But they should also be cheering. We finally have data on which to make decisions regarding the long-term use of hormones. And more data are forthcoming as many studies now in progress come to fruition.

It is scientific data that has allowed this edition to have less hedging and more recommendations. Medicine is always a work in progress—and the progress in this field is reflected in almost every page.

Aside from the dangers of long-term estrogen and progestin use, what have we learned since 1997? For one thing, the connection of cholesterol and heart disease is being questioned. There is increasing evidence that homocysteine and inflammation may be serious components, explaining the value of multivitamins and baby aspirin. The WHI added fuel to this debate when it showed that while Prempro (the commonly used estrogen-progestin combination) did indeed lower cholesterol, it actually increased heart attacks. Does this mean that cholesterol doesn't matter or that something else matters more? In this situation we have drugs (statins such as Lipitor and Zocor) that have been shown in randomized controlled studies to decrease heart attacks, but we are not completely sure we know how they work.

The bone-density test has taught us a lot about osteoporosis. On the one hand, we now have a way of diagnosing low bone density early, while on the other, we don't always know what to do about it. We have drugs that will stop bone loss, but we still don't know their long-term safety. Should we be treating osteopenia (weak bones) with drugs such as Fosamax (bisphosphonates) that stay in the bones permanently? We don't really know since these drugs have been used for only a few years. Concerns based on animal studies are causing a shift in the recommendations. Experts now suggest that women wait until age sixty-five to have a bone-density test, at which point it will be clearer whether they are truly at risk for fractures. In addition, they are suggesting that treatment may be better reserved for actual osteoporosis rather than osteopenia. It is also crucial that the two conditions be defined distinctly: *osteopenia* is often referred to as *osteoporosis*.

Breast cancer treatments and risk determination have changed, with new techniques such as ductal lavage able to help determine which women are at high risk and might benefit from prevention strategies such as tamoxifen and preventative mastectomy. New drugs such as raloxifene (Evista) are being tested as preventative agents. And lots of research is going on to figure out the relationship between estrogen and progestin and breast cancer.

There has been more research on Alzheimer's disease, suggesting that it may be caused by inflammation, and such research should lead us to better ways to help prevent the disease.

Even the ways we understand symptoms of menopause have seen some changes, as studies document women's experiences over time rather than just survey their complaints in the doctor's office. *Perimenopause* is the new term for the unstable time prior to the last period. Is this just increasing PMS as we head toward the end of cycling or a separate biological state? We will talk about our current understanding of the biology and what you can expect. Your options for treating symptoms will be reviewed from drugs to herbs with a discussion of the data that support their use. There are, for example, new nonhormonal approaches identified in randomized controlled studies to treat hot flashes in women who can't take estrogen. These include low-dose antidepressants and herbal remedies. I have reviewed the new dosages and types of hormonal therapies in this edition, including the "relationship-saving" vaginal sustained-release estrogens such as Estring and Vagifem.

With the Women's Health Initiative estrogen and progestin study halted prematurely, the whole notion of the value of long-term hormonal therapy after menopause for prevention of the diseases of aging has been called into question. The best approach continues to be lifestyle changes: not smoking, eating a healthful diet, and exercising regularly. We review strategies for getting your act together and becoming fit.

As the baby boomers move rapidly into midlife, we need to beware of the increased marketing of menopause by both pharmaceutical companies and supplement distributors. Isoflavones like soy are being added to everything with claims that they will solve all of your menopausal problems. Just as with HRT, if something sounds too good to be true, it is. Also compounds that are safe in food may not be as safe as supplements. We have to stay vigilant as new claims come out for all types of products in the wake of the first report of the Women's Health Initiative.

Luckily there are many ongoing studies looking at peri- and postmenopausal women that should guide us going forward. While I can't anticipate all the findings that will come, I can give you the background you will need to understand them, put them into context, and decide how they should affect your life.

All of this is discussed in depth in this new edition of *Doctor Susan Love's Menopause and Hormone Book.* It is my sincere hope that this book will give you the foundation to understand whatever comes along and to join with me in celebrating the fact that we are finally basing women's medicine on evidence rather than on wishful thinking.

(And keep an eye on my website, www.SusanLoveMD.org, for the latest news.)

ONE

WHAT IS MENOPAUSE?

Before we can discuss how to deal with menopause, we need to have a clear understanding of what it is. If menopause means "the time after your periods stop," why are you having hot flashes while you still have periods? What if you have had a hysterectomy—does that count as menopause? What if you never go through menopause: your doctor just puts you on hormones and you still get your periods?

STAGES OF MENOPAUSE

Some of this confusion exists because there are two different stages of the menopausal process. During *perimenopause*, your hormones are winding down, fluctuating, and often creating the mass of symptoms we think of, incorrectly, as "menopausal." (I'll discuss those symptoms in detail in Chapter 3.) In most cases these are self-limiting and will go away in a few years.

Then there's menopause itself—which is, strictly speaking, your last period (the permanent "pause" of your menses). In the aftermath of menopause, you may also experience some symptoms, but these are typically different from the symptoms of perimenopause. (Menopause itself, by the way, probably lasts for only a few days, and you can never be absolutely certain when it's occurred. Menopause is usually identified retrospectively, when it's been a year since your last period. Everything afterward is, strictly speaking, "postmenopause"—though for some reason this term has never existed as a noun.) To avoid ambiguity, in this book I'll comply with popular custom and continue to speak of menopausal women, menopausal symptoms, etc. Keep in mind that I'm referring to the time after that elusive moment when your last period ends.

The reason I'm making such a fuss about semantics is that terminology can cause a lot of needless fear. One of the reasons many women dread menopause is that they confuse the lesser, often nonexistent symptoms of menopause with the symptoms of perimenopause—and so they think that the most difficult, confusing symptoms will last the rest of their lives. In reality, the vast majority of women experience these two stages very differently.

A study done in 1965 found that, with the exception of hot flashes, the symptoms of perimenopausal women were closer to those of adolescents entering puberty than to those of postmenopausal women.[1] When adolescent girls experience weight gain, bloating, and mood changes, doctors assume it's because of high estrogen levels. When women around menopause get the same symptoms, the assumption is that it's caused by low estrogen. Yet it has seemed obvious to me for quite a while that the time right before menopause is the mirror image of puberty. During puberty, this mechanism is starting up. Then, at the other end, when the process is gearing down, the same things happen again. What these two life stages have in common is big hormonal shifts.

Times of hormonal shifts and changes are times of symptoms. Remember the highs and lows of puberty? Your face broke out. You slept half the day. Your brain didn't seem to work the way it used to. You didn't know what was going on with your body. Well, with perimenopause it happens all over again. This, too, is a time of symptoms in many women—hot flashes, mood swings, fuzzy thinking, insomnia, and, most of all, unpredictability. Fortunately, just as with puberty, these symptoms do end. The hot flashes dry up, just as the acne did. Your sleep patterns return to normal; your brain becomes able to focus again. Nothing lasts forever. Overall it takes about three to six years for each transition, until your body is balanced at a new place. (God help those of you who have teenage daughters going through puberty while you are going through perimenopause!)

Acknowledging the parallels between puberty and perimenopause makes the whole process less strange and scary. You've been through puberty. It may not have been fun, but you survived it. And you did it without any of the wisdom and coping skills you now have. Most of you also experienced the enormous hormonal shifts that accompany pregnancy and childbirth, and you got through those as well. There's no reason to fear perimenopause or menopause. It's just hormones again, and we all know how to deal with them.

Biology of Perimenopause: Puberty in Reverse

What exactly is going on in your body, bringing about all this change? In order to clearly define the phases of the menopausal transition, we need to review a little biology. Okay, I know there are those of you who want to skip the technical stuff—"I don't want a biology class—just tell me what to do!" Feel free to skip the next several paragraphs and pick up again on page 16. For those of you who want to know how it works, read on.

It's amazing to realize how little we actually know about the way a woman's body works. We do know, however, that hormones work together in a wonderful and intricate dance.

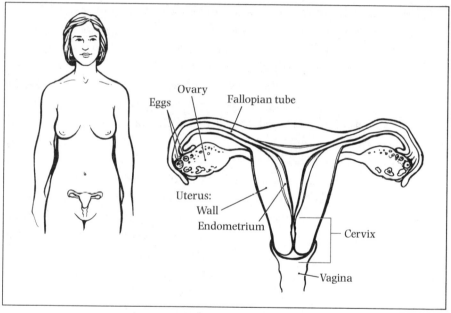

Figure 1.1. Female reproductive organs.

At birth your two ovaries contain all the eggs you'll have throughout your lifetime (Figure 1.1). The eggs sit there comfortably for several years; then you hit puberty and the beginning of your years of menstruation. Your hormone levels begin fluctuating wildly before settling down as you reach maturity. The major hormones involved in this process of puberty are follicle-stimulating hormone (FSH) and luteinizing hormone (LH), which come from the pituitary gland (a small gland that lives near the brain, between the eyes); and estrogen and progesterone, which come from the ovaries. In addition, the hypothalamus (part of the brain) produces gonadotrophic-releasing hormones (GnRHs). (Are you still with me? One friend who read this chapter said it was great until she saw FSH, and then her eyes glazed over. And she is a doctor!)

Now you've left puberty, and you're in your fertile years. Here's basically what goes on for the next three decades. Stimulated by FSH, the follicles (the eggs encased in their little sacs) produce estrogen. When estrogen rises to a certain level, the hypothalamus gets the message and secretes LH-releasing hormone, which tells the pituitary to turn off the FSH and produce a surge of LH. When the LH is at its peak, you ovulate—that is, your body releases an egg from the follicle. The follicle shifts to a new phase (the corpus luteum) and starts to produce progesterone in addition to estrogen. These hormones build up the lining of the uterus. The corpus luteum is short-lived, and its production of hormones soon begins to decline. Once the progesterone in your blood drops to a certain level, you get rid of the uterine lining by getting your period. In addition, these lower levels of estrogen and progesterone tell the hypothalamus to get some FSH going, and the cycle continues. Every month (except for those few months when you're pregnant), your body goes through this familiar dance.

It can take a while for this dance of hormones to get its choreography down (Figure 1.2). One study confirmed that earlier on, girls have longer periods.[2] The follicles don't mature, and there may be a longer time between periods. This seems to be in part because the ovaries aren't yet really producing eggs, and egg production is necessary for a regular "loop" to be completed. Once the whole system gets coordinated, a girl's cycles become regular and her symptoms settle.

This dance, like most dances, has a few variations. In some months, you don't ovulate. Then there's no progesterone, and your period may actually come early and be lighter or later, or you may skip a period altogether. Your body also requires a certain amount of fat to ovulate; if you're very thin or anorexic, or an athlete who is very muscular with very little fat, you will often lose your period and in essence be in temporary menopause. This time it is literally a "pause," because you'll get your periods back once your fat level increases.

So far, so good. But our understanding of the process gets a little fuzzier when you come to the end of your fertile years. The standard line in the textbooks is that when you run out of eggs and you're no longer

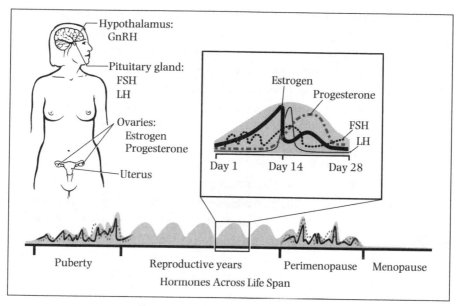

Figure 1.2. The hormonal dance.

ovulating, your body stops making estrogen. This causes your FSH to go up as your pituitary tries to kick start the ovary into producing more eggs. When that doesn't work, everything just shuts down.

Yet often the symptoms of perimenopause (breast tenderness, head-aches, increased vaginal lubrication) are symptoms not of low estrogen but rather of *high* estrogen. Some recent studies have looked more deeply into what may explain this phenomenon. A study in 1989 fol-lowed five perimenopausal women, one of whom had occasional periods every six weeks.[3] Fortunately, the researchers were monitoring her while this was going on. They discovered that she had low estrogen in the beginning of her cycle. Her ovaries were just tired. As a result of the low estrogen, she had symptoms such as hot flashes for a couple of weeks. Meanwhile, her hypothalamus and pituitary responded to these low lev-els by increasing her FSH. Her ovaries woke up in a panic, as though they had been sleeping on the job, and decided to make up for their inat-tention by sending out lots more estrogen—two to three times the nor-mal amount. And then she ovulated. Now her symptoms were those of high estrogen—breast tenderness, etc. Her progesterone went up after ovulation, and her period came exactly two weeks late and was very heavy, because of the extra estrogen. You can see why life at this stage is so unpredictable. (While working on this book, I experienced exactly the same cycle as the woman in the study and was relieved to know exactly what was going on.)

This is often what happens in perimenopause. Sometimes your estrogen levels are high and your progesterone is low, and you might get symptoms of PMS. At other times, your estrogen levels shift and you get hot flashes. Then for several months you're back to normal. So the common explanation—that your symptoms are due to low estrogen—is wrong. Your symptoms are actually caused by *fluctuations* of high and low estrogen.[4]

This also explains why you can't just get a blood test, as some doctors suggest, to tell if you are in perimenopause. Because your FSH goes up with menopause (once your periods have stopped for a year), some doctors will measure your FSH level in perimenopause, hoping to determine whether or not your symptoms are related to menopause. If your FSH is low, they tell you you're not in menopause and they don't know what your symptoms are from. If your FSH is high, they say you're menopausal—even if you're still menstruating.

Are they crazy? No. They simply don't understand perimenopause. A study in 1994 confirmed that perimenopausal women show varying patterns.[5] Some women in the study still menstruated, even with increased levels of FSH. Some had increased FSH and normal to low estrogen. Some continued having cycles and had abrupt fluctuations of both FSH and estrogen. Some had typical postmenopausal levels one month and typical premenopausal levels the next month. So testing FSH isn't a really definitive tool for determining your menopausal status.

If you've stopped menstruating for several months, the FSH test might be a little more useful for determining if you've really gone into menopause. But even then it's not 100 percent accurate. Another study found that 20 percent of women who have no period for three months start having their cycles again.[6] I've had patients with breast cancer who were thrown into menopause by their chemotherapy treatments, missed three or four months of periods, and showed high FSH levels—and then got their periods back. There's no foolproof test to determine menopause. The only way we can really do that is the good old-fashioned way. If you haven't menstruated for a year, you're menopausal.

Biology of Menopause: The Misunderstood Ovary

In a way, you can't blame the doctors for failing to understand what the ovary does in perimenopause. Throughout most of medical history, we have never really understood the ovary itself, and because we haven't grasped the full complexity of this intricate organ, doctors have assumed that after menopause, when the ovary is no longer capable of reproduction, it shrivels up, dries out, and becomes completely useless.

Actually, this misunderstanding can serve as a metaphor for the way our culture sees the postmenopausal woman herself—as nonproductive, dried up, and useless. This is consistent with the common definition of menopause as "ovarian failure." With the assumption that the ovary's sole function is to produce eggs comes an inevitable corollary: when it stops doing that, it's "failed."

In fact, making eggs isn't the ovary's whole function, any more than reproduction is a woman's whole function. The ovary is more than just an egg sac. It's an endocrine organ—an organ that produces hormones. And it produces hormones before, during, and after menopause. With menopause, the ovary goes through a shift. It changes from a follicle-rich producer of estrogen and progesterone to a stromal-rich producer of estrogen and androgen. Stroma is the glue that holds the eggs together. In youth, you have more eggs and less stroma. As time goes on, you have fewer and fewer eggs but more and more stroma. In its hormonal dance with the hypothalamus and pituitary, the postmenopausal ovary continues to respond to the call of the pituitary. It responds to high levels of FSH and LH with increased production of testosterone as well as continued lower levels of the estrogens estrone and estradiol and the estrogen precursor androstenedione.[7] (I'll discuss this in Chapter 15.) The hormonal dance doesn't end; the band just strikes up a different tune.

Testosterone is, of course, a male hormone. But don't panic: you're not going to grow a heavy beard. Every human being produces both male and female hormones; the proportion differs according to your gender. Much of the testosterone and androstenedione is converted to estrone (a form of estrogen) by an enzyme called aromatase found in fat and muscle. This continued production of hormones varies somewhat from one woman to the next and may well explain some of the individual differences in symptoms after menopause. It also explains why women who have both ovaries removed surgically, thereby losing all of these hormones, have worse symptoms of menopause and increased vulnerability to osteoporosis and cardiovascular disease.[8]

Jane Cauley, a researcher on menopause, measured hormone levels in the blood of postmenopausal women.[9] She found a lot of variability, but interestingly, neither age nor time since menopause had much to do with it. Hormone production doesn't automatically dwindle with age. Obesity, defined as being at least 20 percent over your ideal weight, was a major determinant of estrogen levels in postmenopausal women. The estrogen levels of obese women were 40 percent higher than those of nonobese women. This is because aromatase is found in fat. However, obesity wasn't the only determinant. Women who were physically active also had higher blood levels of estrone. Although some active women had lower levels of estrogen (because they were thinner), paradoxically, those with more muscle mass had higher estrogen levels. This is probably because muscle also has a large amount of aromatase. In fact, outside of the ovary, the aromatase in muscle accounts for the conversion of 25 to 30 percent of androgens to estrogens, while the aromatase in fat accounts for only 10 to 15 percent.[10] Other organs that have this enzyme include the brain, skin, hair, and bone marrow. Some organs, like the breast, can make their own local estrogen. Studies show that in postmenopausal women, the fluid in the breast duct can have forty times more estrogen than the blood.[11] So we're not left without hormones after menopause. Our misunderstood ovaries continue to be productive.

In fact, Bruce Ettinger, M.D., of Kaiser Permanente, reported in Boston at the North American Menopause Society Meeting in September 1997 that they had studied estrogen levels in the blood of older women. They found that a number of women had levels between 5 and 25 picograms: these women had half the fracture rate of those women who naturally had levels less than 5 picograms. Not all women are "estrogen deficient," after all.

What this all means is that our ovaries serve more than one function. Reproduction is their most dramatic function, but it isn't the only one. These organs have as much to do with the maintenance of a woman's own life as they do with her role in bringing other lives into the world. The menopausal ovary is neither failing nor useless. It's simply beginning to shift from its reproductive to its maintenance function. It's doing in midlife exactly what many people do—it's changing careers.

PREMATURE MENOPAUSE

Some women go through menopause in their thirties—an unusually young age. This is called premature menopause. Just as you can start your period early (any time after age nine) and still be normal, you can normally stop menstruating early. Like surgical menopause, which we will discuss below, this leaves you at greater risk for bone loss and higher cholesterol levels. So you might want to take hormones until you reach fifty, the average age of menopause. You can then gradually taper off, mimicking a natural menopause.

SURGICAL MENOPAUSE

Up to now, we've been talking about natural menopause—that is, what happens to a woman on her own, as she ages without intervention. But there are other ways to go into menopause. The most dramatic is to have both of your ovaries removed. This is called a bilateral oophorectomy, and it may be done independently or together with a hysterectomy—surgical removal of the uterus. Removing the ovaries will result in an immediate menopause. Not only do you experience an onslaught of symptoms because of the sudden change in hormones, but you lose most of your hormones permanently. You don't lose all of them, however. The adrenal gland also produces androstenedione and a little bit of testosterone. This androstenedione is converted to estrogen in fat and muscle. For some women, particularly those who are obese or muscular, this may be enough to counteract symptoms. For others it is not. In addition, there are some data indicating that women who have their ovaries removed have higher rates of osteoporosis and heart disease, even on hormone therapy.[12]

Sometimes only one ovary is removed. If the remaining ovary continues to function, you'll go through menopause at the normal time. But sometimes the remaining ovary stops functioning prematurely (perhaps because of injury to its blood supply during surgery), and you experience premature menopause.

Finally, you may have your uterus out but still retain both ovaries. In that case, as we discuss in Chapter 11, you may go through menopause earlier or right on time. But how will you know? Since you're no longer menstruating, you won't have any missed periods to show that you're approaching menopause. You may get hot flashes, night sweats, or any of the other symptoms we discuss in Chapter 3. But suppose you don't have any symptoms? Generally, you can figure that you'll have gone through menopause somewhere between ages forty-eight and fifty-three. You can consider estrogen therapy if you're suffering from symptoms. You shouldn't wait, however, to adopt a healthy lifestyle. The sooner you start with that, the more it will help prevent all kinds of diseases, whenever you actually go through menopause.

MEDICAL MENOPAUSE

There are other forms of menopause brought on by forces outside your own body.

Certain drugs block the gonadotropin-releasing factors that stimulate FSH and LH, which can put you into a reversible menopause. They include Lupron and Synarel, which are usually given for short periods of time to treat endometriosis or to shrink fibroids before surgery. Zoladex, too, can create temporary menopause, and it is now being used for this purpose in premenopausal women who have estrogen receptor positive breast cancer. Very often women who have been treated for cancer with chemotherapy go into temporary or permanent menopause. Fifty-seven percent of premenopausal women have hot flashes while on adjuvant chemotherapy. The drugs can create a chemically induced menopause, with hormonal changes, hot flashes, emotional mood swings, and the absence of a period. Many women don't know this ahead of time and are startled and distressed at suddenly having to cope with this unexpected situation in the midst of already distressing treatment. A woman of forty-five who receives chemotherapy has an 80 percent likelihood of going into menopause as a result of the chemicals—a much greater percentage than is the case with tamoxifen. A thirty-five-year-old woman has a 20 percent chance of becoming permanently menopausal.

We don't really know what happens in women who have chemical menopause. Does the chemotherapy completely destroy the ovaries so they never produce anything again? Or does it simply throw the woman into regular menopause, so she gets postmenopausal levels of hormone production? We do know that women around thirty who get chemotherapy often go into temporary menopause and get their periods back. This might mean that the chemicals don't totally wipe out the ovaries' ability to produce hormones but simply push the middle-aged woman in the direction she's already heading. Thus these women who are apparently thrown into permanent menopause may still have some ovarian hormone production. Or it may mean that some of them do and some don't. This is an area we simply need to study more. Chemical menopause has not been well studied. Nonetheless, it appears that with medical menopause the severity of symptoms is somewhere between that associated with surgical menopause and that associated with natural menopause. If the chemotherapy was given for a nonhormonal cancer such as Hodgkin's disease, colon cancer, or lung cancer, then short-term use of hormones may be considered for symptom relief. More controversial is the use of HRT for women with endometrial (uterine) cancer, ovarian cancer, or breast cancer. Although there are a few studies going on to see if this is indeed safe, most clinicians are leary of using hormones in these situations. The increasing use of chemotherapy for premenopausal women with breast cancer has swelled the ranks of medically menopausal women and led to more studies on alternatives to estrogen for symptom relief (see page 192). It is an important area of research that will potentially help all women.

Radiation for colon cancer can also create menopause. In this situation the menopause is permanent.

WHY DO WE HAVE MENOPAUSE?

The Theory That "We Weren't Supposed to Live This Long"

The pervasive assumption that the postreproductive ovary is useless probably ties in with our culture's generally negative attitude toward aging. There is a widely held misconception, based on a misreading of statistics, that old age itself is unnatural—that we're not meant to live long enough to go into menopause. According to this argument, in the old days, before human intelligence created artificial, life-prolonging environments, people died of "old age" at thirty or forty. Since we've artificially extended life, we need artificial tools to help make the extra years bearable. Thus we need hormone replacement to address the illnesses resulting from a life that should have been over long ago.

But "average life expectancy" doesn't mean the age at which people usually die. It means something quite different. It's determined by adding together all ages of death and then dividing them by the number of people who died. If many people die young, you'll have a low average life expectancy. For example, the average life expectancy in 1640 was thirty-two. This was a time of high infant mortality and widespread poverty that caused malnutrition and the deadly exhaustion from constant work with no time for rest. Among the wealthy, those "who survived to twenty-one could expect to live into the early 60s."[13] It appears that a fairly large percentage of people lived into healthy old age, in fact. During the Renaissance, men in most European countries were considered fit for military service until they were sixty.[14] A late-sixteenth-century English chronicler estimated that in most villages 10 percent of the inhabitants were sixty or older. Antonia Fraser, in *The Weaker Vessel*, cites numerous examples of seventeenth-century Englishwomen who lived into their nineties and beyond: "It would not be so much the lack of aged persons as the lack of a large middle-aged group which would surprise us about the seventeenth century," Fraser writes.[15]

"Nature," then, has no particular objection to our living past our fertility.

In the article "Overview on Menopause," researcher Wulf Utian offers a look at some of the history of this stage of life. "Menopause," he tells us, "was recognized as a stage in human life at least as far back as the biblical era. Abraham in Genesis acknowledged the fact of reproductive failure when he pondered the prospect that a couple who were 190 years old would be granted offspring."[16] It's unlikely that people really did live for two hundred years or more, but this does suggest that they routinely lived past their fertility—that women lived past menopause. Further, Utian notes, Aetius of Amida, writing in the sixth century, observed that women usually menstruated until forty-five, rarely continuing past fifty. He said nothing to suggest that it was strange for a woman to live this long—as he surely would have if most women died before forty. He attributed variations in menstrual activity to age, season of the year, the woman's eating habits and other activities, and the presence of complicating diseases.

The fact that the ovary is an organ with two distinct life phases—first as a source of eggs, then as a maintenance organ—also gives the lie to the idea that nature didn't intend us to live this long. If we were all supposed to be dead by menopause, there would be no natural purpose in the ovary's switching gears like this. It would simply stop working—just as popular mythology believes it does. But it doesn't; it simply starts its new job.

The Grandmother Hypothesis

The anthropologist Margaret Lock, among others, has pondered why menopause exists—from an evolutionary perspective.[17] Why, she asks, is women's fertility limited when men's is not? What advantage is created for survival when women live on after their fertility is over? From studying hunter-gatherer societies, anthropologists have come up with the "grandmother hypothesis."[18] Human children need to be cared for over a long period of time, and so women who were fertile their whole lives would not be able to care as well for their later children. In addition, society needed a group of nonfertile women who could serve as teachers and child care workers and gatherers of food while fertile women were busy having babies. These women, the "grandmothers," were the core of a society and served a necessary function in propagating and maintaining the tribe.

But this theory of evolutionarily predestined grandmothers has little currency in cultures that devalue age. In the United States, we've been particularly prone to this. We deny most of what's good about old age. We deny the elderly their sexuality at the same time that we define sexuality as all-important. We pat the grandmother on the head and send her Hallmark cards, without really acknowledging the deep joys she can have both in her role as grandmother and outside of it. We treat old age as a shameful condition, not as a passage in life. Instead of offering respect for old age, we offer illusions of eternal youth.

I am not trying to deny all the problems that come with aging, or to pretend that aging is all fun. You may lose strength as you grow old. You're susceptible to many more illnesses than when you're young—and you're closer to the inevitability of death. But wisdom, life experience, and the ease of having passed through certain phases of your life and knowing who and where you are—all these have their own value.

MENOPAUSE AS A METAMORPHOSIS

Susun Weed, in her book *The Menopausal Years: The Wise Woman Way*, describes menopause as a metamorphosis, a time when you truly change from one person to another, just as you did at puberty.[19] Such a change is never fun, or even comfortable, but the end result in growth and maturity is usually worthwhile. And indeed we are leading new lives, whether they appear so in clear-cut life changes or not. Often a perimenopausal woman will say, "I don't feel like my old self." To the extent that this means she's feeling unwell, or that she's disoriented by symptoms, the feeling will eventually go away as she moves into and past menopause itself.

But on a deeper level, she feels this way because she isn't her old self—any more than the twelve-year-old adolescent is the eight-year-old she was before, or any more than the twenty-year-old is the twelve-year-old or the forty-year-old is the twenty-year-old. Menopause is a transition into a new part of your life: some of your old self will remain—or will return when your symptoms quiet down—and some of it will fade away as it's replaced by new ideas, interests, attitudes, and abilities.

Germaine Greer talks about our truest self emerging from the "chrysalis of conditioning"[20] only after menopause has liberated us from our reproductive bodies. Ursula Le Guin writes that "the woman who is willing to make that change must become pregnant with herself."[21]

I think that's an important consideration when you're thinking about taking hormones—especially if you're considering taking them for the rest of your life. If you never experience this change, something gets stunted. Certainly it makes sense to alleviate any overwhelming symptoms. But it seems to me that at some point, you want to experience the transition, to go through it literally to get to that other place. It's a bit like childbirth. Most of us don't want the drug-induced "twilight sleep" our mothers may have had, where they never knew what happened but simply woke up to find a newborn in their arms. Today, some women choose natural childbirth; others want an epidural to help them along; but most women want to experience giving birth if they can. Even puberty is worth experiencing. I think of the young kids using alcohol, pot, even stronger drugs rather than living through the painful, terrifying, unpredictable experiences of adolescence. You blot out the pain, yes—but at what cost to your spirit? You can create for yourself a state of suspended animation, without pain or confusion, but also without joy, without growth, without discovery.

A NEW PARADIGM

As you can see, how you look at menopause is all in the framing. As long as we refer to menopause as "ovarian failure," "reproductive failure," or "estrogen-deficiency disease," we will have negative feelings and expectations about it. But if we view it as a hormonal shift mirroring puberty, it begins to look much different. As I thought about this concept, I began to see another way to frame women's lives.

Recent studies on young girls have shown that they are full of themselves. (I'm the mother of a fourteen-year-old girl: I didn't need the studies to figure that out!) They have lots of self-esteem and they are on top of the world. Then, when puberty hits, they lose it. They become timid.

They do less well in school. They become insecure about their bodies. They're not the fearless world-beaters they once were.

Meanwhile, at the other end, what happens to postmenopausal women? Occasionally they get worn down by society's devaluation of them, and they end up mirroring the forlorn figures in the estrogen ads. But when they're able to break through that image, they blossom. They feel themselves capable of changing the world. They no longer feel constrained by the dictates of finding a man for reproduction. They come into their own. Margaret Mead called this stage of life "postmenopausal zest." It has often been postmenopausal women who become leaders—Golda Meir, Indira Gandhi, Margaret Thatcher, Eleanor Roosevelt. It was postmenopausal women who helped get us the right to vote.

What does this say? Maybe the problem isn't estrogen deficiency after menopause—maybe it's too much estrogen before. Dare I say "estrogen poisoning"? Maybe the only way women can become docile enough to couple and reproduce is if they are under the influence of domesticating hormones. Biologically, this would mandate forty years of having cycles. But maybe when our biological responsibility is taken care of, we're allowed to be freed of those domesticating hormones and can reclaim our ten-year-old self again, full of beans and ready to take on the world.

I know you're laughing—or at least smiling. Who knows what's true? But doesn't this view make you feel a whole lot better about menopause?

The time has come for us to reclaim menopause from those who try to define it for us—and to look squarely at those who wish to medicalize it.

TWO

THE MEDICALIZATION OF MENOPAUSE

MENOPAUSE AS THE NEWEST DISEASE

We've seen it before. Childbirth was once considered natural. Women gave birth at home, attended by midwives. Then, during our grandmothers' times, childbirth moved from home to hospital, and midwives were replaced by doctors. The results weren't uniformly disastrous: for one thing, infant and maternal mortality were greatly reduced. But better prenatal care would have had an even greater effect while still allowing women to control their own birth processes. And the rate of cesareans went up with hospital births.

As Western culture has become more and more high-tech, so has birthing. Fetal monitors are used routinely. If you don't get ultrasound, chorionic villus sampling (the newest technique for prenatal diagnosis), or amniocentesis, you are made to feel you are somehow neglecting your baby. The medical profession is slowly recognizing that many women don't like this medicalizing approach, and so there has been a boom in birthing rooms, made to look just like your bedroom at home—but all the high-tech machines are still present, carefully hidden from view.

The medical profession even tried to medicalize puberty. Many of us were put on birth control pills during puberty to "regulate" our cycles—but the cycle is supposed to be irregular at that point of our lives.

And in the recent past there has been a strong push to medicalize menopause. Interestingly, as Sandra Coney points out in *The Menopause Industry*, the medical profession's concept of "treating" menopause was shaped by the advent of tranquilizers and antidepressants in the 1950s. These drugs were first used primarily in mental hospitals, but "there was a bigger market waiting to be tapped and the pharmaceutical companies were not slow to realize it. By the early 1960s, psychotropics were widely promoted to doctors as being ideal for middle-aged women and able to 'cure' the 'symptoms of menopause.'"[1] Though the widespread prescribing of tranquilizers for housewives was soon abandoned, a subtle change had taken place in the public's thought process. Menopause was considered an illness to be treated.

The next step was to shift from the mind to the body. These women weren't crazy, just sickly: they just had "estrogen-deficiency disease." One might think that if estrogen deficiency were really a disease, the doctors would have declared all men chronically ill. But no, this disease was a result of a particularly feminine problem defined in the gynecology textbooks as "reproductive failure" or "ovarian failure." Women in midlife were therefore defined as sick failures—and this notion continues to dominate medical thinking.

It's an ugly and dangerous notion, equating a natural stage in a woman's life with illness. It echoes age-old attitudes about the "uncleanness" of menstruation and childbirth. While men go from youth to adulthood to old age, women progress from uncleanness to disease.

To be fair to the doctors of the mid-twentieth century, they were following a misogynist tradition dating back two hundred years. Earlier descriptions of menopause were fairly matter-of-fact. But by the 1700s, according to Wulf Utian, editor of the journal *Menopause,* doctors began sounding gloomy about menopause.[2] By 1845 a man named Colombat de l'Isère was warning postmenopausal women not to allow themselves to have erotic feelings, since no one could possibly respond to them: "Their features are stamped with the impression of age and their genital organs are sealed with the signet of sterility."[3]

This image has never died out. Over a century later, the gynecologist Robert Wilson wrote a spectacularly popular book called *Feminine Forever.*[4] Its cover boldly described the book as a "fully-documented discussion of one of medicine's most revolutionary breakthroughs—the discovery that menopause is a hormone deficiency disease, curable and totally preventable." (I'll discuss this watershed publication in more detail shortly.)

So it's no surprise that F. P. Rhoades, writing in the *Journal of the American Geriatric Society,* in 1967 called menopause a tragedy: "Many women are leading an active and productive life when this tragedy strikes. They are still attractive and mentally alert; they deeply resent what to them is a catastrophic attack upon their ability to earn a living and enjoy life."[5]

In 1985, the International Menopause Society, meeting in France to reach a consensus on how to define menopause, took a less melodramatic approach, describing the climacteric simply as the transitional period from reproductive to nonreproductive status, and menopause as beginning with the final menstrual period, typically occurring around age fifty-one.[6]

Wulf Utian was unhappy with this straightforward medical definition: it lacked the tragic dimension favored by Wilson and company. Menopause, Utian claimed, was an endocrinopathy—an endocrine disease—that had drastic effects on the pelvis and its surrounding tissue. "The longer these effects are allowed to continue without corrective therapy," he warned grimly, "the more likely there is to be an expression of the pathological process."[7]

Today, this controversy continues. Elizabeth Barrett-Connor was one of the first doctors to discover that hormone therapy might protect against heart disease, yet she has consistently warned that "estrogen deficiency is not a disease in the same sense as diabetes or hypothyroidism, because every woman who lives long enough will become estrogen deficient."[8] Other doctors, however, still cling to the notion of menopause as a disease. For example, the physician Theresa L. Crenshaw was quoted in 1996, in an article in the *Philadelphia Inquirer,* as saying that menopause "is not a natural condition; it is an endocrine disorder and should be treated medically with the same seriousness we treat other endocrine disorders, such as diabetes or thyroid disease."[9]

This insistence on viewing menopause as a disease has a number of implications. On a practical level, it implies the need for medication: diseases are treated. On a deeper level, it defines older women as aberrant. Premenopausal women are normal; postmenopausal women are not.

Indeed, if we insist on defining women as hormonally diseased creatures (as distinct from their wholesomely testosteroned brothers), we might just as well look at our reframing again. "Estrogen deficiency" is, supposedly, a disease from a biological standpoint because, as I'll discuss in depth later, it makes women more susceptible to colon cancer and thinner bones. But the premenopausal years also have health risks related to estrogen—too much estrogen. Breast and uterine cancer are both caused, in part, by an oversupply of this hormone. So we could argue that, since nature intended us to have ten or twenty children, rather than the two or three most women have, this constant fertility, unchecked by regular pregnancy, keeps all that estrogen circulating and creates its own disease—let's call it "estrogen-surplus disease." Fortunately, however, it's a disease we can cure. We can put all women into menopause at puberty, and give them drugs to reverse it temporarily when they want to have children. In fact, one researcher, Malcolm Pike, suggests that women at high risk for these diseases be put into a reversible premature menopause and then given very low doses of hormones to maintain their hearts and bones.[10] This idea may sound crazy, but is it any more crazy than putting all postmenopausal women on hormones and trying to keep them premenopausal forever?

In fairness, not all the advocates of hormone therapy believe that every woman should be kept premenopausal. Pieter van Keep describes a "milestone" in the history of hormone therapy—the first meeting on the subject held by the Health Foundation in Geneva in 1971.[11] These European scientists and clinicians defined their therapeutic strategy: "We should not aim at making . . . a postmenopausal woman into a premenopausal woman again," they said, refreshingly. But they still wanted us all on hormones. "We should try to make a bad postmenopausal woman into a good postmenopausal woman."[12] So now, not only are menopausal women diseased—some, at least, are also "bad." But we can become both healthy and good by taking magic little pills.

This depiction of menopause has crept into the thinking of women as well. A study done in 1986 found that 53 percent of women thought menopause was a medical condition and should be treated medically.[13] That was more than ten years ago: the percentage must be far higher now. Studies show that the women most likely to remain on hormones are those who think of menopause as a medical complaint. It makes sense: if you think you have a medical problem, you take pills to cure it. If you think you're going through a normal stage of life, you're far less likely to respond to that by taking medicine.

In the United States, the highest use of hormone therapy is among women who have had their ovaries removed due to hysterectomies. There are two reasons for this. First, hysterectomies are often done on women who are comparatively young—in their mid-thirties or early forties. In this case, the women tend to want to take hormones at least until the time they would have probably gone naturally into menopause. Second, women who have hysterectomies later, at around the time of menopause, generally have a stronger sense of menopause itself as a medical condition, since it's been instigated by a medical procedure. Their symptoms have been brought on by a medical process, not a natural one, and it seems reasonable to treat them medically. (Few postmenopausal women have hysterectomies, and those who do generally have them because of cancer, which usually rules out hormone therapy; see Chapter 8.)

Many other women believed that menopause was a disease because their doctors treated it as a disease, insisting that a woman patient should take hormones simply because she was approaching menopause. I would often discover, in the course of getting a new patient's medical history, that she was taking hormones; she'd be surprised when I asked why. "Well, because you're supposed to be on it," she'd say. When I probed further, some women would indeed tell me they had awful hot flashes, extreme swings of mood, or some other very troublesome symptom. But some would turn out to have had no symptoms at all. Their doctors simply told them they should be on hormone therapy, and they complied. Many of these women have told me they expressed uneasiness to their doctors about continuing the hormones and wanted to stop, only to be told emphatically that they should remain on the medication for the rest of their lives. (This recommendation has been given a big blow with the recent release of results from the Women's Health Initiative; see Chapter 7.) Even people you'd expect to be skeptical about Western medicine often buy into the idea that menopause must be "treated." A forty-five-year-old friend of mine (who eats health food, takes herbal remedies, and avoids doctors like the plague) told me she'd been lucky so far because she hadn't needed any estrogen. But she knew it was in her future and said that when the time came, she'd try to take natural estrogen. When I asked why she was so sure she'd need it, she said, "I'll need it to manage my menopause, of course!" It apparently hadn't occurred to her that she might not need to "manage" anything. I've come across this frequently—people in the alternative medical movement who accept without question the basic premise that all women need estrogen and quibble only about which kind.

CROSS-CULTURAL STUDIES AND THE "DISEASE MODEL"

Looking at other cultures highlights something very important. If menopause is a disease, its worst symptoms seem to be limited to white women in Western cultures. I think this is a crucial point. Until menopause became big business, American women were always told their symptoms were in their heads. With the new business of hormone therapy, there's been a complete flip-flop. Not only have the symptoms become "real," but all women are expected to experience all symptoms, and with the same degree of severity.

Yet individual and cross-cultural differences in women's experience of menopause suggest something far more complex. Diet and reproductive history probably influence what symptoms a woman has, and social factors influence how she interprets her menopause. So we need to look at the whole experience.

Menopause in Japan: Differences in Lifestyle

Margaret Lock did a survey of menopausal symptoms in Japan.[14] She was astonished to find that the Japanese had no word for a hot flash. Instead, they used words that encompassed a range of changes in body temperature, including suddenly flushing after drinking alcohol, a sensation experienced by a large proportion of East Asians of both genders. The most common symptom, experienced by 52 percent of the women in Lock's study, was stiff shoulders: it's almost as if these women literally felt the weight of the world on their shoulders. Twenty-eight percent had headaches. Less than 20 percent had other symptoms. Only 9.5 percent had hot flashes, and only 3.2 percent had night sweats.[15]

Interviews with doctors confirmed these findings. Thirty doctors were questioned for this study, and all said that the symptoms their menopausal patients complained of most were shoulder stiffness, headaches, and dizziness. The equivalent words for hot flashes were near the bottom of their list of symptoms; some didn't even include them at all. "Every Japanese doctor interviewed during the survey and since that time confirms that hot flashes are not symptoms about which Japanese women consult a doctor," writes Lock.[16] Women hadn't been going to their doctors with menopausal symptoms: when they did go, they consulted primary care physicians, not gynecologists or psychologists. Yet Japan is an extremely health-conscious nation with a high doctor-patient ratio and universal health insurance, with easy access to health facilities.

But changes are brewing. For the past two years, the subject of menopause has suddenly been taken up repeatedly in Japanese women's magazines. The supposed long-term benefits of hormone therapy have been emphasized, including its alleged effectiveness against dementia, stroke, heart disease, and osteoporosis. Many articles have indicated that hormone therapy can help women recover their youth. The medicalization of menopause is creeping into Japan.

Japanese women have an average life expectancy of nearly eighty-two years—higher than ours. It's true that, like American women, Japanese women have osteoporosis at twice the rate of men—in part, at least, because they live longer. Yet osteoporosis—a bone-thinning disease that typically affects people in their late seventies and eighties—is only half as common among Japanese women as among American women. What makes this really fascinating is that most Japanese women have lower bone mass than Caucasian women. If osteoporosis were only about bone mass, they'd have more, not less, of it—as you'll see in Chapter 5. As for coronary heart disease, the mortality rate of Japanese women is a quarter that of American women. The mortality rate from breast cancer is a fourth to a third that of North American women. Japanese women drink little alcohol, exercise continuously throughout their lives, and rarely smoke. Apart from a high consumption of pickled foods, they eat a well-balanced diet with a lot of soy products and no milk. (See Chapter 12 for a discussion of the amazing qualities of soy.) It's beyond me why they'd want to interfere with what seems like a winning system by introducing hormone therapy.

Biological Differences

Not all the differences are based on diet, however. Other studies of different cultures demonstrate that at least some cross-cultural differences are biological. Jews from North Africa living in Israel experience few symptoms, while Jews of European ancestry have symptoms similar to those of Americans. In 1990, one study looked at two groups of Indonesian women who experienced few hot flashes.[17] The researchers had hypothesized that the women who migrated and became acculturated into urban life would get more hot flashes, but in fact they turned out to have no increase in symptoms.

The Mayan Indians have no symptoms with menopause, even though they have the same hormonal changes as white women.[18] Since they live in a tropical climate, one might expect them to have hot flashes, but they don't. Even when researchers asked very specific questions, the Mayan women didn't express any familiarity with the symptoms they were being asked about. In fact, like the Japanese, the Mayans have no word for "hot flash."

Cultural Influences

In addition to biological differences, the cultural milieu has a powerful effect on the experience of menopause. One study looked at the Rajput women of Northern India.[19] These women, who are kept in strict purdah during their fertile years, are restricted far less once they reach menopause; they are then permitted to move freely about the village. They experience no unpleasant menopausal symptoms. The study concluded that the two facts were related: if menopause improves the quality of your life, either you experience no symptoms or those you do experience are so minor compared with the rewards that you don't mind them.

The studies of Mayan women confirmed this view. Like the Rajput women, they also look forward to menopause, which frees them from constant pregnancy and childbirth. Is that why they have no hot flashes? Several studies conclude that menopause is actually a biocultural event: lifestyle differences like diet and reproductive histories as well as cultural views of older women play a large role in how women experience menopause.[20]

This biocultural effect was demonstrated in 1994, in a study of women and their physicians in a village in Thailand.[21] The interviewer was a native, which was important because the researchers wanted to be certain they understood the nuances of the language. In this village, the women all saw both menopause and menstruation as a natural part of life. Their word for menopause translates roughly as "no more babies." They tend to welcome it, since it relieves them of the burdens of menstruation, pregnancy, and childbirth. Since it signals the beginning of old age, they feel they are now able to free themselves from the menstrual taboos that accompany fertile years in their culture. They have greater independence, and most of the premenopausal women interviewed were looking forward to menopause.

Perimenopausal women in this study did report symptoms, but for the most part they didn't find them very troublesome. About a quarter of these women experienced hot flashes—a condition for which they, like the Mayans and Japanese, don't have a specific word. They described it as a burning sensation inside the body or on the skin. It made them uncomfortable, and they became irritable. Dizziness and headaches were the most common symptoms, and the headaches sometimes kept them from concentrating, which affected their work—this was the symptom that most bothered them.

Most believed their symptoms were temporary and didn't seek medical help, feeling comfortable with letting nature take its course. On the infrequent occasions when a woman's symptoms were so severe that she wanted help, she went to a healer, an herbalist, or a village elder.

Their doctors, however, had a different attitude. A middle-aged gynecologist in the village, Dr. Chaaj, told the interviewers that menopause should not be treated as a natural event but as a state of estrogen deficiency that causes heart disease, osteoporosis, and other illnesses. He wanted to persuade these women, who did not even "treat" menstruation with sanitary napkins, to treat their "deficiency" with estrogen pills. "Hormone replacement therapy is used to promote quality of life in the industrialized countries," Dr. Chaaj explained, "and its use in Thailand will ensure that women have a happy postmenopausal life."[22] He attributed this belief to the medical literature he'd read, mostly from the West. The fact that the women in his village were already having perfectly happy postmenopausal lives without hormone intervention didn't seem to faze him.

He was not alone in his attitude. Altogether fifteen Thai gynecologists were interviewed, and all saw menopause as an estrogen-deficiency disease that should be treated with hormone therapy. They felt that Western technology was superior to traditional village values.

The Experience in England

Lest I leave you with a biased view—that all women in other countries are going through menopause happily but are being badgered by doctors to take drugs—we should look at the other side of the coin. In 1983, a book about hormone therapy called No Change by Wendy Cooper was published in England.[23] It set off an explosion among Englishwomen who had long been complaining about menopausal symptoms. After Cooper's book came out, more and more Englishwomen began to seek out hormone therapy. Unlike women in the United States, who were having hormones thrust on them, the British women asked for hormone treatment but were often denied it.

The experiences and views of 3,117 women receiving hormones at 21 menopause clinics in the United Kingdom were cited in an epidemiological study in 1988.[24] The article quoted one woman who was grateful for "the chance to talk to an understanding doctor about the symptoms that were physically and mentally draining but didn't seem important enough to take to an ordinary doctor. My own doctor gave me the impression that I had to live with it.... The very fact that some interest is being shown in the distressing symptoms I was suffering and someone was trying to do something about it was very comforting." Until then, she had been convinced that "the medical profession thinks that middle-aged women are neurotic idiots with hypochondria."[25] This suggests an interesting possibility. It may be that some women need support during perimenopause and menopause and that the medical profession interprets this as a need for drugs. Hormone therapy is still used less in the United Kingdom than in the United States: only 7 to 10 percent of women in the United Kingdom take it, as compared with 32 percent in the United States.[26]

BIG BUSINESS

If so many cultures experience menopause as a natural stage of life, why is it being turned into a disease? As I've said, this is at least in part because diseases need treatment and treatment costs money. Unfortunately, the medical world is no freer from the manipulation of big business than the rest of us are—and the pharmaceutical industry is very big business indeed.

Although we might like to think of the medical profession as pure and the drug industry as altruistic, we live in the real world. Drug companies want first and foremost to make money. They are expert at marketing to us as well as to doctors. If corporations can make us believe that smoking will make us sexy and that waxing the kitchen floor will save our marriages, they can make us believe anything. Doctors are as susceptible to marketing as the rest of us. Drugs and diseases go in and out of fashion, just as lipstick shades and car models do.

We also cling to the idea that because medicine is "scientific," doctors are always right. But science itself is never pure: it changes with new discoveries and with new social values. Tonsillectomies, which were so popular when we were kids, are done rarely today. Ulcers, once thought to be caused by stomach acid, are now treated with antibiotics, because we've learned that they're caused by a bacterial infection. And the use of hormone replacement therapy to prevent heart disease has been shown to be ill conceived—even counterproductive.

One of the most powerful marketing techniques used to influence both doctors and patients is the manipulation of fears of aging and death. In our youth-oriented culture, we tend to act as if we can stay young forever as long as we do everything right. We think that death is optional. Time challenges that illusion. In spite of all the hair coloring, wrinkle creams, and miracle vitamins, we do age. Menopause, that undeniable harbinger of middle age, eventually comes to any woman who's lucky enough not to die young. You start to get hot flashes or rushes of heavy bleeding—often disruptively severe, always a reminder that youth is gone. And then you're offered a lovely little pill that can make it all go away.

That little pill has been around since the 1940s, and for many women, it has been lovely. For years it was given to patients who suffered from hot flashes and vaginal dryness, offering real relief for extreme symptoms. But during the past several decades, pharmaceutical companies have seen an opportunity here and have tried to capitalize on it: why confine their pills to the relatively few women with severe symptoms, when they could offer them to all women in menopause?

Marketing Eternal Femininity—and More

The drug companies began by creating a fancy name: "hormone replacement therapy." This was a nice touch, suggesting that something should be there but has been taken away, and that they can give this something back to you. The idea of "hormone replacement therapy" is consistent with the language that marketing has created everywhere: you can smell "naturally fresh" by using an artificial deodorant; you can have "home-baked goodness" by buying a packaged food; you can prolong youth by "replacing the hormones nature has taken away."

Getting all women in menopause to take hormones required identifying a purpose for the medication beyond simply alleviating severe symptoms. It meant mythologizing those symptoms, and, more, it meant creating new claims for hormone therapy. The pharmaceutical industry began to encourage the idea that estrogen could do more than relieve present symptoms—that it could also prevent a large range of problems, from wrinkles to heart disease.

Paula B. Doress-Worters, in the preface to *The Menopause Industry*, called hormone therapy "a product in search of a market."[27] Part of the strategy, she says, was to promote hormone therapy "not simply as a palliative for the discomforts of menopause but also as a panacea for 'psychological problems' supposedly related to the change of life. Such claims were unproven but were treated as common knowledge." The postmenopausal older woman was depicted as "asexual, neurotic, and unattractive."

The pharmaceutical companies were incredibly lucky to discover a spokesman for this view, a gynecologist in Brooklyn, New York, named Robert Wilson. His book *Feminine Forever* (1966), written for laywomen, was heralded for years as the book that was changing women from dried-up relics of their lost youth to vibrant, joyful, perennial twenty-year-olds.[28] Wilson told the story of his mother's menopause: "I was appalled at the transformation of that vital, wonderful woman who had been the dynamic focal point of our family into a pain-racked petulant invalid. I could feel the deep wounds her senseless rages inflicted on my father, myself, and the younger children. It was this frightful experience that later directed my interest as a physician to the problem of menopause." He went on to describe a second crucial event. A local woman had drowned herself in the reservoir because, the "town gossips" told him, she had "gone mad" with the change of life. Wilson apparently accepted the diagnosis of the town gossips; it did not occur to him that there might have been reasons other than menopause for a middle-aged woman's suicide.

In his book, Wilson also told how he had confirmed that estrogen could keep women looking eternally young. He examined a fifty-two-year-old patient and was struck by how youthful she seemed. He asked her her secret, only to find that she was still using birth control pills because she was still menstruating. Wilson was amazed and immediately became a zealot about the wonders of estrogen. "I therefore believe that menopause prevention far transcends the purely clinical aspects of the subject. It even transcends any narrow view of sex as such. What is really at stake is a subtle and almost metaphysical factor—a woman's total femininity."

Wilson's book became a best-seller, first in the United States and later in Europe, selling more than 100,000 copies in a few months. In 1969 a survey conducted by the International Health Foundation of four hundred women in five European countries found that the popularity of *Feminine Forever* directly influenced the extent to which hormone therapy was used in each country.[29] "The more publicity there had been in a country, the higher the percentage of perimenopausal women who had heard that medical treatment existed to lessen the problems of the climacteric." Although estrogen was being prescribed for short-term, self-limited symptoms, the implication was that if you stopped taking it, the symptoms would all come back. To remain feminine forever, you had to stay on estrogen forever.

Sales of Premarin, the most popular formulation of estrogen, soared as women sought this fountain of youth. Dr. John Lee, a gynecologist in San Francisco, tells of being given a free copy of Wilson's book by a pharmaceuticals representative.[30] In fact, the makers of estrogen soon started funding Wilson's lectures to women's groups. Barbara and Gideon Seaman, who are experts on estrogen, have written about Wilson's private trust, the Wilson Foundation, established to promote the use of estrogen.[31] Wilson's foundation received $1.3 million in funding from pharmaceutical companies. In 1964—two years before Wilson's book was published—the foundation had received $17,000 from Searle, $8,700 from Wyeth-Ayerst Laboratories, and $5,600 from the Upjohn Company, all of which made hormones that Wilson promoted for the treatment of menopause.

While Wilson proselytized menopausal women, the pharmaceutical companies continued their barrage on the doctors. Medical journals ran ads showing dour old women who perked up immediately on estrogen. Combinations of estrogen and the tranquilizer Librium were formulated and advertised "for the problems that bother him the most." Presumably the job of the doctors was as much to keep husbands happy as to make women patients feel better.

Wilson shared this focus. He saw "estrogen-deficient" postmenopausal women as the source of most of society's woes: "The transformation, within a few years, of a formerly pleasant, energetic woman into a dull-minded but sharp-tongued caricature of her former self is one of the saddest of human spectacles. The suffering is not hers alone—it involves her entire family, her business associates, her neighborhood storekeepers, and all others with whom she comes into contact. Multiplied by millions, she is a focus of bitterness and discontent in the whole fabric of our civilization."[32] Reading his book, one wonders why he stopped short of blaming the sinking of the *Titanic,* World War II, and the fall of the Roman Empire on postmenopausal women.

The Worm Turns—For a While

But even with all this hype, sales of Premarin have still been subject to the vicissitudes of medical knowledge. The ups and downs of prescriptions for estrogen reflect the flip-flopping advice in medical books. A study done in 1993 examined changing information in gynecological textbooks, internal medicine textbooks, a pharmaceutical text (written by

Goodman and Gilman), and the *Physicians' Desk Reference* (PDR) over the last sixty years.[33]

Until the mid-1970s, as we've seen, estrogen was used mostly to treat existing menopausal symptoms—hot flashes, mood swings, etc. In 1975, 28 million prescriptions for Premarin were written in the United States. Then, in 1975, suggestions appeared that women were at risk for heart disease and that hormone therapy could help lower the risk. (Studies in the 1950s had suggested that estrogen could prevent atherosclerosis in animals fed a high-fat diet.)

As a result, a study was launched—of men. Don't ask me why the first effort to determine the effects of estrogen on the heart was done with men; the logic eludes me. But the fact remains that the first randomized controlled study of estrogen and heart disease was done on men who had had heart attacks or angina, the crushing pain that indicates heart disease.[34] (The more recent studies on women will be discussed later.) The men were given high doses (2.5 milligrams and 1.25 milligrams) of Premarin in the hope that it would lower their risk of repeat attacks. It didn't—in fact, it was correlated with more heart attacks. The doctors became concerned that the same effect would occur with women, so they decided that women who were at risk of heart disease should not receive Premarin. (It's too bad we didn't stick with that notion.) Other studies were starting to show that use of estrogen could lead to endometrial cancer.[35] Doctors immediately stopped prescribing estrogen for women, except for those who had had hysterectomies and therefore did not have uteruses that could be harmed. (This fact, as you'll see in Chapter 4, becomes important when we look at the pool of women who have been studied to see the effects of long-term use of Premarin.) By 1980, sales had fallen to 14 million.

The decline in prescriptions for Premarin was only a temporary lull. The drug companies once again had an answer: add another drug. In the early 1980s, gynecologists began to prescribe estrogen combined with an oral progestin called Provera, which was shown to protect the uterus. (They had no idea whether the progestin had any effect on heart disease, because there were no studies on this, but naively assumed that its only effect was on the uterus.)

With the successful addition of Provera to the mix, estrogen sales began to rise again, hitting 16.6 million by 1983—an improvement, but still a plummet from the levels of 1975. The makers of Premarin needed a new approach to counteract the bad publicity from the association of estrogens with cancer—and to add even more women to their lists. The baby boomers might not all embrace the promise of eternal youth, but they were increasingly health-conscious and concerned with preventing disease. So the drug companies picked up on another aspect of Wilson's theory: without estrogen, all women were doomed to osteoporosis.

There had been some preliminary studies suggesting that estrogen therapy could decrease the risk of osteoporosis if taken over the long term. Marketing on this basis might be just what was needed to rehabilitate the drug before the baby boomers reached menopause. The pharmaceuticals industry was savvy enough to recognize that marketing a disease is the best way to market a drug. Osteoporosis suited their needs: it has no symptoms until you have fractures, which means you can have it for years and not know until it's too late. If the baby boomers could be convinced that without drugs their bones would slowly and silently deteriorate, they'd be more likely to take drugs at the first hint that menopause was approaching. The pharmaceutical companies started placing ads in the medical journals, showing wheelchairs, X rays of crooked spines, and pathetic-looking women with dowager's humps. They funded medical meetings and lectures about osteoporosis.

These scare tactics were extremely successful. In less than ten years, women and doctors were viewing osteoporosis as a "female disease" (although it occurs in men and women), the inevitable fate of women who did not take estrogen after menopause.

This approach continues into the present. Merck, the company that makes Fosamax (a nonhormonal treatment for osteoporosis), stated in its annual report of 1995: "Consumer research shows a growing level of awareness and knowledge about osteoporosis. We have been aggressively working to educate consumers about the disease and the importance of early diagnosis and appropriate treatment with organizations such as the National Osteoporosis Foundation, the Older Women's League, and members of the European parliament. We have established the Bone Measurement Institute, a nonprofit organization, to increase the accessibility and affordability of bone measurement technologies. Merck has also provided funding for the first world summit of osteoporosis societies."

And Merck funded more studies. It even ran commercials on television, aimed at the public rather than just doctors. One showed a healthy-looking grandma who's just been diagnosed with osteoporosis looking wistfully at her grandson and wondering how long she'll be able to play with him. Another commercial showed wishbones being pulled, just on the verge of breaking.

These public education efforts have been very successful. On June 15, 1995, the *Wall Street Journal* reported that "Charles H. Chestnut, a researcher [on osteoporosis] and Professor of Medicine at the University of Washington, says that when he gave presentations of his work at scientific meetings two decades ago, 'there would be three or four people in the audience, and most of them were the next speakers.'" Now the disease is hot.[36] Chestnut said that research funding had increased dramatically and that his presentations drew hundreds of scientists. Researchers credited media coverage of the disease in the early and mid-1980s for generating public awareness, along with efforts of the NIH and other scientific groups.

In spite of all this media blitz, messages to doctors about who can benefit from estrogen, and who is at risk, have kept changing. These mixed messages are demonstrated in one gynecology textbook.[37] In 1961, the authors cautiously advised that estrogen therapy might protect against cardiovascular disease, adding in the editions of 1965 and 1971 that it should be given to women who have a family history of heart disease. In the 1975 edition, however, as a result of the studies on men, they said that it should not be given to women with a history of heart disease. In the editions of 1981 and 1988, they went back to their earlier position: "Women with a family history of heart disease should be treated with hormone therapy." With the new data the books will be changed again.

Because of all the changes of attitude—often based on bias rather than on hard evidence, as I'll explain in Chapter 4—doctors are getting, and giving, mixed messages. Further, when they want to update their information, they don't always turn to the latest scientific studies. Instead, they often turn to sales representatives for drug companies or to medical meetings that may be funded by drug companies. In 1995, meetings sponsored by pharmaceutical companies rose 31 percent. Pfizer, which doesn't make any HRT products, led the industry in promotional expenditures in 1995, spending $364 million on sales representatives and $93.7 million for events. Pfizer made 2.7 million sales calls to doctors in 1995; American Home Products, the parent company of Wyeth-Ayerst (the makers of Premarin), was second in the total number of sales calls (mostly to doctors): 2.4 million.[38]

Medical journals are replete with ads selling doctors on the wonders of particular drugs. *Menopause,* the official journal of the North American

Menopause Society, has ads for hormone therapy scattered among its articles, proclaiming the benefits of various hormone therapy drugs. A doctor is as susceptible to advertising as the next person, especially if he thinks that a treatment will make a patient younger, happier, and healthier. I'm not saying that doctors are lazy. At a time when doctors must struggle to keep current with a vast and proliferating body of research, it's easy for them to let their attention be drawn to information that's neatly packaged for ready absorption. At any medical meeting, one of the most popular spots is the exhibits area, where drug companies put up elaborate booths and give away anything from cappuccino to tote bags stuffed with information about their latest products. In fact, many of the speakers at these meetings are also provided, or at least paid for, by the drug companies' representatives. A drug company doesn't tell a speaker what to say, but a recent study showed that a medical audience is influenced by a sponsoring company; one month after a talk, most members of the audience prescribed more of a drug produced by the drug company paying for lunch than other drugs for the same purpose.[39] In most teaching hospitals, the main teaching rounds provide lunch courtesy of local drug representatives.

THE RISE OF THE GYNECOLOGIST

Along with changes in the profile of estrogen have come changes in the profile of the doctors prescribing it. In 1971, 27 percent of the doctors prescribing estrogen were gynecologists. In the 1980s, that percentage started to increase, and by 1991, 60 percent of these prescriptions were given by gynecologists.

Probably because of this, advertisers are marketing hormones most heavily to gynecologists. And gynecologists derive some benefit from putting you on hormones, so they're more likely to buy into the advertising. Once you stop having babies, you don't often need to see a gynecologist—unless you're on hormone therapy. Not only do you have to see the gynecologist every six months for a refill, but, as you'll see later, women on hormones are more likely to need many more revenue-generating gynecological procedures such as endometrial biopsies, D and Cs, and of course hysterectomies. (I thought I might be unduly cynical about this until a gynecologist friend of mine wrote me that she'd come up with the same theory; she ruefully added, "And to think I prescribe this pill daily.")

THE MEDIA

The drug companies and the medical profession are not the only sources of mythology and misinformation. The popular media have certainly contributed their share. On the nightly news, tentative new findings in small studies become transformed into miracle cures. The media often confuse news stories and advertising, touting a new product's claims as if they had been proven. As recently as December 1995, the cover of *Reader's Digest* boldly touted Premarin as "the pill that keeps women young." Meanwhile, the package insert for Premarin says, "You may have heard that taking estrogens for long periods (years) after menopause will keep your skin soft and supple and keep you feeling young. There is no evidence that this is so and such long-term treatment may carry serious risks."

The media have been aided and abetted by the corporations who produce the drugs and devices used in medical interventions. When a new study comes out that might call the safety of hormone therapy into question, the pharmaceutical companies send out a news release to the media offering expert spokespeople who will discuss the flaws in the study. For example, in 1995, when a study from Harvard validated earlier studies showing that postmenopausal estrogen might increase the risk of breast cancer, American Home Products lined up a prestigious crew of scientists to attack the Harvard results. One of them, Leon Speroff, a professor at Oregon Health & Science University in Portland, immediately sent out a letter to the media urging caution in interpreting the study. "As a physician/researcher who treats and studies menopausal women, I've witnessed firsthand the hysteria that can be generated as a result of unbalanced study data—particularly related to breast cancer." Speroff wasn't paid to write this by American Home Products, but he has done clinical work for the company. American Home Products also distributed its own meta-analysis rebutting the Harvard study.[40]

On the other hand, when a study showing a beneficial effect of hormone therapy comes out, the drug companies make sure it gets a lot of press: they'll hand out copies of the study to doctors and the media and offer to pay the authors of the study to speak at national medical meetings and press conferences. They rarely pass out the less favorable studies. This means that doctors and the media get an unbalanced impression. Before you know it, interesting preliminary data become accepted as dogma.

The claims that the pharmaceutical company experts make are often belied by the products' own package insert (which is required to use language approved by the FDA). Take a look at the small print in the ads in women's magazines for Premarin, Prempro (a combination of estrogen and progestins by the maker of Premarin), or any other estrogen—or, if you're already taking one of the drugs, at the insert that used to come with your own pills. The Prempro insert reads in part: "Some research has shown that estrogens taken without progestins may protect women against developing heart disease. However, this is not certain. The protection shown may have been caused by the characteristics of the estrogen-treated women and not by the estrogen treatment itself. In general, treated women were slimmer, more physically active, and were less likely to have diabetes than the untreated women. These characteristics are known to protect against heart disease."

Although this label is now being revised in light of the new studies, we didn't see any drug companies step forward earlier to set straight the public misconception that a proven connection between hormones and preventing heart disease existed. They haven't actually lied, but they haven't actually told the truth, either.

As I've pointed out earlier, there are many competing interests in this business. Researchers want to get more research money and more fame, and so they have a tendency to make their own studies sound better and more important than those of their colleagues. The university where a study is done wants more donations from its wealthy patrons, so it, too, wants to make all of its discoveries sound bigger and better. The media—and the medical journals, for that matter—would rather publish studies that show positive results than negative results, and they would rather publish studies on drugs than on changes in lifestyle. Take, for example, the journal *Maturitas:* from 1978 to 1985, this international journal for the study of the climacteric had ninety-six articles related directly to hormone therapy, but only seven on nonhormonal medication.[41]

In evaluating research in this area, you need to question what hasn't been studied as well as what has been. If most research on treating menopausal symptoms is based on evaluating the role of hormones rather than of, say, lifestyle, it isn't surprising that doctors and consumers develop a bias toward hormone therapy.

Further, experts who don't follow the party line are often not published. Jerilynn Prior, an endocrinologist, tells of having a colleague call and ask her to do a chapter in a book on menopause.[42] When she told him that she didn't believe all women needed to be on hormones, she was told that they'd find another author. Barbara Seaman, an expert on estrogen who is often cautionary, found that "in the 60s, 70s and 80s most discussions of menopause permitted several points of view. As a result of the vested interest pharmaceutical advertising supports, the conservative view on hormone therapy is no longer admitted on talk shows and is rarely seen in magazines that seek advertising. . . . In the 90s I have given interviews to scores of magazine writers, only to have my comments removed from the final copy. In the 90s I have been called by and booked on all three network morning programs, only to be canceled out with some lame excuse."[43]

Women's magazines are encouraged to run stories on osteoporosis and heart disease, and they run plenty of ads for hormone replacement therapy. It's probably not a coincidence. In 1997, when the first edition was written, *Prevention* magazine, a popular health monthly, had run at least two major articles in favor of hormone therapy. They also ran ads for Premarin in the same issue. When they ran an article discussing the use of soy protein as an alternative to estrogen for decreasing hot flashes, there were no Premarin or Prempro ads in the issue.

The women in the ads for hormones keep getting younger and younger. The drug companies aren't actually saying that you'll look thirty-five forever if you take estrogen, but having a woman who looks thirty-five in the ad says it without words. Cigarette companies don't say that smoking will make you sexy, either—they just show very sexy women smoking.

Is it any wonder that you can't figure out what's really going on? Obviously a lot of people are invested in this "disease" and its treatment, and it's important to be aware of all of them. It's unfortunate that corporate profits and media fads should determine anyone's medical treatment—or lack of treatment. But they do, and just as consumers need to distrust the glittering promises of car companies and perfume manufacturers, they need to question the promises of the pharmaceutical industry, filtered through the agency of well-meaning doctors and superficial media coverage.

WHY PREMARIN?

From the earliest days of estrogen "replacement" therapy, one product—Premarin—has dominated the market in the United States. You'll hear more about Premarin in this book than about any other kind of estrogen. The fact that so many doctors have been persuaded that their patients need estrogen doesn't explain why, in the United States, one brand of estrogen dominates all others. The credit for that goes to drug companies' "positioning." The story of Premarin is perhaps the best example of the power and influence of pharmaceutical companies.

Remember that in 1975, 28 million prescriptions were given for Premarin in the United States. After the dip following bad publicity linking estrogen with endometrial cancer, sales of Premarin slowly climbed again. By 1992, there were 31.7 million prescriptions; in 2000, prescriptions had gone up to 46 million. It had become the most frequently dispensed brand-name pharmaceutical in the country. And a further 22.3 million prescriptions were written for Prempro. Thirty-eight percent of postmenopausal women took hormone replacement therapy in the year 2000, and the vast majority of them took Premarin.[44]

Premarin was studied initially because it was more readily available than other preparations and because the manufacturer, Wyeth-Ayerst, provided it free to researchers. Wyeth-Ayerst also sponsored research using its product. Premarin is the subject of nearly 90 percent of the estrogen studies (more than three thousand studies to date). Now doctors argue that they prefer to prescribe Premarin because it's been studied more than the others. This is true, but the situation has become highly self-perpetuating. When new studies were planned, such as the Women's Health Initiative (see page 74), they tended to study Premarin and Prempro because they want to concentrate on drugs in common use and, again, because the pharmaceutical companies would provide the drugs free. Wyeth-Ayerst agreed to donate more than 100 million tablets of Premarin and medroxyprogesterone (a progestin) or placebo to the National Institutes of Health, which funded the Women's Health Initiative. Wyeth-Ayerst has also funded the $40 million study called the Heart and Estrogen-Progestin Replacement Study (HERS), which investigated Premarin for women with preexisting coronary artery disease. In both cases it backfired: rather than give them the data they needed to market Premarin and Prempro for the prevention of heart disease, the studies showed an increase in heart attacks and strokes in the women taking the drugs. Wyeth-Ayerst is also funding a $16 million study to investigate whether Premarin can prevent or delay Alzheimer's disease. It will be very interesting to see how that comes out. This strangle hold on the research being done means that we do not know now whether other formulations of hormones are safer or even more dangerous.

The maker of Premarin has done other things to maintain its dominance. Premarin reached $1 billion in sales in 2000.[45] Premarin (or conjugated equine estrogen, as it's formally called) comes from the urine of pregnant horses, a fact its manufacturers have used for twenty years to block FDA approval of any generic equivalents that have been developed. (A generic CEE was approved in Canada in 1996.) They argue that Premarin contains six dominant estrogenic compounds (horse estrogens), including one that is missing from the proposed generic equivalent. They contend this is a key factor in the drug's effectiveness. The manufacturers of the generic versions claim that their product is just as effective, but they've been unable to include this particular horse estrogen. Regardless of the truth of the matter, the difficulties in mimicking horses' urinary estrogen has kept Premarin on top.[46]

Interestingly the dominance of Premarin is weakening as more and more pharmaceutical companies have brought out alternatives such as estradiol and patches, and "designer estrogens" with fewer side effects have begun to hit the market. Further, the recent studies showing that Prempro and Premarin don't prevent heart disease have allowed the alternatives to try to position themselves as the safe ones. It is important to remember that the absence of data does not mean that they are any safer.

I don't mean to make either the drug companies or the media sound like the Evil Empire. They're all doing their jobs, and in many ways we benefit from that. The fact that 90 percent of new medicines are discovered by drug companies doesn't mean that these medicines aren't valuable, and the media do provide the public with important information about diseases and treatments. But the limitations built into what both institutions are doing mean that you, too, have a job—to be as fully informed as possible, to be aware of biases in research and reporting, and to make up your own mind.

THREE

"What Does It Feel Like?"

IDENTIFYING SYMPTOMS

Problem 1: Variations—We Are Not All the Same

Perimenopause, the three to six years before the last period, is extremely individual: each woman experiences this transition in her own way. This is not surprising. Each of us had her own experience of puberty. Some of us have had PMS while others have sailed through our years of menstruating. Some of us had morning sickness with pregnancy and others didn't. I know some women who claim they knew they were pregnant from the moment of conception, and there are stories of women who never knew they were pregnant until they went into labor. Hormones and hormonal shifts affect each one of us in their own unique way, so it's only natural that perimenopause and menopause will be experienced highly individually. There's a wide range of possible symptoms, limited only by your imagination.

Women are usually able to recognize which of these symptoms are actually related to their hormones and which aren't. Doctors are not always so perceptive. One of my patients, a lawyer, was in the midst of a fairly humdrum meeting with a client one day and suddenly got palpitations and shortness of breath. She covered as best she could, and as soon as the client left, she called her husband, a doctor. Could this be the start of menopause? she asked. He asked if she'd felt hot or had turned red, and when she said no, he said it couldn't be menopause; it was just nerves. When it happened again later in the day, she started to get scared and went to an emergency room. She ended up seeing a team of specialists and having a battery of tests, none of which turned up anything. She asked the doctors several times whether this episode could be related to menopause. And to a man, all the doctors were adamant. These were not menopausal symptoms. Absolutely not. When she finally got home that night, she told her Latina housekeeper about her symptoms. "Oh, señora, that's just your change," the woman laughed. "It happened just like that to my sister." And, of course, the housekeeper turned out to be right. What my patient had experienced was, as she herself had suspected, a variant of a hot flash. As I was writing the update of this book, Oprah Winfrey did a show on menopause. She described having palpitations and seeing several doctors in an attempt to figure out what was going on. As she said, "Not one of them considered that it might be related to menopause—and I'm Oprah!" I guess things have not improved much.

Women remain the experts about our own bodies. Your intuition about symptoms at this time of life is probably right. You've been living in your body for almost fifty years and you know it pretty well. Though some symptoms are more common than others, the range is enormous. My experience of the menopause transition included hot flashes, palpitations, and restless legs. As I told the young female cardiologist I saw for the palpitations, "It just feels like my whole body is unstable." I have listed in Table 3.1 some of the symptoms that have been reported by various women at various times to Janine O'Leary Cobb, who wrote a newsletter on menopause for twelve years.[1] I would add to her list jiggly legs, fuzzy thinking, blurry vision, and swollen joints. This list should show you that whatever you're feeling is probably normal. But don't be alarmed if your symptoms don't appear here. It doesn't mean that you're crazy or that you've really got some deadly, exotic disease. You'll want to check with your doctor to rule out anything serious, but it probably just means you've got a particularly unusual symptom.

On the other hand, you may not have any unusual symptoms—or even any of the usual ones. Ten percent of women don't experience perimenopause at all. They just stop menstruating. And this can seem the weirdest "symptom" of all, because we're so conditioned to think of menopause in terms of hot flashes, vaginal dryness, and wild mood swings. When one of my friends, an intelligent woman in her mid-forties, was told by her gynecologist that she seemed to be in menopause, she denied it. It was true she hadn't had a period in months, but she wasn't having flashes, her mood was fine, and nothing else in her body had changed. The poor doctor had an awful time convincing her that she wasn't premenopausal; she was just lucky.

The duration of perimenopausal symptoms also varies, although they rarely go on for more than a few years. Sonja and John McKinlay, Boston

TABLE **3.1**

Perimenopausal and Menopausal Symptoms

Menstrual irregularity

Hot flashes and/or flushes; night sweats

Dry vagina

Insomnia and/or weird dreams

Sensory disturbances (vision, smell, alterations to taste)

Funny sensations in the head

Lower back pain (crushing of vertebrae)

Waking in the early hours of the morning

Onset of new allergies or sensitivities

Fluctuations in sexual desire and sexual response

Annoying itching of the vulva (area around vagina)

Sudden bouts of bloat (waistline expands by two to three inches for an hour or two)

Chills or periods of extreme warmth

Indigestion, flatulence, gas pains

Rogue chin whiskers

Overnight appearance of long, fine facial hairs

Bouts of rapid heartbeat

Crying for no reason

Aching ankles, knees, wrists, or shoulders

Waking up with sore heels

Thinning scalp and underarm hair

Graying scalp and pubic hair

Mysterious appearance of bruises

Sudden inability to breathe (air hunger)

Frequent urination

Urinary leakage (when coughing or sneezing, or during orgasm)

Prickly or tingly hands with swollen veins

Lightheadedness, dizzy spells, or vertigo

Weight gain, and in unusual places (on the back, breasts, abdomen)

Sudden and inappropriate bursts of anger

Sensitivity to being touched by others (touch impairment)

Inexplicable panic attacks

Tendency to cystitis (inflammation of the bladder)

Vaginal or urethral infections

Anxiety and loss of self-confidence

Depression that cannot be shaken off

Painful intercourse

Migraine headaches

Easily wounded feelings

Crawly skin (formication)

Disturbing memory lapses

Table adapted from J. O. Cobb, *Understanding Menopause* (New York: Plume, 1993), p. 20, with permission of author.

researchers, were critical of most of the studies of women's experience of menopause because the studies looked only at women in medical settings. Women who go to doctors are usually having symptoms—that's why they're there. So the McKinlays did their own five-year study in Massachusetts, following 2,570 perimenopausal women. They found that the average length of the perimenopausal or transition period for these women was about three and a half years. About 10 percent of the women went from pre- to postmenopausal in a very short time—less than six months. They had fewer symptoms, particularly hot flashes, than the average woman in the study, and about 20 percent of naturally menopausal or surgically menopausal women reported that they never had hot flashes at all.[2]

According to most studies, about 5 percent of women continue to have hot flashes well into menopause or even for the rest of their lives; the rest have them off and on over about two to five years. Other symptoms of perimenopause are also usually short-lived. Even vaginal dryness can be transient. Generally, the body gradually rebalances at a lower level of estrogen. Menopausal symptoms, on the other hand, are usually persistent. These include symptoms that really come from living at a new level of hormones rather than just adjusting to the shift. They include vaginal dryness that persists or occurs several years after the last period and persistent decrease in libido.

It's interesting to note the degrees to which women are troubled by symptoms. In the McKinlays' study, only 16 percent felt that their hot flashes were really bothersome, 12 percent were upset by night sweats, 7 percent by problems with menstrual flow, and 3 percent by vaginal dryness. More women rated their symptoms as somewhat bothersome: 33 percent for hot flashes, 25 percent for night sweats, 5 percent for problems with menstrual flow, and 10 percent for vaginal dryness.

Some situations affect the severity of symptoms. You'll recall from Chapter 1 that surgical and medical menopause are more likely to give you abrupt and more disturbing symptoms. But of course none of this is carved in stone. You may have your ovaries removed and sail through your postmenopausal years symptom-free; you may have a natural menopause and flash till you're ninety.

Problem 2: Are You Perimenopausal or Just Getting Older?

Another problem with delineating perimenopausal and menopausal symptoms is that so many other things are happening at this stage in your life. Thus it's not always easy to sort out what causes what. You go through major life changes at middle age: your children leave home, your parents become ill and die, and your body begins to sag, wrinkle, and otherwise remind you of your lost youth and your own mortality. Stress can cause depression, and it can also throw your hormones out of whack.

Further, your body goes through other physical changes at middle age. Many symptoms attributed to menopause are actually just symptoms of aging. A doctor named Bungay in England sent a questionnaire to 1,120 women and 500 men.[3] Never mentioning menopause, he listed a number of symptoms and asked each respondent to note how many of them she or he had ever experienced. Much to his amazement, he found that the only symptoms that affected women more than men were hot flashes and vaginal dryness. All of the other symptoms, including many that we think of as perimenopausal, affected men as much as, or more than, women. Many of these symptoms turned out simply to be signs of aging. For example, loss of appetite, crawling or tingling sensations in the skin, headaches, and difficulties with intercourse affected men and women about equally.

Other experiences did appear to be related to menopause, however. While both men and women had crises around midlife that involved loss of confidence and difficulties in making decisions, perimenopausal women seemed to have more trouble with these than did men or post-menopausal women.

PERIMENOPAUSAL SYMPTOMS

Perimenopausal symptoms are usually transient, but they are often more troubling than menopausal symptoms. You can have any of these symptoms in varying degrees of severity or mildness, and you may experience the same symptoms differently at different times.

Let's look in depth at some of the more common perimenopausal symptoms. Later, in Chapter 11, I'll discuss how you can cope with them.

Hot Flashes

Hot flashes aren't confined to perimenopause, or even to women. Men with prostate cancer who are treated with estrogen sometimes get hot flashes when the treatment stops. And men who have had their testicles removed will also experience hot flashes, as will men put on tamoxifen to treat breast cancer. Niacin, too, can cause hot flashes in both men and women. However, since hot flashes are so frequent in perimenopausal and menopausal women, they are inevitably associated with menopause in people's minds.

The usual description of a hot flash goes something like this: you're sitting there minding your own business when all of a sudden you get a strange feeling and then your whole face and neck are hot, and maybe sweat breaks out on your upper lip or the nape of your neck, or even all over, and your heart starts racing. You pick up something to fan yourself with, or you think about tearing off your clothes—but before you know it, it's gone and you're drying out. Not a terrible experience when you're alone at your computer, but an extremely disorienting one in the middle of a presentation to the board of directors or a class of sixth-graders.

Hot flashes are the most common symptom of perimenopause in the Western world. We know they're related to estrogen, because estrogen medication gets rid of them—though the relationship is probably more complicated than simply a question of low estrogen.

Studying them hasn't been easy for researchers. They can't schedule you for a 2:30 lab appointment, then sit you down and say, "Okay, will you have a hot flash now, please?" They have to draw blood while you're there, hoping you'll have a hot flash or two while they're doing it.

In spite of this obstacle, some good studies have been done. One important study found that the flash is initiated not in the ovary but in the hypothalamus—the part of the brain involved with the pituitary and menstrual cycling.[4] That makes sense. The hypothalamus is located next to the thermoregulatory center, the thermometer in the brain that regulates your body's core temperature.

This gave researchers a clue about how exactly a flash works. Apparently what happens when you get a hot flash is that the normal mechanism overshoots. Normally, if you get hot, how do you cool down? Your face gets red, because blood rushes to the vessels nearest the surface so that they can release heat more easily, and you sweat. A hot flash is misnamed: it's really an attempt by your body to cool down. Researchers think that hot flashes happen when the set point of the thermoregulator gets abruptly shifted. It's as though somebody has walked by and pushed the thermostat in your head down to 55 degrees. Your brain says, "Uh-oh, you're 98.6 degrees now—that's too hot!" and immediately tries to cool you down by increasing your heart rate and the blood supply to your skin so that you blush and sweat. You may not have actually been too hot, but you will cool down.

One study documented that 30 percent of women have hot flashes within three years before menopause.[5] By one year before menopause, almost 50 percent of women have had at least one hot flash. By four years from their last period, however, only 20 percent of women were still having hot flashes. And 50 percent of women never experience hot flashes at all.

Howard Judd, an endocrinologist at UCLA, recorded the hot flashes of twenty perimenopausal women for two weeks.[6] Of a total of 1,041 hot flashes, the average flash lasted about three and a half minutes, but they ranged from five seconds to sixty minutes. On average, each woman flashed three or four times a day.

The menopause researcher Ann Voda questioned women about their flashes.[7] Most women in Voda's study described an aura or premonition before a flash started. Either a woman's heart rate went up or she felt a sensation in one spot—for example, behind one ear—just before it happened. (I get a prickly feeling on the backs of my hands.) The average age at which the flashes began was forty-five in women who had had surgical menopause and forty-eight in those whose menopause had occurred naturally. (This reflects the fact that a surgical menopause usually occurs earlier than a natural one.) There was no particular predilection for day or night flashing. The number of flashes varied greatly. One woman had 241 hot flashes in a two-week period; another had 2. One woman who had had 59 flashes in two weeks had 51 of them between 10 A.M. and 10 P.M.; another had all of hers between 4 P.M. and 2 A.M. There were two women who just had long flashes. The flashes lasted between thirty seconds and four minutes; the women who had the most flashes had the briefest ones.

The researchers were surprised at where women felt their hot flashes. Over half of the flashes started in the neck, head, scalp, and ears; 68 began in the neck or breasts; 59 below the breasts; 114 all over; 19 in the neck and above the breasts. Not all these women experienced flashes consistently in the same areas, though some did. One always had her flashes in her earlobe and cheek.

With regard to intensity, 455 flashes were rated as mild, 358 as moderate, and 116 as severe. *Mild* meant that a flash was barely noticeable, was quick, and didn't interfere with anything. *Moderate* meant that it was warmer, noticeable (with obvious perspiration in certain areas), and longer lasting; often the woman tried to end it by taking off some clothes. *Severe* meant that a flash was intensely hot and caused the woman to stop what she was doing immediately, remove as much clothing as she possibly could, and seek a way of cooling down. It caused profuse perspiration, often over the entire body.

When women in this study were asked what they did to relieve the flashes, they said that they fanned themselves or drank cold liquids, but nothing really helped much. There was no single common trigger event. Many of these women got flashes when they were asleep; some got flashes chiefly when they were very emotional. One woman's flashes responded to the temperature of the air around her: when it got hotter, they lasted longer.

Many had considered themselves "cold-blooded" before the onset of hot flashes. They had usually been colder than the people around them. They'd always had to dress warmly, especially before going to sleep; they wore socks to bed. When the hot flashes began, their overall body temperature changed. They now slept in light nightwear or in nothing. They disliked skin-to-skin contact with other people because they felt uncomfortably warm. They cut back outdoor activity during the hot summer months and used more air-conditioning than they had in the past.

This study and others confirm that there seem to be as many variants of hot flashes as there are women who have them. Some women experience waves of heat and drenching sweats followed by chills, but sometimes the chills come first. For some it's nothing more than a transient sensation of warmth; for others it's a perpetual heat wave. Sometimes flashes are accompanied by feelings such as tension, anxiety, heart palpitations, and nausea. Sometimes they aren't exactly flashes, but rather an overreaction to a normal stimulus. You're doing an exercise that usually makes you sweat a bit, and suddenly you're pouring sweat. Or you're in a room that's slightly stuffy and you suddenly feel as if you're in the Amazon forest.

Hot flashes aren't always awful. Many women don't mind them at all. Since I started writing this book, I've been getting frequent hot flashes myself, and I'm rarely bothered by them. Sometimes there will be a band of sweat across my upper lip. I have managed to have a hot flash while being interviewed on TV (triggered by the lights), while giving a talk about menopause, and in church (I always wondered why all those women made fans out of the program when I was a kid). My study is always strewn with sweatshirts and jackets that I have had to rapidly remove to cool down. On rare occasions, I have to rip off as many layers of clothes as I can without getting arrested for indecent exposure. Once I was heading toward downtown Los Angeles on the freeway and found myself pulling clothes off as I drove. (Luckily it *was* L.A., so no one noticed.) When I do something that would normally make me a little warm, like running across campus because I'm late for a lecture, I become very hot and sweaty. I often end up lecturing with my jacket off.

I don't find my hot flashes particularly distressing. In a way, I like having them: they're a badge of honor, a sign that I'm a perimenopausal (and now almost postmenopausal) woman. (Of course, if they were more severe, I might feel differently!) I never hide the fact that I'm having them. If someone asks why I've just removed my jacket in this cool room, I say, "It's okay—I'm just flashing." I now wear a button stating boldly THESE ARE NOT HOT FLASHES I AM HAVING, THEY ARE POWER SURGES.

In *The Menopausal Years: The Wise Woman Way*, Susun Weed describes hot flashes as useful—a way to get extra heat out of your body now that you're no longer menstruating.[8] Some women said they were actually happy about having hot flashes. To them, flashing signaled a quick, easy transition into menopause—almost as though they were flushing themselves out, allowing themselves to get on quickly with their lives. Without hot flashes, they believed, menopause was a longer, less comfortable process.

There are even cases of women enjoying the actual sensations of hot flashes. Sadja Greenwood, author of *Menopause Naturally*, interviewed a large group of women about hot flashes and found that between 2 and 3 percent liked "feeling the heat as energy traveling through their bodies."[9] My coauthor's aunt had hot flashes during a cold winter and appreciated the extra warmth.

Night Sweats and Insomnia

Night sweats are hot flashes that occur in the middle of the night. Typically, you wake up in a pool of sweat, having soaked your nightclothes and bed linen. Sometimes your heart is racing, and it is very difficult to get back to sleep. At other times you can change your nightclothes and go right back to sleep. Or you may not even wake up at all. I find that I just wake up a little damp in the morning, having slept through the whole thing. Sometimes a flash wakes me and I have to urinate, and then go right back to sleep Needless to say, if your night sweats keep you awake, you will grow increasingly tired. This can lead to mood swings and anxiety.

Some clinicians have attributed all of the insomnia of perimenopause to night sweats. But there probably is something else going on as well. While most night flashes cause waking, 40 percent of wakening is not associated with hot flashes. Most people awaken once or twice in the night, but they usually go right back to sleep. The perimenopausal woman often can't. It's this lack of sleep rather than the hot flashes or night sweats that drives many women to seek relief, medical or other. Hot flashes can usually be dealt with (see Chapter 11), but it's hard for a sleep-deprived woman to go to work or take care of her family.

Heavy Bleeding and Fibroids

Perimenopause brings changes in your menstrual cycles. For one thing, your periods often become irregular. The most frequent sign of the coming change is shorter periods. During your fertile years you usually have a cycle of about twenty-eight days. But in perimenopause, as in puberty, it's very normal to have wildly irregular cycles—twenty-one to twenty-five days between cycles and then sixty days before the next cycle. This can be confusing and alarming. Your period is late, and you wonder if you're pregnant. Or you're sitting in your office, and you suddenly feel that telltale dampness...but it's been only a couple of weeks since your last period. Once you've gotten used to the irregularity, and remember to take tampons or pads with you everywhere, irregular periods are usually not too much of a problem, though they can still be annoying.

Heavy bleeding, however, is a different story. It's the most distressing symptom most women report, the symptom that usually has them running to the doctor—and rightly so. Often, it's transitory. You may have a couple of heavy months and then stop, or have a heavy flow one month and a light flow the next and then a heavy flow again the next.

Other women are bothered by bleeding between periods. This can range from slight spotting to flooding, and it can last for a few days or continue without stopping.

Ann Voda is one of the first researchers to ask women about their experiences of perimenopausal bleeding, rather than telling them what they should be feeling. She describes how a woman goes through four stages. First you notice changes in your menstrual cycle. As these patterns change, you find you can no longer use your previous experience of your periods to predict what to expect. Of course, when your pattern of bleeding is so changed that you don't know when to expect a period, you're likely to feel anxious, annoyed, concerned, uncomfortable, or frustrated. Soon you find yourself checking with other women and your doctor to see whether this is "normal." If you find this happening, you realize you always have to be prepared for surprises, and you start to take precautions. (There was a time when I never left the house without a stash of tampons close at hand.) Finally, you reach the stage of wanting it to end. After all these years of menstrual periods, you get tired of wearing pads and tampons. The last straw is the unpredictability and uncertainty of perimenopausal bleeding, which reinforces your desire to just get it over with.

Sound familiar? It sure helps to know you are not alone. Most women can get through all of these changes as long as they know they are okay. Sometimes, however, even these normal changes are more than we can take.

Heavy bleeding can interfere with your life: it can make you anemic; it can make it nearly impossible to leave the house. Most alarming is the fact that though it's usually associated with hormonal shifts, you can't be certain that that's the case. It could be a symptom of something more serious. You should always check with your doctor and make sure. One of my old friends, a college professor, had heavy bleeding that she ignored because she assumed it was menopausal, and she ended up dying of endometrial cancer—cancer of the lining of the uterus.

You should consult a gynecologist if your periods come more than every twenty to twenty-one days, if they last more than seven to eight days, if you bleed between periods, or if your periods become much heavier than they used to be. To pinpoint the cause of abnormal bleeding, you'll need an endometrial biopsy. This is an office procedure in which a catheter the size of a straw is passed into the uterus and a small "bite" is taken from its lining. This is usually uncomfortable but not too painful. Some women will have uterine cramps or bleeding as a result. This is the easiest and most cost-effective way to make sure your bleeding isn't caused by endometrial cancer or hyperplasia (see Chapter 8). The biopsy can also indicate if you're ovulating. If it doesn't confirm that the bleeding is caused by hormonal shifts, then you'll need further evaluation. Your gynecologist may then do a vaginal ultrasound (putting a specially shaped ultrasound probe into your vagina to get a picture of the uterus) or hysteroscopy (putting a pencil-thin instrument into the uterus that allows the gynecologist to see the endometrium, the lining of the uterus). The traditional D and C (dilation and curettage) is hardly ever used for diagnosis anymore, because it isn't necessary.

Cancer, fortunately, is the least common cause of abnormal nonhormonal bleeding. Other, more likely, suspects are polyps and fibroids, which are anatomical problems.

Polyps are small outgrowths of the lining of the uterus. The surface of a polyp can erode and lead to bleeding. Polyps can be seen on ultrasound and snipped out easily through a hysteroscope.

Fibroids are also outgrowths of the uterus. They're very common: over 30 percent of women have them by the time they reach fifty. Nothing needs to be done about fibroids unless you're having symptoms. They are self-contained balls of uterine tissue that can grow quite large. They can be found under the surface of the uterine lining (submucosal), in the middle of the uterine wall (intramural), or on its outer edge (extramural, or subserosal) (see Figure 3.1). If they are on a stalk, they are called

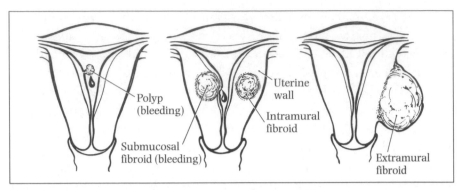

Figure 3.1. Anatomic uterine problems.

pedunculated. Where they're found determines the symptoms they cause. The surface of submucosal fibroids will sometimes erode and cause bleeding. This bleeding may be hormonally related, in which case it will get worse with your period. Taking hormones won't usually help the bleeding, however, because it is basically caused by an anatomical problem. Submucosal fibroids can be identified by vaginal ultrasound or hysteroscopy and can usually be removed at the time of hysteroscopy with an instrument called a resectoscope. Unless a fibroid is unusually large, there is no need to have a hysterectomy (see page 199).

Even if fibroids don't bleed, they can create other problems. Sometimes they can become enormous—even as large as a basketball. If that happens, you get symptoms because they take up so much room. They lean on your bladder, so you have to urinate constantly. They can cause indigestion. They're not cancer, and they're not going to spread—it's purely a question of discomfort.

Fibroids tend to get bigger as you get closer to menopause, and then they usually shrink after you go through menopause. So if your symptoms start at around forty-eight, you might want to try to hold off two or three years, till your body gets rid of them for you. I know many women who are playing a waiting game, hoping they'll reach menopause before their fibroids become so bothersome that they're driven to drugs or surgery.

The most common cause of heavy bleeding or abnormal periods in perimenopausal women is hormonal fluctuations that result from an imbalance of estrogen and progesterone. When you have an anovulatory cycle (one in which no egg was released), you don't produce any progesterone. The estrogen causes a buildup in the lining of the uterus, which then sheds irregularly as your estrogen levels go down. It's too much estrogen that leads to heavy bleeding in this situation. This problem can sometimes be diagnosed by vaginal ultrasound but is more commonly diagnosed by endometrial biopsy. It's actually a process of elimination. If it's not polyps, fibroids, or cancer, it's probably hormonal. And if it responds to hormonal treatments, it's probably hormonal.

Mood Swings

You know the image: the middle-aged woman is suddenly sullen and bitchy; her friends are aghast and her long-suffering husband explains sadly, "She's going through the change." It was this notion of the distressed, anxious menopausal woman, so prevalent in the 1950s, that inspired a popular drug called Menrium, a combination of the tranquilizer Librium and estrogen (variants are still available today).

Menopausal mood swings do occur, but not everyone gets them, and they're not always overwhelming. Many women describe perimenopause as similar to PMS. If you have mood swings—or just moods—right before your period, then you'll probably experience them during perimenopause.

Serious psychological problems such as depression and deep emotional distress are another matter. Several different studies suggest that these are not a common symptom. Major studies of a total of 13,000 women in Norway, Canada, and Massachusetts found that perimenopausal women did not experience an increase in psychological symptoms.[10] In the McKinlays' study, women who had a long and symptomatic perimenopause were more likely to feel somewhat depressed—which is hardly surprising. Other studies also suggest that mood changes are minimal. But women's experience of menopause varies widely, and what studies call minor symptoms may not be so minor to the women who have them. I think that there probably are some women whose brains are very sensitive to hormonal fluctuations. They're the ones who get postpartum depression and terrible psychological PMS, and they might also react to menopausal hormone changes, particularly if their menopausal situation comes on suddenly rather than gradually; for example, if they have had their ovaries removed. Studies show that women who have had hysterectomies are more likely to experience menopausal-related depression. That may be caused by a reaction to losing a body part, or by the sudden loss of hormones. It also occurs in women who have received chemotherapy for breast cancer. Women who have been on estrogen therapy and quit abruptly—rather than tapering off slowly—are also more likely to experience mood swings. Sometimes drugs like Lupron, which throws you into artificial menopause, can have that effect. The brain reacts to many chemical neurotransmitters that are related to the hypothalamus and thus to the menstrual cycle. We all know that there is a correlation between your hormones and your moods (ask any woman or anyone who has lived with one), but we really don't understand it. What tends to happen in these cases is an interaction through which outside emotional stress becomes exacerbated by internal chemical events. The hormonal changes don't actually cause the depression, but they change your body's equilibrium, so that a situation that would normally upset you a little upsets you a lot, and a situation that would normally upset you a lot devastates you. (This is similar to the change in temperature set point we saw with hot flashes.) For example, my coauthor, before her hysterectomy, was taking Lupron to stop her heavy bleeding. She was going through a family crisis and was already anxious and depressed. On the Lupron, she suddenly found her depression deepening and found herself becoming furious over small irritations. After the hysterectomy, she stopped taking Lupron and went on estrogen. Her mood went back to the level it had been at before, though the family situation remained the same.

Since we have so few studies on it, I can't prove this, but I'd be willing to bet that this is also what happens with puberty: the erratic hormonal activity intersects with outside issues in a girl's life and intensifies her moods. (I should note here that, while the infamous "swings" are usually discussed in terms of negative moods, they can also happen with positive moods: the mildly funny television show is suddenly hilarious, or the pleasant evening of bowling is wonderfully exciting.) I doubt that these subtle variations in mood are easily detected in large cross-sectional studies that are usually able to pick up only diagnosable psychological problems, such as clinical depression. Nonetheless, many women do experience this sense of imbalance in their moods.

My coauthor's situation illustrates the difficulty in identifying emotional states connected to menopause. Even at the level of clinical depression, this isn't easy to ferret out. As I've said, menopause occurs at a time when stressful changes are often taking place in people's lives. Children are growing up and leaving home—or staying at home as adults because of problems with marriages, finding jobs, or other troubles. Parents are elderly, growing more feeble, facing lingering illnesses, and dying.

Spouses or lovers may leave or become ill. The loss of youth can be devastating to middle-aged people in a culture that idolizes youth. The fact of oncoming menopause, quite apart from any of its physical effects, can be distressing, signaling the end of your fertile years and the end of an era in your life. Whatever combination of these things a woman is going through can cause periods of depression, just as it does with men.

The British researchers J. Greene and D. Cooke carried out an investigation of how a range of stresses affect postmenopausal women.[11] They found that stressful events in a woman's life accounted for more psychological and physical problems than did her menopausal status. Of course, life stress may have a direct biochemical effect on estrogen levels. There is some evidence that women who are depressed have lower estrogen levels, which go up when the depression lifts. In fact, a recent study showed a lower bone density in women who were depressed, another sign of decreased estrogen levels. It may be that feeling distressed triggers hot flashes in some women. Certainly we've all experienced hormonal changes with anxiety: you worry that you might be pregnant, and then your period is late.

Different women have different coping abilities before menopause, and those differences remain during and after this stage. If you're good at coping with stress, you won't suddenly lose that capacity with menopause. And often the anticipation of menopause is far worse than its reality. One study showed that premenopausal women had more negative attitudes about menopause than did women who had already been through menopause.[12] Seventy to eighty percent of the women in the study said they were relieved to reach menopause.

There is also a danger in underestimating the degree of psychological distress you're experiencing. Mood swings and fluctuations can be uncomfortable and unnerving, but actual psychological problems are disruptive and can take over your life. These can be triggered by menopause or can become intolerable with the additional stress of menopause. If you're in doubt, consult a therapist. Just as you don't want to take drugs unnecessarily for a normal life transition, you don't want to suffer needlessly from a treatable disorder—and emotional distress is treatable.

Fluid Retention

Fluid retention is another common symptom of menopause, and it can be very frustrating. You diet and exercise rigorously, step on the scale, and find you've gained five pounds! This happens premenstrually to many women of all ages, but often it begins in perimenopause in women who have never experienced it before. We don't know why this happens: I wonder if the body is trying to make sure it has enough fluid on board to take care of extra bleeding and sweating.

Like bleeding, fluid retention can happen one month and not again for the next several months, or it can happen for several months until you're convinced it will go on forever, and then suddenly it will stop.

Memory Problems and Fuzzy Thinking

You go upstairs to get something, and by the time you get there you can't remember what it is. You run into an acquaintance in the supermarket and can't for the life of you remember her name. Your brain just doesn't seem to be working right. Often your doctor will attribute this to lack of estrogen, but the evidence that menopause causes memory loss and fuzzy thinking is hard to quantify.

Some of the memory loss experienced around the time of menopause is caused by age, not hormones. When women over forty experience it, doctors tend to attribute it to menopause. In one study, a range of men and women were shown a list of things and then asked to repeat them.[13] Younger people did better than older ones, but nobody looked to see how much this differed between genders, if at all. Men have memory loss as well, and there are no studies indicating that their loss is less than women's. We do know that as people age, long-term memory remains better than short-term memory. You'll forget the name of someone who works in your office today; you'll remember the name of someone who worked in your office thirty years ago.

Again, it's hard to separate any effects of hormones on your ability to think clearly from the effects of the stresses of midlife. We do know that some aspects of perimenopause contribute indirectly to memory problems. Loss of sleep, stress over heavy bleeding, or constant severe hot flashes can bring on or exacerbate forgetfulness.

Fuzzy thinking is not uncommon in times of hormonal flux in general. Remember when you were pregnant? With big hormone shifts, there are certainly changes in your ability to concentrate and remember things. We all expect it. Postpartum fuzzy thinking can even be worse, although we chalk a lot of it up to lack of sleep. But rest assured that it all evens out again, and your brain does go back to normal.

The menopause researcher Barbara Sherwin found that even at different points in the menstrual cycle women have different levels of memory.[14] When your hormones are low, you do better at spatial, "male" things; when they're high, you're better at verbal, "female" things. But we're talking about really subtle changes. You may not notice them at all, or if you do, you'll think it's part of PMS. There's no reason to believe, for example, that your verbal memory is actually impaired in the phases of the menstrual cycle marked by low levels of estrogen.

Estrogen activates and progesterone apparently depresses the central nervous system. But although few studies have really looked at the effect of estrogen in normal women, those that have have shown no association between lower hormone levels in general and cognitive functioning.

We've all seen the headlines: ESTROGEN HELPS MEMORY! and ESTROGEN HELPS YOU THINK! These are mostly from a number of small studies (usually looking at only twenty women at a time) on memory loss in menopausal women. There have been two kinds of studies. In one type, the researchers take women who are on hormones and women who aren't, give them a battery of tests, and then compare the results. They find that women on hormones do a little better on some of the tests. It's hard to know what this means. The women on hormones are usually healthier, better educated, and of a higher socioeconomic status than the women who aren't. So it may not be the hormones causing the difference.

The other approach to studying this problem is to look at women who are about to have hysterectomies in which their ovaries are to be removed. Barbara Sherwin did one such study.[15] First she tested the women a month before the surgery. After surgery, she divided them into two groups. Half got estrogen and androgen; half got estrogen alone, androgen alone, or a placebo. Three months later she tested them again. The ones who got hormones did better on the memory tests than did those who got a placebo. Though these findings are interesting, it was a very short study. We don't know if the effect of hormones on someone thrown abruptly into menopause is the same as on someone who has a natural, more gradual, menopause.

Also, each of these studies used a combination of different tests. For instance, Elizabeth Barrett-Connor studied a group of women in the community of Rancho Bernardo.[16] The women who had used estrogen for at least twenty years had higher scores on one test but lower scores on the other tests. This suggests that estrogen might help maintain some aspects of short-term and long-term verbal memory, but it does not improve, and might even be bad for, visual spatial memory. It's certainly not a cure-all for memory problems. This was supported by the recent randomized data from the HERS study (see page 133), which showed that there were some tasks that were done better by the women on estrogen and, more interestingly, some that were done worse. The Women's Health Initiative has several studies that will be looking at this issue more closely.

In any case, the studies don't seem to be turning up differences in women's own awareness or experience. For example, a study by Jerome Yesavage and others at Stanford looked at seventy-two women who were on estrogen and seventy-two who weren't.[17] The women were given a list of sixteen names and asked to memorize them. On average, the women on estrogen could remember four names, and the others could remember three. Yesavage called that a "significant difference." In terms of statistics, he's right. But it's probably not too significant in terms of the women's lives. None of the women could remember ten names, as they probably could have done when they were twenty.

Such memory problems as exist are probably fairly short-term, even among women whose ovaries are gone. Animal studies appear to confirm this. In one study, researchers removed monkeys' ovaries, then put half of them on estrogen. They found no difference in the monkeys' memory, but the monkeys on estrogen had slightly better attention spans when tested.[18] However, the differences lasted for only a short time: within three months, the monkeys who were not given estrogen had caught up to the others. So either the monkeys got better at the test with practice, or some attention deficit comes from abrupt change of hormones and then evens out.

My conversations with postmenopausal women lead me to think that most of the fuzzy thinking and memory changes are short-term. We may not be able to avoid the toll the years take, but we're certainly as good as the monkeys at compensating. As we did with puberty and pregnancy, we do get back on an even keel.

Headaches

Migraines are definitely related to hormones, but exactly how and why they strike is unclear. Some migraines—particularly the kind that are related to the menstrual cycle—tend to go away after menopause. Some women have their first migraine during perimenopause; in some others, migraines become worse after menopause. Generally, a migraine has to do with blood-vessel constriction in the brain. Most commonly you notice an aura: this may cause a change in your vision, a blind spot, or even difficulty talking. This will be followed within about twenty minutes by a headache.

We know that migraines are more common in women than in men and that they start at puberty, so there's obviously a hormonal element. But it doesn't seem to be consistent. Nor do we know whether estrogen or progesterone is the culprit. Both affect blood-vessel constriction in the brain. Estrogen tends to dilate vessels; progesterone has the opposite effect. Hormone therapy sometimes alleviates the problem, but at other times it makes migraines worse. Obviously, we don't really understand migraines.

Many other kinds of headaches are related to hormones; these may well increase during perimenopause.

MENOPAUSAL SYMPTOMS

Though the majority of symptoms that have been called menopausal occur right before menopause, during the perimenopausal years, some do occur afterward. They may be short-term, but in some cases they last for the rest of a woman's life.

Vaginal Dryness

The image of the postmenopausal woman as "drying up" and becoming asexual refers to the common notion that with menopause you will lose all sexual lubrication and therefore all interest in sex. Although this is thought to be a universal symptom of menopause, it actually isn't. One study of 1,109 women showed that only 20 percent of postmenopausal women reported vaginal dryness, and only 15 percent of those were bothered by it.[19] Another study reported that 45 percent of postmenopausal women and 25 percent of pre- and perimenopausal women complained of vaginal dryness.[20] Some of the differences may have to do with how many surgically menopausal women were in each study. But in either case, this problem occurred in fewer than half of the women.

Vaginal dryness is not unique to menopause. Furthermore, it's not always a big problem when it does occur: one study showed that 80 percent of women with vaginal dryness felt satisfied with their sexual relationships.[21] (Since the study didn't include questions about whether or not the women were sexually active, it may be that at least in some cases this answer reflected the fact that the women didn't have or want a sexual relationship.) What I find most interesting is the fact that vaginal dryness also seems to be transient in many women. As with many of the other symptoms we have been discussing, it often improves when your hormones come into balance again. Unfortunately, though, this isn't always the case. For some women dryness continues after menopause, and it tends to worsen with age.

Vaginal dryness probably results from changes that occur in the genital area at lower levels of estrogen. The vagina and surrounding connective tissue can lose elasticity. The vagina can get smaller, thinner, and more fragile. It bleeds more easily if it's scratched, and it can get very sore and raw.

In addition, the acidity of the vagina can change, increasing the possibility of infection. The cervix gets a little smaller, and you can experience less lubrication with sexual arousal. This tends to be particularly true of women who are not very sexually active—the old principle that "if you don't use it, you lose it." Regular intercourse stretches out the vagina and increases blood supply and lubrication. Even regular masturbation will decrease symptoms of dryness and irritation.

I think vaginal dryness (sometimes called vaginal atrophy) is often overdiagnosed. It can be extremely alarming to a woman who has no symptoms to be told by her gynecologist in the middle of a pelvic exam that she is "drying up down there." One woman I know had a vague sense of something being different in her vagina and went to her gynecologist. He examined her and found nothing wrong but decided she was a candidate for vaginal dryness and gave her estrogen cream to prevent it. While it's true, as we'll discuss in Chapter 15, that the dosage of estrogen in vaginal cream is low, it's still medication, and I think it's foolish to use it when you don't need it.

Studies show that women who have had a surgical menopause and women who undergo menopause as a result of chemotherapy have more problems with vaginal dryness than women who undergo a natural menopause. This again is probably caused by the lack of the testosterone and estrone that the ovary provides.

Skin Changes and Wrinkles: Is It Menopause or Age?

As part of their effort to sell youth, the drug companies often imply that estrogen keeps your skin young. They use young-looking models to sell the product, intimating that these are menopausal women made youthful by estrogen, and that if you use estrogen, you'll look like these near-nubile women. As with many other ads, the actual language doesn't lie—they never say that estrogen will prevent wrinkles. As I mentioned in Chapter 2, the package insert for Premarin clearly states that it does not help your skin and even lists as one of the side effects "a spotty darkening of the skin, particularly on the face." But the picture does the lying for them: that smooth-skinned, youthful beauty isn't saying, "My mom uses estrogen."

Loss of estrogen doesn't cause wrinkles and sagging. Age does that, in both women and men. Too much exposure to the sun, and smoking, will hasten the process. The most important factor for youthful skin, however, is your genes. If you are born with the right genes and stay out of the sun and don't smoke, you'll have the best chance at staying youthful looking for a fairly long time.

There are only a handful of scientific studies on estrogen and skin changes, and they show little or no relationship between the two. One study from Spain showed that estrogen didn't prevent the expected loss of collagen with age.[22] Another study looked at collagen content in the skin of women who were taking estradiol and testosterone.[23] The ones who were on hormones had slightly more collagen in their skin than the ones who weren't. There was one other, larger study looking at collagen in both bone and skin. These researchers found differences in bone, but not in skin.[24] Although these studies are interesting, they don't tell us anything immediately useful, since we don't know exactly how collagen is related to wrinkles, sagging, and aging skin. One theory is that estrogen doesn't actually prevent wrinkles and sagging but rather causes the skin of your face to retain fluid, making it a bit more puffy and thus filling out some of the lines you've earned over the years.

A large observational study in 1997 gave more credence to the claims that estrogen helps prevent skin aging. It showed a decrease in dry skin and skin wrinkling in the women on estrogen compared to the women who were not. This study, of course, has all of the limitations of observational studies, since healthy women are more likely to take hormones. Nonetheless, it is interesting and needs further research.[25]

Weight Gain

One of women's greatest fears is that menopause will cause them to gain weight. In a society that's neurotic about being thin, women panic at the thought of weight gain. In fact, women usually do put on some weight with menopause, but it's hard to determine the exact cause. As we discuss in Chapter 12, you need fewer calories to maintain your weight as you grow older. If you also decrease your activity, as people often do in middle age, then you're bound to gain weight. But more important, you're likely to see your weight shift. It's as if all those years of gravity finally take their toll, and you find that your hips, lower abdomen, and bottom are bigger than you remember. Although you can't stop gravity, you can keep your weight stable with exercise and a reasonable diet.

Urinary Problems

Since there is a larger elderly population today than in the past, we're hearing more about incontinence (leakage of urine). As you can see from all the television commercials for Depends, this is a problem that comes with aging, and it can happen to both women and men. It's more common in women, however, and in many cases is probably related to menopause.

There are many kinds of urinary problems. You may have pain when you urinate (dysuria). Sometimes you'll have a sense of urgency—you feel as though your bladder is desperately full—but when you try to urinate, only a little comes out. You might also experience frequency, a constant need to urinate. These symptoms are related to infection and irritable bladder and are best treated by a urologist. The more common symptoms can be described with two questions: Do you lose urine when you cough? Do you sometimes lose urine because you can't get to the bathroom in time? These symptoms have been linked with menopause. In fact one study did show that the vast majority of urinary problems after menopause were in women who had had hysterectomies.[26] Whether the urinary problems came from the surgery itself or from these women's lower hormone levels is not clear, however.

There are two kinds of incontinence. One is *urinary incontinence,* which affects 10 percent of postmenopausal women. The urethra, the tube that carries urine from the bladder out of the body, has estrogen receptors. After menopause, the urethra gets thinner, and some of its tissue shrinks. This causes it to lose strength. When you need to urinate and feel a lot of pressure in your bladder, you tighten up the muscles that hold it in till you can get to the nearest toilet; but a weakened urethra can't help hold it in as well, and you'll get leakage.

Stress incontinence is probably the most common urinary problem in women between ages sixty and seventy-five. It occurs when you lose a little bladder control if you laugh, cough, jump, sneeze, or bear down. This tends to be related to muscles and to having had children, rather than to low estrogen levels. In rare cases, there's a loss of sensation: you don't know you have to urinate and aren't tightening the muscles, so the urine comes out. There are of course factors other than the urinary tract related to stress incontinence. You may be bedridden and unable to get to a bathroom. Or you may have arthritis in your hands that's so severe you can't get your underpants down in time.

In the HERS study, which randomized women to Prempro and placebo, researchers were surprised to find that women on HRT had an *increase* in urinary incontinence and uterine prolapse (where your uterus drops).[27] One more incidence where HRT has not fulfilled its claims.

Not all incontinence is permanent. As with vaginal dryness, some women have a temporary problem while their hormones are readjusting and then are fine again. Studies have tried to determine if women on hormones have fewer urinary tract infections, but until recently they hadn't found any connection. Finally, in 1993 a randomized controlled double-blind trial was done on postmenopausal women with recurrent urinary tract infections who used intravaginal estriol cream. After eight months, the women treated with estriol had a statistically significant reduction in urinary tract infections. This is good news. Estriol is less potent than estradiol and much less is absorbed from the vagina into the rest of the body, making this a good choice for women whose only problem is urinary tract infections.[28] Keeping a record or diary of all the fluid you drink, and when and how much you urinate, can be a useful tool for diagnosing urinary tract problems.

Libido

Does menopause quash or quicken your love life? We all know that the most important sex organ is the brain. It's a little difficult to judge what the effect of menopause is on sexual interest and sexual behavior because they appear to be relatively independent of natural estrogen levels. No correlation has yet been found between estrogen levels and sexual interest.

What is the origin of the idea that after menopause you lose interest in sex? It comes from small, widely reported studies. Most of the sexual problems studied have come from clinical samples—women who had gone to the doctor because of some health concern and so had problems of one sort or another already. There have been very few well-designed studies of sexual interest in healthy people. The famous sexologist Alfred Kinsey and his colleagues interviewed women throughout their life cycles, and they found that there was a decline with age in incidence and frequency of marital intercourse and of intercourse to the point of orgasm. But there wasn't a decline in women's solitary sexual activity until well after sixty.

A study done in 1972 showed also a gradual decrease in sexual activity with age, particularly between forty-five and fifty-five, in both men and women.[29] A British study in 1985 showed that men reported a greater sexual loss of interest in their late forties and fifties than women did.[30] This would suggest that loss of sexual interest and reduced sexual activity are signs of age or of a partner's lack of interest, not signs of menopause. And maybe this is why some of those women engaged in solitary sexual activity.

One study of sexual behavior in sixteen women over the course of their menopause found small but significant decreases in sexual activity, sexual thoughts, and vaginal lubrication, but not in frequency of orgasms or in sexual enjoyment.[31] In another study, 70 percent of women between forty-five and fifty-six reported being sexually active, with no differences between the pre-, peri-, and postmenopausal women. Women between fifty-five and sixty-five were less sexually active than younger ones. And the major physical problem they discussed was vaginal dryness, which can cause discomfort with intercourse and thus affect sexual behavior.

In Chapter 2, I mentioned a study of women in a village in Thailand.[32] This research looked at sexual behavior in a different cultural context. Some women in the study experienced a decline in libido, but they didn't see that as a disadvantage: they felt released from having to worry about sex.

So while it seems that menopause either contributes to or coincides with some lessening of sexual desire, not everyone experiences that, and not everyone who does experience it considers it a problem.

Sometimes menopausal symptoms, rather than menopause itself, contribute to sexual problems: vaginal dryness, night sweats, hot flashes, etc.

Again, surgical menopause may affect sexual desire and attractiveness. After hysterectomy, whether or not her ovaries have been removed, a woman can lose interest in sex. She may also lose a degree of sexual desirability. There seems to be some biological basis for this. Studies of monkeys show that the male is no longer attracted to a female who has been hysterectomized.[33] But when the vaginal secretions of nonhysterectomized female monkeys are rubbed on the one who had the hysterectomy, the male regains interest. These secretions contain pheromones—aromas that are sexually stimulating. After hysterectomy they are no longer produced in the female. We do need to be careful about drawing conclusions about human sexuality from animal studies, since so much of our sexuality is psychological and sociological. But we can't rule out the possibility that the loss of pheromones affects male sexual responsiveness—or, for that matter, female responsiveness—to a woman.

In addition, hysterectomy alters the relationship of the vagina to the surrounding tissues. (Once something is taken out, the other organs shift to fill in the space.) This may affect how intercourse feels to both partners.

Another consequence of hysterectomy and removal of the ovaries has been postulated by the researcher Barbara Sherwin, who thought that a lack of testosterone may be what causes problems with libido.[34] In 1985, Sherwin and her colleagues found that giving testosterone to women who'd had their uteruses and ovaries removed enhanced the intensity of their sexual desire and arousal and the frequency of sexual fantasies. However, there was no evidence that testosterone affected the women's physiologic response or interpersonal aspects of their sexual behavior. The effect appeared to be more on motivation than on activity. Most of the articles about the effect of testosterone on libido are not scientific studies, just theories. This hasn't stopped one writer, Susan Rako, from writing a popular book—*The Hormone of Desire*—about the wonders of testosterone.[35] She writes about herself and many women she has consulted with (see Chapter 15), but she lacks the scientific data that might prove her case. The recent data on the significant increased risk of breast cancer in women with high testosterone levels make this approach more questionable.[36]

As I've pointed out before, menopause is a major change. You're unlikely to "feel like your old self" and more likely to feel like a new self. This may include new ways of being sexual and intimate. Some women feel more able to have sex with abandon, since they no longer have to worry about birth control; others feel less driven by their hormones to have sex. Everyone is different, and everyone's response is different. The most important point is that you feel comfortable with yourself and your libido. If you don't, then give yourself permission to explore ways of changing the situation. I'll discuss a few of these ways in Chapter 11.

FOUR

PREVENTION AND RISK: UNDERSTANDING RESEARCH

Once upon a time, you went to the doctor because you were sick. If you felt okay, you didn't worry; you assumed that nothing was wrong and you went about your business. But in the past twenty years, there's been a strong focus on stopping disease before it starts. With this emphasis on preventive medicine, the concept of health has been redefined. As one cynic has said, "If you think you're healthy, you just haven't had enough tests done yet." Prevention has saved lives and forestalled needless suffering. But it has also fostered a boom in medical technology that has made health care decisions more complex and confusing. We have far more options about health care than our mothers and grandmothers ever had.

This hasn't been an unqualified boon. We started to realize this when daughters of women who had taken DES to prevent miscarriage in the 1940s showed an increased rate of vaginal cancer, while the mothers themselves had a disproportionate incidence of breast cancer. The original high-dose birth control pill caused strokes. The radiation therapy given to cure acne of the chest in the 1950s caused breast cancers that began to emerge in the 1990s. Understandably, though, the medical industry has preferred to focus on the more positive aspects of scientific progress.

Nowhere has the concept of preventive medicine caused more confusion than in the area of menopausal hormone therapy. In Chapter 3 we talked about the short-term symptoms of perimenopause and menopause. When treatment of such symptoms is called for, it is, for the most part, used for only a few years. Taking hormones for three to five years for the symptoms that you're having now, and then tapering off over six to nine months, may well make sense. For symptoms such as vaginal dryness that can sometimes be lifelong, very small doses of hormones, applied locally, may be the right choice (as you'll see in Chapter 11). But when we move into prevention, the issue gets trickier. Do you want to take hormones for the rest of your life to prevent diseases that you may or may not get? This question hinges on several others. Can hormones really prevent osteoporosis and heart disease? Is it safe to take these drugs for twenty or thirty years? Do we really know whether they cause breast cancer?

When I wrote the first edition of this book, there were no large prospective randomized controlled studies of postmenopausal women and hormones. That kind of "gold standard" research, which I'll explain shortly, just hadn't been done. And therefore there were no real answers. The first of many randomized controlled studies have since been done, prompting this update. First were the studies on secondary prevention. That means we are studying women who already have a disease and are trying to prevent recurrence or further events. The initial studies have been in heart disease and osteoporosis, but several studies on Alzheimer's disease are ongoing. It is usually the case that interventions that work in secondary prevention will have a lesser but real effect on healthy women. An example would be lowering cholesterol in women who have had a heart attack in order to prevent a second heart attack (which is secondary prevention) and lowering cholesterol in healthy women with high cholesterol but no heart disease (which is primary prevention). The good news is that we also have a very large study of primary prevention underway.

The Women's Health Initiative (WHI) was designed to define the risks and benefits of strategies that could potentially decrease heart disease, breast and colorectal cancer, and fractures in postmenopausal women. It is really a set of clinical trials including a low-fat diet, calcium, and vitamin D supplementation, Premarin alone (in women who have had hysterectomies), Prempro, and an observational study with no intervention. It started in 1993 and has recruited 161,809 women over five years in forty different clinical centers. Although the plan was to give the first results of these studies in 2006, one of them was stopped early because the risks of Prempro outweighed the benefits (see page 80).[1] The good news is that not only do we have some answers about the use of Prempro but that there will be lots more data coming out of the WHI over the next ten years. It is likely to be the defining study of menopause and will finally give us some of the answers we have been craving. Until then we will review all the data we have on each topic, observational and randomized. Remember as you read this that the unrandomized data are circumstantial evidence and like all circumstantial evidence, it's flawed and subject to interpretation.

In this chapter I'm going to try to explain the evidence: how the studies are done and what their limitations are. My goal is not only to help you understand what weight you should give the studies that have been done, but to help you evaluate the ones that you'll hear about after this book comes out. In other words, I'm going to help you become a more discerning consumer of health news. My goal is to help you understand how we could have been so wrong about HRT and heart disease. I want to warn you now, however, that many of you will find this boring. If you want to, you can skip to Chapter 5. My feelings won't be hurt. And you'll be in good company—most doctors don't understand these nuances, either. Those of you who want to be one up on your doctor and want to really understand how to analyze one of these studies, read on. And those of you who aren't sure, come on in. Read what you want and skip what you don't.

There are many ways to conduct studies. But doing a completely accurate, comprehensive study is next to impossible. There are too many variables in studying even the simplest disease or life stage. To understand how accurate a study is, you need to be able to look at all its elements. It may be weak in one area, stronger in another, and excellent in a third. It's sort of like comparing the different grades for a school composition. One composition may get A for spelling, B for handwriting, and C for content. Another might get B for spelling, C for handwriting, and A for content. Although the average grade is B in both cases, the composition graded C for content may not be half as good as the one graded A for content. There are different aspects of a study that make it more or less credible.

Unfortunately, most doctors don't really understand study design. (Statistics and epidemiology are the courses most students sleep through in medical school.) And doctors are as prone to self-deception as the rest of us: they tend to believe the studies that feed their biases and discount the ones that don't. Further, as we discussed in Chapter 2, their source of information is often a drug company—which means that their bias is usually in favor of hormone therapy. Thus their overall tendency has been to overestimate the benefits and underestimate the risks of long-term use of hormone therapy.

This same tendency is reflected by the media—whose relationship to corporate interests is strong ("Tonight's weather is brought to you by . . .")—and they are even less able than doctors to critically analyze the strengths and weaknesses of studies. We've all had the experience of reading in a newspaper that some study shows that drug X causes disease

Y, only to read in the same paper a few days later that a new study proves it doesn't. The reporters often don't understand the nuances of the study, and the researchers have their own bias in presenting the results. Rarely do news reports point out flaws in the design of a study. And even when they do, we often hear what we want to hear. Recently I read an article in the *New York Times* about a study that had been started, looking at the effect of estrogen on Alzheimer's disease. The article clearly stated that the current data were preliminary and thus a big, well-designed study was necessary. That day at lunch a friend of mine overheard a woman in a restaurant saying to her companion, "Did you hear that estrogen can cure Alzheimer's disease?" All of these factors create widespread confusion about hormones and their effect on the prevention and risk of disease.

KINDS OF STUDIES: WHICH ARE MOST RELIABLE?

There are two main categories of studies, each with its own strengths and weaknesses. One is the observational study. In an *observational study* the researcher observes people doing what they might normally do but doesn't intervene. The second is a *clinical trial,* or *interventional study,* whose purpose is to test a certain drug or treatment, so the researcher has the subjects change their behavior (by taking a pill, perhaps) and records the results. There are a few varieties of each of these studies.

Observational Studies

Observational studies can be cross-sectional studies, cohort (follow-up) studies, or case control studies.

In *a cross-sectional study,* a large number of people are asked about their symptoms at a given moment in time. One study might survey a number of fifty-year-old women who have had bone-density tests and find that 50 percent of them have low bone density. That will provide a sense of the usual bone density of a fifty-year-old. It won't, however, provide any idea about why they have a given bone density—and, as you'll see in Chapter 5, there are significantly different possible reasons.

In a *cohort,* or *follow-up, study,* a particular group of people is observed over time. For example, a study could look at a hundred forty-five-year-old women and measure their bone density for the next ten years. This is sometimes also called a longitudinal study, since the women are followed over time. This would provide a better idea of whether all the women lost bone density at menopause or whether only some did. On the other hand, the data would be limited to those one hundred women, who might or might not be representative of the population as a whole. If a cohort is large enough, the researchers can compare people with a given condition and people without it. The Nurses' Health Study in Boston, Massachusetts, is a cohort study that has carefully followed a group of 121,700 nurses since 1976.[2] The nurses fill out questionnaires about their health every two years. The researchers periodically analyze different diseases or risk factors in this group. Because the number of subjects in this study is so large, the data obtained are very powerful, but the study still has limitations. The researchers have no control over the behavior of the women in the study. They can't, for example, decide who gets hormones, or who gets mammograms; they can just ask questions. So the study might include some women at risk for breast cancer who aren't getting hormones or who are getting more frequent mammograms, and this will skew the results.

Cohort studies can be either retrospective or prospective. *Retrospective studies* look at the medical histories of a certain number of people, some of whom have a particular condition and some of whom don't. The researchers then try to determine how many of them had a certain risk factor. For example, they might look at women diagnosed with Alzheimer's and find out how many of them took estrogen at menopause.

Prospective studies start on the other end. They take a group of subjects and follow them forward over a period of years. For example, a prospective study might take a group of women who have been on estrogen at some time in their lives and compare them with a group who haven't, to see how many develop breast cancer in the next ten years. Prospective studies are generally thought to be more accurate than retrospective studies, which depend on the participants' memories: depending on memory is chancy at best, and the difficulty is compounded when the subject being studied has a disease like Alzheimer's. But prospective studies are more difficult to conduct, and more time consuming.

A *case control study* looks at a group of people with a certain condition, comparing them with another group of people who don't have the condition but who are similar to them in other ways. For example, you might take a group of people recently diagnosed with lung cancer and match them up with people of the same age and sex chosen randomly out of the phone book to see how many people in each group carried cigarette lighters when they were in their thirties. And you might learn that, indeed, more people who carried cigarette lighters got lung cancer. But there's always the chance that factors you don't know about or don't understand will enter into the equation. For instance, you might conclude that the plastic in cigarette lighters causes lung cancer, completely missing the fact that people who carry cigarette lighters use them to light cigarettes, and it's the cigarettes that cause the cancer.

This, of course, is a fanciful example, invented to illustrate my point. But there are many actual cases of such mistaken leaps of logic. And it is similar to what we think did happen with HRT heart disease and breast cancer. We've noted that women who have hysterectomies are more likely to be on long-term estrogen therapy and also that most women with hysterectomies have also had their ovaries removed. This was particularly true in the 1970s and 1980s, when the fact that estrogen increases the risk of uterine cancer had just been proved. It was for this reason that 60 to 80 percent of the women in the large studies of estrogen therapy were those who had undergone surgical menopause: they no longer had uteruses at risk from estrogen. But women who have had surgical menopause tend to be fairly young—in their early thirties or forties—so the women in these studies are often younger than women who experience menopause naturally. Thus the subjects in the studies are at lower risk for breast cancer to begin with, and the increase that we find from estrogen may be underestimated.

A particular group may be chosen for an observational study because of convenience—e.g., researchers might question all the women who live in the same retirement village to study the relationship between estrogen and breast cancer. But this creates some limitations. It may not be clear why some women were put on estrogens and others weren't. Asking them would be of limited use, because they themselves may not know—many patients simply do what the doctor tells them to without asking questions. This can introduce enormous bias, as you'll see when we look at one such study in more detail later on.

Clinical Trials or Interventional Studies

Clinical trials, or interventional studies, are actually studies of treatment. (By definition, clinical trials are prospective.) Everyone in such a study is given a certain treatment to see what happens. The problem is that in order to tell if something works, you need a *control group*—people who haven't been given the treatment—for purposes of comparison. Sometimes researchers will use "historical controls," meaning that they'll look at what the results of a previous treatment were and see if a new treatment makes a difference. The problem with this type of study is that you don't really know what made your patients different from those in the past. For example, the survival rate of women with breast cancer has improved, even with conventional treatment. So if you tried a new treatment and saw a small improvement, you wouldn't know if that was from the treatment or whether it was just another instance of the fact that women do better now.

Our hypothetical study of a retirement village would be even better if researchers gave the "experimental" group estrogen and the "control" group a placebo (inert pill). This would be a *controlled study*. You could compare the results in one group with the results in the other, but you wouldn't know if the two groups themselves were really comparable. For example, if by chance all the women with a family history of breast cancer were in the experimental group, the results could be inaccurate.

It would be a much stronger study if researchers could take the women in the retirement village and randomly pick a number of them to take estrogen, and then follow them for ten years to see who got breast cancer. That way we could be sure that the women given estrogen weren't by coincidence those at low risk for breast cancer, thus biasing the results. The study would then become a *randomized controlled clinical trial.*

Randomization is a concept that most people don't understand. *Randomized* doesn't mean "accidental" or "capricious"; it means that each person in a given group, large or small, had an equal chance to be chosen for a study, or that each person had an equal chance to be chosen to receive one treatment or another. In a randomized study, each subject's treatment is picked randomly, usually by a computer, to eliminate the possibility that subjects will be chosen on the basis of situations they're already in, skewing the results. If all of the women who exercise were put on one treatment and all the couch potatoes on another, the first treatment would end up looking a lot better than it really was.

If neither the researchers nor the subjects know who's taking which pill, there will be no temptation to treat one group differently, perhaps by performing more mammograms on the group taking estrogen. That type of study is called *double-blind* because both the researchers and the subjects are in the dark as to who's getting what treatment.

A *prospective randomized double-blind controlled study* is the "gold standard" of studies. It has the fewest flaws and is thus the most reliable.

There's still the problem that women who choose to participate in such a study may not be like the rest of us—most people, after all, prefer to know what treatment they're getting and don't want to risk being given nothing or a placebo. But it's the closest we can get to good data.

The first large randomized controlled study on HRT and heart disease is the HERS study. This study took women who had heart disease, or angina, and randomized them to take Prempro or placebo. The results of this study surprised everyone. The women on hormones had more heart attacks and strokes than the women on placebo. This is exactly the opposite of what had been demonstrated in the observational studies, which indicated a decrease of 50 percent in heart attacks in women on HRT. This finding was substantiated in healthy women when the Women's Health Initiative halted the estrogen and progestin randomized control study early. They also found an increase in heart attacks and strokes (29 percent and 41 percent, respectively).[3] How can we explain this difference? In the observational studies the women on hormones tended to be healthier, wealthier, and more likely to be prevention-minded. The observational studies could not distinguish whether hormones make you healthy or healthy women take hormones. The randomized studies now suggest that it is the latter. Observational studies can only suggest hypotheses but cannot prove cause and effect. We need well-designed, randomized studies to do that. Luckily, there will be much more data coming out of the Women's Health Initiative as well as many other randomized controlled studies that are ongoing.

WHO'S IN WHAT STUDY?

Aside from knowing what kind of study you're looking at, you need to be aware of who's in the study. In this case, you need to know how a study defines "hormone use." Some studies take into account how long a woman has used hormones; others don't. Some simply compare women who have taken hormones with women who have never taken them, without considering how long the hormones were taken. Such a study ends up lumping together someone who took hormones for three months and someone who took them for thirty years. Other studies lump together women who have taken different doses and preparations of hormones. Some studies compare women who are currently taking hormones with women who took them in the past.

All of these studies may have different results, depending on how estrogen relates to the particular disease being studied. If estrogen prevents heart disease by lowering levels of the cholesterol that gradually clogs arteries, you'd expect that taking it for ten years would put off your risk of heart disease for ten years. On the other hand, if its effect is mostly on dilating clogged coronary blood vessels at the time of a heart attack, you'd expect that only a woman who was taking it at the time of her heart attack would get any benefit.

We also need to be aware of *selection bias*. A study is biased if the people in it are not typical of the general public. As you'll recall from Chapter 2, the approach to giving estrogen therapy to women with a risk of heart disease has been contradictory over the years. Originally, there were two things that worried researchers about using estrogen to prevent heart disease. One was the study we discussed in Chapter 2, in which estrogen was given to men who had heart attacks.[4] Not only did the estrogen fail to reduce their likelihood of further heart attacks; it actually seemed to make their risk of future heart attacks a bit worse, and doctors feared that it would have the same effect on women with heart disease. Doctors were also concerned when it became clear that the early high-dose birth control pills, especially when used by women who smoked, caused an increase in heart disease and strokes. They feared that estrogen treatment for menopause would have the same effect.

These two concerns made doctors reluctant to give estrogen to women who had high blood pressure or were otherwise at risk of heart disease. So until fairly recently, they didn't. Nor did they give estrogen to women who were at risk of breast cancer, because of a suspicion that the hormones would promote the cancer. This is why the women getting hormones have been at low risk for heart disease and breast cancer to start with. This selection bias—studying women at low risk to start with— means that all observational studies are likely to end up *overestimating* any benefits in terms of controlling heart disease and *underestimating* dangers in terms of contributing to breast cancer.

Perhaps most important, we need to understand the *"healthy woman" effect*. As I mentioned, studies have shown that the type of women who take hormones are the type who also do other things to take care of their health.[5] They go to the doctor frequently. If they have high blood pressure, they take care of it. They exercise; they eat a good diet; they don't smoke. They tend to be better educated and to have a higher socioeconomic status. It's these motivated women, with a healthier lifestyle, who get put on hormones and studied. They read the magazines; they go to the doctor and say, "I read about high blood pressure in this article. How do I prevent it?" In fact, women who take estrogen therapy have a decrease in all causes of death, even those that have nothing to do with estrogen, like injuries.[6] Women who aren't on hormones, on the other hand, tend not to go to the doctor till they're sick, not to exercise, not to reduce fat in their diets, etc. They therefore tend to be less healthy. As I mentioned, the "healthy woman" effect has proven to be the explanation for much of our inflated vision of the benefits of HRT.

In addition, there is the *"compliant woman" effect.* Women taking estrogen replacement therapy are by and large compliant people—they do what the doctor tells them to do. A study of men and women who had heart attacks showed that participants who were compliant about taking their prescribed placebo had the same reduction in the risk of heart attack as those who took drugs—and both groups did better than those who didn't take their placebos regularly.[7] We don't really know what this means. It isn't just the well-known placebo effect, which shows that to some extent what you believe is happening to you influences what actually does happen. The compliance effect is more like the "healthy woman" effect. If you're someone who follows the doctor's orders, you not only take your pill religiously every day, but you also exercise religiously, avoid high-fat foods, and generally do the other things your doctor tells you to do. Also, because most women don't stay on hormones (only about 25 percent of the women who start on estrogen are still taking it five years later), those who stick with them over the course of many years in a given study are a select group for that very reason.[8]

I myself fell into this trap of not looking at who was being studied when I stated in the first edition of this book that "under age seventy-five, more women die of breast cancer than of heart disease." Critics pointed out that according to U.S. Public Health Service statistics, there are more deaths from heart disease than from breast cancer in women over sixty. I was basing my remarks on the Nurses' Health Study. In this study there is less heart disease than in the general population, since nurses, in general, take better care of their health. Therefore, this may not be the best group to use. My point that breast cancer occurs at a younger age than does heart disease is valid, but it got lost when I didn't pay enough attention to who was being studied.

WHAT IS THE STUDY STUDYING?

Since women who are on hormones are more likely to go to the doctor, they're also more likely to get mammograms and other screening for cancer. It's possible, therefore, that when these women get breast cancer, they're more likely to be diagnosed earlier, which means that they'll get treated earlier and have a higher survival rate. Thus a study might turn up an increased incidence of breast cancer, but not an increased death rate. These are two different things. One study might look at how many women on hormones get breast cancer, while another might look at how many women on hormones get breast cancer and die from it. It's very important to know what a study has been set up to determine. This is known as its endpoint. When you're looking at the results of a study, you need to ask yourself what its endpoint is. That endpoint may or may not be relevant to your life.

There's a well-known example of this. A study examined the benefits of hip replacement surgery versus simply nailing back together a patient's broken hip. The endpoint was to determine how many days patients from each group had to spend in the hospital. The researchers found that patients who had hip replacements had longer hospital stays—which, given the study's endpoint, meant this procedure was not as good as the other. If they'd looked at which procedure gave the patient a better chance of walking, however, they'd have come to the opposite conclusion. No one asked the patient with a broken hip—who probably would be perfectly happy with an extra day or two in the hospital if that meant being able to walk out of it. This is why it's so important to look at exactly what the endpoints of a study are, and to make sure that they're as relevant to you as they are to the researchers.

Sometimes a study on one disease can also give us some information about other diseases. For example the MORE (Multiple Outcomes of Raloxifene Evaluation) trial, which looked at raloxifene (Evista) as a treatment for women with osteoporosis, also noted effects on breast cancer and heart disease. It is important to mention that the randomization is done for the primary disease. In this case it was women's risks for fracture that were balanced, and a similar effort was not made for the risks of breast cancer or heart disease. We can look at the effect of the drug on these other diseases, but we can't prove that it works except in that limited population. So the fact that raloxifene decreases breast cancer significantly in that study means only that it decreases it in women with osteoporosis. We need another study (luckily it is being done: the STAR study [the Study of Tamoxifen and Raloxifene]) to see if this is also true in women at risk for breast cancer.

HOW SERIOUS IS "INCREASED RISK"?

When you hear the results of a study on preventing a disease, you need to know how common the disease is, at what age it's likely to occur, and what your personal risk is.

For example, ovarian cancer can be very deadly, but it's not very common: about one in eighty women over forty will get it. If you are at double that risk, your chance is one in forty. Breast cancer, by contrast, has a lifetime risk of one in eight. Doubling that risk gives a chance of one in four—a much higher probability of developing the disease. A greatly increased risk of a rare disease may have less overall effect on a woman's health than a modestly increased risk of a more common disease. It's easy to get overly alarmed when a headline blasts that a certain treatment doubles your risk of a deadly disease if you don't take into account how common or uncommon the disease is.

It's also critical to look at the average age of people who get a disease. You may not want to take a drug like estrogen for thirty years to prevent a disease like osteoporosis that you're not likely to get till you're eighty, especially if you're at risk for other life-threatening medical conditions.

WHEN SHOULD PREVENTION START?

There are two ways to approach prevention, and they have very different implications. *Primary prevention* means treating people to prevent a disease that they may or may not get. The idea is to try to keep the disease from happening at all. This is the rationale for giving all women over fifty hormones to try to prevent them from developing heart disease.

Secondary prevention means treating someone who already has a disease, in order to prevent the problem from recurring or worsening. For example, a woman who has had a heart attack at sixty-five may be put on estrogen to try to prevent a second heart attack.

Primary prevention has its advantages: obviously, you're better off not getting the disease in the first place. But it involves subjecting people to new risks in order to prevent something that may not happen at all. Thus, many women with osteopenia (low bone density, which is not in itself osteoporosis: see Chapter 5) who would never have had hip fractures may take a drug like Fosamax and may suffer from long-term side effects from the treatment that we aren't even aware of yet. With secondary prevention we're treating only those we know will benefit, such as women who have had a fracture. But there's the risk that people will suffer more severely because they developed the condition in the first place: some women will die from the original fracture, or be seriously weakened by it.

Since each approach has its risks, doctors often try to reserve primary prevention for those who are at higher risk for the disease—those for whom there is likely to be more benefit than risk. Therefore, one of the major questions about hormone therapy is whether to take it now or wait until later, and that brings us to our next question.

CAN WE PREDICT WHO IS AT RISK?

Risk factors are conditions that increase your likelihood of getting a particular disease—for example, smoking increases your likelihood of getting lung cancer. Having a risk factor doesn't necessarily mean that you'll get a disease, nor does not having any risk factors mean that you're home free. In fact, few risk factors are as dramatic or as clear-cut as the connection between smoking and lung cancer. Knowing your risk factors is just a tool for making an educated guess.

It's also important to realize that having a risk factor for a disease doesn't necessarily mean that you're going to get it sooner than anyone else. If most people have a one-in-ten chance of getting a disease at age fifty and you have a factor that doubles the risk, this means that you have a one-in-five chance of getting the disease at fifty—not that you'll get it at twenty-five. Certain risk factors do, however, mean you're more likely to get a disease prematurely—for example, hereditary breast cancer often strikes younger women than the more common, nonhereditary kind.

This is something you need to be very clear about when making a decision. You may feel very different about an increased risk of a life-threatening illness that will hit you when you're fifty, when you could reasonably hope for another twenty-five or thirty years, as opposed to one that will strike when you're eighty, when you're more likely to die of other causes anyway.

It's sometimes hard to apply these numbers to yourself, since your issues are rarely just about one factor. You might have a history of breast cancer and also have low bone density, or you might have a lot of both breast cancer and osteoporosis in your family. We will talk more about how to weigh your individual risks in Chapter 16.

DISEASE OR RISK FACTOR?

Sometimes, instead of studying a disease itself, researchers study a risk factor for that disease. For example, instead of trying to learn how many children who see the Joe Camel billboards will end up dying of lung cancer (a study that could take decades to complete), we could look at how many of the kids who see the billboards start smoking. We know that not all of those children will die of lung cancer, but we also know that many more smokers than nonsmokers get lung cancer, and that most people who get lung cancer die of it. A risk factor used as the endpoint of a study is called an *intermediate marker*—we're looking at an early stop along the road to the disease.

But we need to be careful not to confuse these two kinds of endpoints. It's important to know what affects risk factors, but it's equally important not to confuse risk factors with diseases. Even with something as clear-cut as cigarettes and lung cancer, the equation isn't exact: not all smokers get lung cancer, and not all people who get lung cancer smoke. With less clear-cut risk factors, this is even trickier. Are we measuring how many women get fractures of the hip, or what happens with their bone-density tests? Are we measuring heart attacks or cholesterol levels? Not everyone with high cholesterol will get a heart attack. In addition, if a drug improves heart disease because it dilates clogged blood vessels rather than lowering the cholesterol that causes the clog, the studies looking at cholesterol alone might misinterpret the drug's effect on heart disease. In fact the women in the HERS study and also in the WHI saw their cholesterol go down significantly but did not have a corresponding decrease in heart attacks. Even with a good study like the Postmenopausal Estrogen/ Progestin Interventions (PEPI) study, which I'll discuss in depth in Chapter 6, this is a problem.

HOW BIG IS THE STUDY?

Finally, we need to know the size of the study. If there's a big difference in the effect of a treatment, it will show up in a relatively small study. If, for example, a treatment decreases the death rate from stroke by a third, that will become obvious after studying one hundred women, with fifty getting the treatment and fifty a placebo: three times as many women in the treatment group will be alive after, say, ten years. But if the effect is smaller, it will take a larger study—a study of more women—to demonstrate that. For example, the Nurses' Health Study, looking at 121,700 women, reported in the summer of 1995 that estrogen and progesterone therapy increased the incidence of breast cancer by 70 percent in women between sixty-five and sixty-nine.[9] (This doesn't mean that 70 percent of women on hormone therapy got breast cancer; it means that 70 percent more women on hormone therapy got breast cancer than women not on hormones.) Within a week, a second study came out from Seattle, stating that there was no increased risk of breast cancer in women taking estrogen and progesterone.[10] The media took these parallel studies as showing that scientists can't make up their minds. In fact, the second study was too small to show a 70 percent effect—it included only 1,029 women. It could only have shown a 250 percent difference (2.5 times as many) between the two groups.[11] It didn't contradict the Nurses' Health Study at all.

All of this isn't meant to confuse you, but to demonstrate why data can be confusing. Needless to say, those who believe in estrogen for everyone will be inclined to quote the studies that feed their bias and ignore the weaknesses in those studies. The same is true of those who feel that estrogen is dangerous. Doctors don't often have the time to analyze studies closely, and so they may accept uncritically the results they want to believe.

In the next chapters, we'll discuss the diseases that have been related to menopause in women, how common they are, what their risk factors are, the age at which they occur, what it's like to have them, and what the studies show about preventing them. We'll address the strengths and weaknesses in all the studies, to help you decide the issues for yourself with the best information available.

FIVE

Osteoporosis: Are We All Going to Crumble?

Osteoporosis (defined as brittle bones—a definition I'll get into later) is one of the new "in" diseases. Although it has been around forever, no one paid that much attention to it because there was no way to prevent it and no good way to treat it. The advent of the bone-density test and several drugs that prevent bone loss have moved it into the forefront.

In an attempt to increase awareness, however, we have gone overboard with ads on TV showing women fearful of breaking their bones or losing height. Osteoporosis is no fun, and I'm not making light of it. But our fear of it is out of proportion to its reality. Only about 25 percent of women will ever develop osteoporosis.[1]

Because we thought that osteoporosis was caused by low estrogen, it got a reputation as a woman's disease. But men, too, can get osteoporosis, if they live long enough. As with heart disease the focus on menopause as the sole cause of osteoporosis has obscured the real issues in this disease. In fact, a recent article by John Kanis from the United Kingdom called attention to this with its title: "Are oestrogen deficiency and hormone replacement a distraction to the field of osteoporosis?"[2] He notes that the incidence of hip fracture is the same in men and women at age fifty. Bone density decreases in women from ages fifty to seventy and then stops decreasing. It would be great to blame all fractures on this differential, but, in fact, hip fractures are most common just when things stabilize out. It probably is not the lack of estrogen that causes these fractures, but other factors. This is substantiated by looking at different countries and their risk of hip fracture. They range from very high in Sweden to one fifth that rate in Germany, implying that more than low estrogen is involved.

THE BONE-HOUSE

To understand osteoporosis, it helps to know a little about bone itself. Bone isn't static. It's continually being added to and remodeled. How this process works is fairly complicated, but I'll try to explain it using a metaphor (itself rather complicated) borrowed from the Old English epic Beowulf, in which the body is called the bone-house. (In medicine, we speak of the bones' "microarchitecture," implicitly accepting this powerful image.)

In the beginning, your skeleton is like the first small house a couple moves into when they're just starting out. It's perfect for two people, but soon the kids start coming and it begins to get cramped. So our young couple, being fairly prosperous, decide to remodel. First they have to do some demolition. Then a cleanup crew comes. Next, a construction crew builds a playroom for the kids. This whole process takes at least six months (see Figure 5.1).

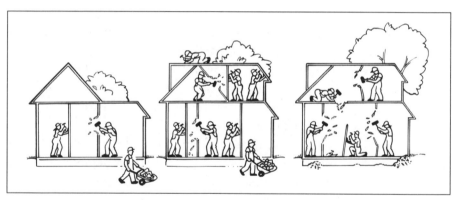

Figure 5.1. The "bone-house."

Your skeleton remodels itself much the same way. There are bone-remodeling units, called *osteons,* which function like the construction crew. These osteons consist of *osteoclasts* (the demolition crew), *reversal cells*—also called *mononuclear cells*—(the cleanup crew), and *osteoblasts* (the rebuilders). Once an area of bone is activated (a process we as yet don't understand, in which the bone is tagged for remodeling), the osteoclasts arrive and spend the next couple of weeks resorbing a predetermined amount of bone in that spot (see Figure 5.2). When the osteoclasts

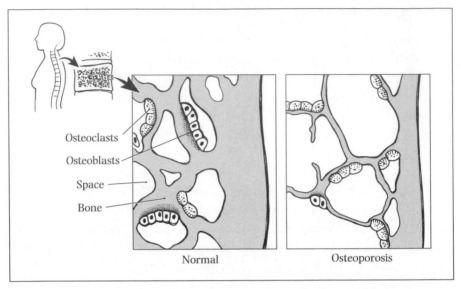

Figure 5.2. Osteoclasts and osteoblasts in *(left)* normal bone
and *(right)* osteoporosis.

have finished, the mononuclear cells come and clean up the surface to prepare it for new bone formation. Then come the osteoblasts. They begin to
fill the newly cleared-out area with new organic matrix, called *osteoid* (a
jellylike substance that frames the new bone). After a delay of twenty-five
to thirty-five days, this osteoid becomes mineralized—it turns to bone. A
complete remodeling cycle takes several months.

This bone remodeling continues throughout your life. During the first
twenty to thirty years of life, there's more building than demolition (as in
the first twenty years of our couple's marriage—they might tear down the
garage to build a kid's room and a playroom). There may be a crisis now
and then that calls for more remodeling, such as a fracture or broken
bone (just as a house might get damaged in a hurricane). By about age
thirty-five, you have all the bone you're ever likely to have.

BONE DENSITY

Peak Bone Mass

The amount of bone that you have by thirty-five is called your *peak bone
mass*. Although you'll continue to remodel when it's necessary, from here
on you'll be losing more bone than you build.

Your own peak bone mass will depend on a variety of factors. One factor is your genes; identical twins raised in different circumstances tend to have very similar peak bone masses.[3] We might compare this genetic component of peak bone mass to the amount of money the couple had in the bank to buy the house in the beginning.

Your diet is another factor. If you take in enough calcium and vitamin D in your early years, you'll build more bone than if you don't. This dietary factor could be compared to investments made by our couple to increase the money available for the house.

Exercise also plays a role. The more you exercise, the more bone you'll build—just as our couple might put in overtime hours in order to earn more money for the house.

Turnover and Bone Loss

Bone turnover never stops completely. In fact, after about age fifty, it increases, though it's not quite coordinated. The building team (the osteoblasts) becomes less and less capable of completely refilling the holes left by the demolition crew. Some women (though not all) experience more rapid loss of bone around menopause; this is thought to be due to increased activity from the osteoclasts, which become hyperactive and penetrate too deep into the bone, perforating it and making it brittle. This results in a less stable structure, disrupting the microarchitecture, which can lead to fractures. Basically, it's like having termites eating away at the framework of your house and weakening it.

The peak amount of bone you started with and the rate of this loss will determine the density of your bones. Density will be very different in different individuals, cultures, races, and sexes.

Low bone density is only one factor in osteoporosis and the fractures that result from it. Another factor is the microarchitecture of the bone. As the osteoclasts demolish or resorb more bone than is rebuilt, the architecture becomes more fragile. Just as a flimsy house is more drastically damaged by a hurricane than a sturdier house, a fall or some other injury will do worse damage to a fragile bone than to a sound one.

Some kinds of bone are more susceptible than others to turnover and loss. As they weaken, the wrist and the hip become more vulnerable to fractures. Vertebral bone—the bone in your back—doesn't really fracture or crack but rather collapses on itself. This makes you lose height and, if enough vertebrae are crushed, gives you a dowager's hump. It usually takes four to five crushed vertebrae before you notice a difference (see Figure 5.3 later in this chapter).

As with everything wise in life, any imbalance tends to be bad. If you stop bone resorption but keep on building bone, you risk having over-mineralized bones—which are also more fragile.

Hormones and Bone

What do hormones have to do with bone? All of these stages of bone maintenance we've been speaking about need fine-tuning. Hormones help do this job. What's interesting about the hormones that affect bone is that they appear to regulate calcium metabolism rather than bone remodeling itself. Calcium is important throughout the body, and the body has a precise mechanism for making sure that there's enough calcium for the heart and other cells. The major hormones involved in the process are parathormone (from the parathyroid glands), calcitonin (from the thyroid gland), and vitamin D (from the skin). (You usually don't think of vitamins as hormones, and most aren't, but vitamin D actually is, in that it's secreted by one organ and travels through the bloodstream to affect another organ—which is the definition of a hormone.)

There are other hormones that influence calcium less directly: thyroid hormone, adrenal hormones, estrogen, progesterone, and testosterone and other androgens (male hormones). These are set in motion by the parathyroid glands—tiny structures in your neck, behind the thyroid. These glands monitor the amount of calcium in the blood. If it goes below a certain level, they go into action and secrete parathormone. This tells the kidney to hold on to calcium and not let it flush out in the urine. They convert inactive vitamin D to active vitamin D (see below), which helps you absorb more calcium from your food. And they tell the osteoclasts to resorb more bone and release the calcium into the bloodstream. Since calcium in the blood is used by every cell in the body to maintain its integrity, they decide to sacrifice calcium in the bone in order to maintain calcium in the blood—somewhat like burning the furniture to keep a cabin warm when you run out of firewood. This becomes important to older women (and men) who may not be getting enough calcium or vitamin D in their diets. The resulting lower blood level of calcium sends the parathyroid glands into action and starts increasing bone loss. Getting enough calcium and vitamin D in your diet can prevent this type of bone loss. A three-year study done in Boston looked at the effects of dietary supplementation with calcium and vitamin D on bone density and fractures in healthy men and women over sixty-five. They found that there was a moderate reduction in bone loss and a decrease in the risk of vertebral fractures.[4] Interestingly continuous high levels of parathormone are bad for bone, but intermittent increases have been shown to build bone and form the basis for the use of this hormone in women with severe osteoporosis.

The thyroid gland produces calcitonin and the imaginatively named thyroid hormone. Calcitonin inhibits osteoclasts and slows down remodeling, maintaining adequate bone mass. Unfortunately, this helpful hormone decreases with age and with menopause. (One of the new treatments for osteoporosis involves a synthetic form of this hormone—see Chapter 15.) Thyroid hormone can cause increased breakdown of bone if it's too high. This can result from having an overactive thyroid or from taking thyroid medication for many years at too high a dose. (If you've been on a thyroid hormone such as Synthroid, you should have periodic blood tests to monitor your thyroid function and make sure the dose isn't too high.)

Vitamin D is always present in our skin, in an inactive form. Sunlight will activate it. It can also be obtained through certain foods. Vitamin D helps the intestine absorb calcium from food; it also helps the kidneys reabsorb calcium from urine. Thus it's an important regulator of blood calcium levels. If you don't get enough sunlight, you'll get rickets, a disease in which the bones soften. This sometimes happens in nursing homes in the Northeast, where sunlight is limited in winter and residents have little need to go outside. However, if you get too much vitamin D (more than 1,000 milligrams a day), it will leach calcium from your bones and so increase bone loss.

Adrenal hormones called *glucocorticoids,* or *steroids,* help your body deal with stressful physical events. They're also sometimes taken as drugs. Steroids make bone overly responsive to parathyroid hormone and vitamin D so that calcium can be mobilized in an emergency. This, of course, increases bone loss.

As far as we've been able to determine, estrogen has a less direct effect on bone. It blocks the bone-resorbing effect of parathormone and stimulates the release of calcitonin and vitamin D. Progesterone also seems to have some effect on bone—possibly by blocking the effect of the adrenal hormones. Finally, androgens like testosterone, produced in women by the postmenopausal ovary, stimulate osteoblasts and can build bone. (This is in part why men have a higher peak bone mass to begin with— they have much more androgen, produced by their testicles.)

There's still a great deal about bones that we don't understand. What tells the remodeling to go on in one place and not another? Why do black women have denser bones than white women? What determines the microarchitecture that is so critical to fracture prevention? As we discover more about the active maintenance of strong bones, we'll be much better able to prevent the problems that occur when they go awry.

So, What Is Osteoporosis?

The definition of *osteoporosis* has gone through many permutations over the years. In the old days, osteoporosis meant fractures caused by thin bones. The current definition—agreed on by an international consensus panel of medical experts in the field—has changed the focus. (These panels are generally funded by government agencies, sometimes with the help of drug companies.) Osteoporosis is now "a disease characterized by low bone mass and microarchitectural deterioration of bone tissue, which lead to increased bone fragility and a consequent increase in fracture risk."[5] In other words, you've got brittle bones that are more likely to fracture. The problem with this definition is that the "disease" is not an actual fracture but only an increased risk of fracture. This is like defining heart disease as having high cholesterol rather than having a heart attack. Needless to say, this new definition has increased the number of women—and men, for that matter—who have "osteoporosis."

Although this new disease has two components—bone mass and microarchitecture—one of them is virtually ignored: the bone's micro-architecture. There's a reason for this. Microarchitecture is ignored because we can't measure it; we can measure only bone density. And if the microarchitecture is strong, you'll be less likely to get fractures. So the definition is beginning to shift again: we're hearing *low bone density* itself, without microarchitectural deterioration, referred to as *osteoporosis*. It's true that people with very high bone density don't tend to get fractures unless they receive a serious blow to the bone. But not everyone with low bone density gets fractures. By these new standards, you could live a perfectly comfortable life for thirty years after menopause with a "disease" you never knew you had.

This might be funny, except it can cause patients needless fear. I got a frantic call once from a patient who'd just learned she had "severe osteoporosis." I asked if she had any broken bones, or was hunched over, or had any other symptoms. No, she said, she was fine. But she'd just had a bone-density test that showed low density, and the doctor had told her she had this terrifying disease and needed to stop playing sports. The poor woman was devastated.

I have serious problems with this whole business. Why not define low bone density as a risk factor for osteoporosis, rather than as osteoporosis itself? That puts it in perspective: it's a warning sign that might be useful so you can begin to consider ways to keep fractures from occurring.

Measuring Bone Density?

As you can see, the ability to measure bone density has changed the way we look at osteoporosis. In the past, the only tool available was the X ray, which couldn't identify low bone density until it was at least 30 to 50 percent below normal. But now we have techniques that can measure density with far more accuracy.

There are a couple of tests used for screening women for low bone density. Both are painless. *Single-proton absorptiometry* was developed first and is still used by many doctors. Now there's *dual-energy X-ray absorptiometry* (DEXA). This is a better tool for gauging bone density (though not necessarily twice as good, as its name might suggest). DEXA can measure the bone density of the hip and spine, the areas usually involved in fractures. It can detect a loss of as little as 1 percent of bone mass from year to year. But this may be misleading. Because there is an error rate of from 1 to 2 percent, bone mass would have to have increased approximately 5 percent in order to be detected by a bone-density test repeated one year after treatment. Even the best treatments take two to three years to achieve this much change. So an unchanged bone-density test after one year does not mean that nothing is working. Despite this fact, many doctors erroneously use annual bone-density tests to monitor osteoporosis.

It has several other limitations. It measures only the lumbar spine—the lower back. It can't measure the thoracic, or upper back, which is the part involved in vertebral crush fractures. It sometimes overreads bone density when there are benign calcium deposits in the area (such as those that result from arthritis). And it can't detect fractures. This is a serious limitation, since spontaneous fractures in the vertebrae are the basis for a lot of real osteoporosis—dowager's hump and loss of height.

To detect crush fractures, doctors take a standard X ray of the upper back. Crush fractures are irreversible, and with two or more of them you fit the original definition of osteoporosis. Even then, however, you might not actually feel anything—as we said earlier, it takes four to five of these fractures for you to notice any difference in your posture.

In addition to DEXA measurements of the hip and spine, bone density can be determined by quantitative CT of the spine, forearm, or hip; by DEXA of the forearm, heel, and fingers and by quantitative ultrasound of the heel, fingers, forearm, and tibia. Although they are all appealing, their exact role has not been determined. This is because the rates of bone loss are not the same in all bones. The T scores (see page 97), thresholds for treatment, and response to treatment are all based on the DEXA of the spine and hip and can't be transferred to these other approaches. In addition, these devices are not good for screening because a significant proportion of women with osteoporosis of the spine and hip are missed. What they are good for is determining fracture risk in older women. This is because the risk of fracture is not based on T score but age and bone density.[6]

Far more useful than any of these would be a test that could measure microarchitecture as well as bone density; with such a test, we could more accurately diagnose the risk of fracture. To date, though, we don't have it. It would also be helpful if we could measure the *rate* of bone loss or turnover.

The key to determining the risk of osteoporosis will be a combination of all these factors—how much bone you have, how strong it is (microarchitecture), and how fast you're losing it. At the moment doctors can learn this only by repeating a bone-density test after three or four years to estimate the rate of loss. Obviously, you'd like to have a much better way to gauge your danger of fracture if they could predict the loss in advance.

There are now two urine tests that can monitor bone resorption (the demolition crew). During resorption, bone breaks down into small collagen fibers, some of which are released in the urine. When you're breaking down bone rapidly (regardless of whether you're also building it up at the same time), the level of portions of these collagen fibers in the urine increases. One urine test, Osteomark, measures one such type of fiber in the urine; CrossLaps measures another. Other blood and urine tests of resorption are being developed. These tests can't detect osteoporosis per se. (You could have very low bone density and not be actively losing bone and thus have a normal test; or you could have temporarily high bone turnover as a result of a healing fracture and thus have a high test.) The reproducibility of bone resorption markers is even poorer than that of bone-density tests, with day-to-day variations on the order of from 40 to 50 percent. Although they are being promoted to monitor the effects of treatment, the tests are not actually accurate enough for this role.[7]

These new tests are just the beginning. Expect to see many more sensitive ways to monitor bone formation and bone loss in the near future.

"Normal" Bone Density

We don't in reality know what "normal" bone density should be. For women, "peak bone density" has been defined as the typical bone density of a thirty-five-year-old. Anything else is defined as abnormal. But that may not be a reasonable definition. Smooth skin is "normal" for a thirty-five-year-old. Does this mean that wrinkles are "abnormal" for a sixty-year-old? Is gray hair abnormal? The rest of your body changes, so why should bone be the same in your sixties as it was in your thirties?

The way experts came up with the definitions of osteopenia (low bone mass) and osteoporosis was by going backward. They measured the bone densities of women who had developed fractures due to osteoporosis. Then they looked at the data and saw that 90 percent of the fractures occurred in women whose bone density was below a certain number.

This number is called the fracture threshold.[8] Researchers determined that between ages forty and forty-nine, 5 percent of women are below the threshold; between ages fifty and fifty-nine, 20 percent are below it; between sixty and sixty-nine, 45 percent are below it. The goal of the osteoporosis researchers is that everyone should maintain bone density above the fracture threshold. To do this, 50 percent of seventy-year-old women and 75 percent of eighty-year-olds would need treatment.

The *T score,* which is reported on a bone-density test, is the number of standard deviations (level changes) between a given bone density and the density of a normal twenty- to twenty-nine-year-old who worked for the company that makes the bone density machine. According to the current definition, set by the National Osteoporosis Foundation and others, *osteopenia* is 1 standard deviation (that is, one step away) from the bone density of a normal young woman. *Osteoporosis* is defined as more than 2.5 standard deviations from the density of a young woman. *Severe* or *established osteoporosis* is bone density more than 2.5 standard deviations from that of a normal young woman plus one "fragility fracture."[9]

So when you hear that *x* women have osteoporosis, what you're often finding out is that *x* women have a bone mass that's 2.5 standard deviations below that of a young woman. Likewise, when you hear that there are now many more women with osteoporosis than there were in the past, part of that increase is nothing but a change in definition. Needless to say, the broader the criteria used to define osteoporosis, the more women will fall into that category. It's as if you were deciding on a definition of *tall*. If you define *tall* as "over six feet," you'll have far fewer tall people than if you define it as "over five feet." This will be very useful to you if you have an investment in the existence of a lot of tall people. The level of bone density that defines osteoporosis has been set rather high, with the result that most older women will fall into the "disease" category—which is very nice for the people in the business of treating disease.

If you define osteoporosis as more than 2 standard deviations below the bone density of a normal young woman (a slightly looser definition than the figure I mentioned above, 2.5 standard deviations), then fully 45 percent of white women over age fifty have the condition at one or more sites.[10] (As I noted earlier, black and Asian women have different degrees of bone density than white women—and most studies, predictably, are done on white women.[11] Interestingly, because Asian women have low bone density, being Asian is often listed as a risk factor for osteoporosis—in spite of the fact that they actually have far fewer hip fractures than white women.)

J. A. Kanis, in an analysis of T score, noted that the effect of age is eleven times stronger than the effect of bone mineral density.[12] For the same level of bone mineral density, the fracture risk is much greater in older than in younger women. Osteoporosis experts are starting to address this dilemma by suggesting other ways to use the bone density data. Best would be using the bone density and age of the woman to predict her actual risk of fracture. This would give you the absolute risk or the risk she has to have a fracture today, rather than her risk in comparison to a twenty- to twenty-nine-year-old. A second approach would be to determine her risk in comparison to the average risk of fracture rather than the risk of young women.

All agree that too much emphasis has been placed on one test. "Bone density is only one part of a complex part of risk factors that indicate whether someone will have fractures in the next few years, and I put it last on the list," says Bruce Ettinger, M.D., a senior investigator at Kaiser Permanente in Oakland, California.[13] "I begin with the more important risk factors, and the number one risk factor is age." If two women have the same bone density, Ettinger explains, and one is sixty and the other is seventy-five, it is the older woman who has a much greater risk of fracture. Next, says Ettinger, he learns whether a woman has had a fracture of the wrist, upper arm, or spine already, because that is the next strongest risk factor, quadrupling the risk for future fractures. He then takes into account whether the woman is thin, smokes, or has a family history of osteoporosis, all of which increase risk. "After looking at all of these things," Ettinger says, "adding bone density modifies risk a little bit, but it doesn't change it all that much. So by starting with the DEXA scan, we've been kind of doing it in reverse."

An even bigger problem is the misunderstanding of osteopenia. The osteoporosis experts "didn't want women who have a lower score to think that they are okay; they wanted them to be aware that their bone density is low," explains Steve Cummings, M.D., a professor of medicine and epidemiology at the University of California, San Francisco School of Medicine.[14] "So how did they decide to motivate women to pay more attention to low bone density and to motivate the government to understand that there are more women with low bone density than the number who have osteoporosis? They decided to make up a word, and that word was *osteopenia*. And then they made up another number, and that was minus one."

There was no real medical basis for choosing that number, though, and "what no one noticed," Cummings adds, "is that now half of all postmenopausal women would be called abnormal and be told that they have osteopenia."

The diagnosis of osteopenia probably has led more women to pay more attention to their bone health. But it also may lead them to worry more than is necessary. What doctors need to point out to women, says Ettinger, is that "osteopenia is not a disease, does not indicate a high risk of fracture in the next five to ten years, and is really almost a variant of normal." If a woman learns she has osteopenia at age fifty-five, he explains, it means she is just around average. "What I tell women in their fifties," he says, "is that having osteopenia means their bones are different than those of a twenty-five-year-old—and I note that there are probably many things about them that differ from when they were twenty-five. And I let them know that it is nothing to be alarmed about."

Kanis agrees, saying that "the use of the threshold for osteopenia is associated with only modest increases in hip fracture risk compared with that of the general population. Indeed, for postmenopausal women at the age of fifty years at the threshold for osteopenia, the fracture risk is *less* than that of the general population at the same age" (emphasis mine). The reason is that the T score is comparing these women with twenty- to twenty-nine-year-olds. He concludes that, "If this range is to be used, then it is inappropriate to use the threshold of osteopenia for clinical decisions even in menopausal women."[15] Osteopenia is not something that should be treated, because we don't even know what it means to young women or women in their fifties. We should keep our eyes out for a new and better definition of fracture risk and not panic with a diagnosis of osteopenia.

MENOPAUSE AND OSTEOPOROSIS

It used to be thought that all women have a considerable decrease in bone at menopause, when their estrogen levels shift—and so "estrogen deficiency" was said to be the cause of osteoporosis. This was based on cross-sectional studies of bone density in women of all ages. It's now becoming clear that the process isn't this simple. Longitudinal studies following individual women's bone density over time have shown that although some women lose a lot of bone with menopause, others lose comparatively little; also, some bone loss starts earlier.[16] One Danish researcher did a study using urine tests to measure calcium loss and concluded that some people are naturally "fast losers" and others are naturally "normal losers."[17] About 35 percent of women are fast losers and will indeed lose a lot of bone with menopause, while others will lose bone more gradually. A longitudinal British study did repeated bone-density tests on a group of women at four-year intervals and found that there was a great variety in the rate of loss from woman to woman.[18] In addition, there was a wide variation in which bones suffered the loss. The researchers also noted that they had been unable to predict from their initial study who would be fast or slow losers.

Some studies have shown that people tend to start losing bone more quickly when they get to their seventies.[19] If these studies are correct, it may make more sense to focus on bone density when a woman is seventy, rather than when she's fifty. Undoubtedly there's a range of loss from woman to woman, as well as from age to age. Anyone who presents osteoporosis as a single, inevitable disease that occurs in all women at menopause is oversimplifying enormously.

There's another problem with the studies on osteoporosis that have been done on women—the same problem that exists in virtually all studies of menopause. Studies of both animals and humans have used subjects whose ovaries have been removed. This castration creates an environment far different from that of the body of a woman who has had a natural menopause. We can't simply assume that what is true for one group applies to the other.

Women and animals who have had surgical menopause have twice as much bone loss as those who have had natural menopause. As we noted in Chapter 1, the ovary produces much more than just estrogen, and it continues to produce hormones after menopause. And at least one study has shown that even women who retain their ovaries after hysterectomy have lower bone mass than women who haven't had hysterectomies.[20] This may be because the uterus produces vitamin D as well as prostaglandin, which seems to be important for bone health.[21] (Prostaglandin is a fatty acid that acts like a hormone.)

All of this tells us that estrogen is only one of several factors connected with bone density. Women with the same hormone levels have different degrees of bone loss. Some get osteoporosis and others don't. Even some women on estrogen get fractures. It doesn't add up to a neat little scenario in which women who don't take estrogen get osteoporosis and women who do take estrogen keep their strong bones.

There are other studies that bear this out. The Mayan women discussed in Chapter 2 live for thirty years after menopause, but they don't get osteoporosis—they don't lose height, they don't develop a dowager's hump, and they don't get fractures.[22] At first the researchers thought this must mean that these women had higher levels of estrogen or androgen, or possibly that they had higher peak bone density, than white American women. So they studied fifty-four postmenopausal Mayan women, analyzing their hormone levels and bone density. They found that these women's estrogen levels were no higher than those of American white women—in some cases, they were even lower. The bone-density tests showed that bone loss occurred in these women at the same rate as in white American women. The only significant difference the researchers could find was that the male hormones produced by the ovaries were less affected by menopause in these women: pre- and postmenopausal women had the same levels of testosterone. This suggests that testosterone may also have a role in bone loss.

If loss of androgen is indeed a factor, that would also explain why women whose ovaries have been removed have more osteoporosis, since the ovaries produce some testosterone, and why having your ovaries removed before age thirty-five strongly affects bone loss, even if you're taking estrogen.[23] In one experiment mentioned in Chapter 2, Malcolm Pike, a researcher at the University of Southern California, placed a group of premenopausal women who were at high risk for breast cancer on a contraceptive regimen that included chemical (and reversible) menopause, with replacement of estrogen and periodic progesterone. After six months, they all showed bone loss. When he added a small amount of testosterone to their regimen, the bone loss was reversed.[24]

All this underscores the fact that the story of osteoporosis, just like the story of heart disease, isn't about estrogen alone.

RISK FACTORS FOR OSTEOPOROSIS

What's Your Risk of Low Bone Density?

How does this all apply to you? How can you figure out how likely you are to get osteoporosis? To some extent, this depends on your own life history.

In your early years, your risk factors for low bone density are those that would lead to low peak bone mass (see Table 5.1). If you start with less bone, you're likely to drop to a dangerously low level sooner when you start to lose bone. Peak bone mass, as we mentioned, is probably largely genetically determined. A recent study showed that daughters of women with osteoporosis had lower bone density than is normal for their age.[25] Large-boned people have more bone mass than small-boned people and are less affected by bone loss, since they have more to spare.

Whether you reach your genetically determined peak, however, can depend on other factors. Chief among them are a diet with adequate calcium and vitamin D, and adequate exercise. If you're sedentary, you lose bone. Even if you're sick in bed for as short a time as a week, you'll lose bone—though it will grow back when you get back to normal, especially if "normal," for you, involves standing and walking a lot. Bones need gravity to grow. (That's one of the things scientists are worried about with astronauts: weightlessness in space may look like fun, but it isn't doing their bones any good.)

Other lifestyle issues that will affect both your peak bone mass and your subsequent bone loss are use of tobacco, alcohol (more than three drinks a day), and caffeine, all of which decrease bone density. Being

---

TABLE 5.1

Risk Factors for Low Bone Density

Thinness

Small frame

Advanced age

Family history of osteoporosis

Early menopause

Abnormal absence of menstrual periods (amenorrhea)

Anorexia nervosa or bulimia

Diet low in calcium

Use of certain medications, such as corticosteroids
and anticonvulsants

Inactive lifestyle

Cigarette smoking

Excessive use of alcohol

Caucasian ancestry

---

overweight, as we have mentioned, actually enhances bone strength, perhaps because it puts more stress on the bones. In addition, fat converts androgens to estrogen, thus contributing to higher bone density. Weight-bearing exercise (for example, jogging and walking) and strength training (lifting weights to increase your muscle mass) will help to increase bone. It might be that the Mayan women, who have worked in the fields their whole lives, have developed strong muscles, and that may be more crucial than their thinning bones.

There are certain medications that can affect your peak bone mass and subsequent bone loss. Taking steroids such as prednisone or cortisone for a long time is likely to decrease bone mass. Steroids are commonly used to treat diseases such as asthma, rheumatoid arthritis, lupus, Crohn's disease, and ulcerative colitis. (These last two diseases can create additional problems of their own, because they're intestinal diseases that affect the absorption of calcium and vitamin D.) Insulin-dependent diabetics generally have lower bone mass. People with heart disease who take Lasix (furosemide), a diuretic that causes more calcium to be excreted in urine, also have lower bone mass. (Not all diuretics have this effect, however; in fact, Thiazide actually helps the body hold on to calcium.) Aluminum-based antacids also decrease calcium absorption. (Calcium-based antacids, on the other hand, are themselves excellent calcium supplements—we'll discuss this in Chapter 12.) So read the label on any antacid very carefully.

As we mentioned earlier, thyroid replacement medication, if given in too high a dose, decreases bone strength.

What You Really Want to Know: What's Your Risk of Fracture?

The factors we've discussed so far are all risk factors for low bone density. But remember that low bone density is itself only an intermediate end-point, and it doesn't automatically mean you'll end up with broken bones. Risks factors for *fractures* are a different matter (see Table 5.2).

TABLE **5.2**
Risk Factors for Fracture

Maternal history of hip fracture before age eighty

Previous fracture after age fifty

Tall at age twenty-five

Health fair or poor by your own rating

Previous hyperthyroidism

Current use of long-acting benzodiazepines (tranquilizers)

Current use of anticonvulsants

Ingesting high doses of caffeine

Spending less than four hours a day on your feet

Inability to rise from a chair without using your arms

Poor depth perception

Poor contrast sensitivity

Rapid heart rate at rest (greater than 80 beats per minute)

Current weight less than at age twenty-five

An ongoing longitudinal cohort study, by the Study of Osteoporotic Fractures (SOF) Research Group, has shown the complex interaction of various risk factors that lead to fractures.[26] This study is looking at 9,703 nonblack women, age sixty-five and older, who have had measurements of bone density in the heel and wrist. The study is planned to go on for several years, but there are some early data. After one and a half years, fifty-three of the women had fractures. As might be expected, the number of hip fractures was inversely related to the bone density: the women with lower bone density had more hip fractures. But bone density turned out to be only part of the problem. Even after it was adjusted for, the researchers found that the risk of hip fractures doubled for each ten years of a woman's age.

The study showed that some of that risk had as much to do with frailty, weakness, and falls as with low bone density. If you don't spend time on your feet, you're not getting the weight-bearing pressure your bones need. If you can't get out of a chair without using your arms, your leg muscles are weak. Poor depth perception and other vision problems are independent risk factors—probably because they mean that you trip more easily. If you have low bone density but you never fall down, you probably won't break your hip. To repeat, then, some of the risk factors have to do with the likelihood of falling rather than with bone density.

How likely you are to have fractures depends on how many risk factors for fractures you have as well as what your bone density is. Compared with a woman with no risk factors, women who had only two of the above risk factors had a risk of about 1.1, essentially normal. Women with no more than two risk factors but normal bone density for their age had hardly any risk of fractures. But women with five or more risk factors and low bone density had twenty-seven times the risk of getting a fracture.

Since there are other, equally important risk factors for osteoporosis and fractures, why is there such an intense focus on bone density? Why aren't we hearing about the other problems?

First, since bone density is (unfortunately) the only risk factor we can easily measure, it's the one we try to control. And it does make sense to try to control bone density; the problem is that you end up with an inflated view of the value of bone-density tests, and of medications that can affect bone density. A medication that slows down bone loss may stabilize your bone density but may not keep you from getting life-threatening fractures in your old age. And some treatments, such as calcitonin, have been shown to decrease spine fractures without increasing bone density. A recent analysis of the raloxifene (Evista) study showed that only 4 percent of the reduction in vertebral fractures could be explained by an increase in bone density.[27] Second, we're not hearing about other factors because there's not much money to be made on them. For instance, I recommend that women with low bone density monitor their use of alcohol and tranquilizers, consult a doctor, start a weight-bearing exercise program, improve their diet, make their houses fall-proof, correct failing vision, and possibly put pads on their hips to cushion a fall—but none of these approaches offers much chance for profits.

WHAT IS IT LIKE TO HAVE OSTEOPOROSIS?

Most women today who are considered to have osteoporosis have no symptoms at all. Brittle bones per se don't usually cause pain or disability. The problems come when a woman with osteoporosis has a fracture. But even then, not all fractures are the same. Different types of fractures vary in terms of how common they are, the age at which they appear, and the disability they cause.

A white woman at age fifty has a 17 percent chance of having a hip fracture at some point in her life. (With white men, it's 6 percent.) The chance of a vertebral fracture is 15 percent in women (5 percent in men). The chance of a wrist fracture is 16 percent in women (2 percent in men). If you add up these figures and factor out the women who get more than one fracture, the chance of getting one of those three fractures is 39 percent for women. That figure is often used as the risk of fracture from osteoporosis.[28]

But there's a big difference between these fractures—both in the age at which you're likely to get them and in the amount of disability they cause. If you fracture your wrist, it's painful and inconvenient, but it isn't the same as breaking your hip.

Wrist Fractures

Wrist fractures typically occur when you fall on an outstretched hand. The average age for a wrist fracture is sixty-seven. Of the women who sustain a wrist fracture, only 1.9 percent are estimated to become dependent as a result.[29] One of the main studies on wrist fractures was done on women from Olmsted County in Minnesota,[30] which has a cold winter climate; but since most wrist fractures occur when people fall outdoors, often when it's snowy and icy, this study may well overestimate the chance of getting a wrist fracture in, say, Los Angeles.

A wrist fracture isn't very painful. Your wrist is put in a cast for several weeks, and you usually recover full mobility. The major importance of a wrist fracture is that it may be an early indicator of decreased bone density, giving you time to do something before a more disabling fracture might occur.

Vertebral Fractures

When you have a vertebral fracture—a disruption of one of the bones in your spine—you typically don't even know it's there at first. Such fractures are usually diagnosed when a woman in her seventies has a chest X ray for some other reason, and the film shows a wedging or crushing of the vertebral body (see Figure 5.3). In Denmark, about 55 percent of seventy-year-old women are found to have a crush fracture of at least one vertebra on a routine chest X ray.[31] In Rochester, Minnesota, about 40 percent of white women have at least one wedge fracture by the time they're eighty.[32]

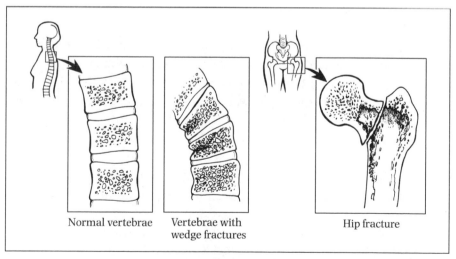

| Normal vertebrae | Vertebrae with wedge fractures | Hip fracture |

Figure 5.3 Osteoporotic fractures.

An acute vertebral fracture may cause severe back pain, but that pain seldom lasts more than three months and can usually be managed with an over-the-counter pain reliever such as aspirin or Tylenol. Many vertebral fractures cause no pain at all. In a random sample of seventy-year-old Danish women, those with wedge fractures had no more pain than those without them.[33] The fracture rarely requires hospitalization. This kind of fracture can cause problems, however. Because fractured vertebrae never regain their normal shape, multiple vertebral fractures may lead to a humped-over posture, loss of height, and some functional limitations such as difficulty in reaching a top shelf, cleaning house, and finding clothes that fit.

Depending on what study you read, the lifetime risk that a fifty-year-old woman will get a vertebral fracture ranges from 5 to 15 percent; and 7 to 15 percent of vertebral fractures will cause significant pain. About 1.5 percent of women who get these fractures will become dependent as a result.[34] This variation may be in part a result of the different lifestyles, diets, and genes of the women involved in the different studies.

Loss of height may occur from vertebral fractures, but these fractures aren't the only cause of the loss of height that comes with age. Muscular atrophy, vertebral remodeling, disk deterioration, and poor posture all contribute to loss of height. In fact, we're all shorter by about an inch at the end of the day. (I guess everything settles.)

Hip Fractures

Hip fractures are the ones that cause most problems. The average fifty-year-old white woman has an 18.4 percent lifetime chance of having at least one hip fracture; the average age for a hip fracture is 79. In 13.7 percent of cases, a woman will have another fracture, either in the other hip or in the same hip. This explains why you sometimes see the figure 33 percent reported as the risk of hip fracture. Of women with hip fractures, 19.3 percent will require a long stay in a nursing home, and 10.2 percent will become functionally dependent, needing help with the activities of daily living. On average, this 10.2 percent will remain dependent or will need to stay in a nursing home for seven to eight years.[35]

Again, all these statistics are for white women. Black women have a lower risk. That may be because of their genes, their body-fat composition, the more stable angle of their hips, their degree of physical activity throughout their lives, or any combination of these factors.

Among Asian women there is a different, and intriguing, pattern. Though they show low bone density on tests, they have fewer hip fractures than white women. This may be because they're short and their hip and leg bones come together at a different, more stable angle.

The difference in the extent of impairment that fractures, even hip fractures, entail is amazing. I have two very good examples from within my own family of how variable the problems can be. My stepmother was seventy-seven years old in 1993 when she went traveling in Cambodia with my father. During the trip she fell and broke her hip and elbow when she was pushed down by a thief trying to steal her handbag. She flew back to Los Angeles, where we arranged for her to have her hip fracture nailed. She recovered promptly and a year later went back to Cambodia to finish the trip that had been cut short. She suffered some short-term disability from the fracture, but it hasn't really affected her life.

On the other hand, when my mother-in-law was eighty-four, she broke her hip when she suddenly fell one day while washing the dishes. She had a hip replacement and a short rehabilitation in a nursing home. She returned home but was never able to be totally independent. A year later she broke the other hip, and after a second hip replacement went to a nursing home, which she has never left. In her case, however, she was becoming more and more frail, and the hip fracture was the last straw. (She subsequently developed Alzheimer's disease and died in the spring of 1997.)

Fractures and Aging

Hip fractures don't occur in a vacuum. They're related not only to bone density but also to whether you fall. Your likelihood of falling is influenced by how good your balance is, whether you get dizzy, and whether you're particularly frail. Also, it's inaccurate to blame all of the subsequent disability and dependency on the hip fracture alone.

More than 90 percent of hip fractures occur in people over seventy, and the average age is eighty. You'll often hear that by ninety, one out of three women has a hip fracture. Although this is true, most of us won't live long enough for that to happen—the average life expectancy of white American women is 78.9 (that of white American men is 72).

I'm not trying to dismiss the danger of osteoporosis, or to suggest that we shouldn't try to prevent it. But I question the assumption that you should try to prevent it by taking a drug for twenty to thirty years that may significantly increase your danger of dying earlier of another disease.

PREVENTION

Should You Have a Bone-Density Screening?

Currently many women are being sent for bone-density tests to see whether they are at high risk for fractures later in life.

In fact there's a lot of talk now about screening women routinely for bone density—like getting regular mammograms to detect early breast cancer. But such screening is of limited usefulness unless it leads to appropriate therapy. If you discover at fifty or so that you have low peak bone mass, it may encourage you to take calcium and start a good program of weight-bearing exercise—things you should be doing anyway, but sometimes you need a little push. The risk, of course, is that it could push you in the direction of long-term hormone or drug therapy without enough data to know the long-term outcomes or risks. It's important to understand the limits of the information such a test can give you. First of all, you should be careful about how you interpret the results of a single bone-density test. There have been some good longitudinal studies showing that these tests are far from conclusive. One five-year study of women's wrist and vertebral density showed no relationship between original bone density at age forty-five or fifty and rate of bone loss, so we can't assume that the people with low bone density are "high losers": low bone density and high loss of density are two separate problems.[36] If you start out with $100 in your piggybank and never spend it, you'll still have $100 in ten years. On the other hand, if you start out with $1,000 and spend a $100 a year, you'll have none of it left ten years later.

If you're someone who turns out to be a high loser, you could have normal, or even high, bone density at age fifty, before the accelerated loss of bone has begun. If that's the case, you might well end up with fractures in your seventies. On the other hand, if you show low density in your original test, you still may not be a high loser, and you might never have a fracture. So all a screening test can do when you're forty or fifty is give you an idea of where you are starting from.[37] (Your bone density may have some relationship to your risk for breast cancer; see page 140.) It is important to remember that the World Health Organization (WHO) criteria for osteoporosis and osteopenia were designed for postmenopausal women—not younger healthy women. We do not know what T scores mean in women from age forty to fifty.

You should look at your personal risk factors for osteoporosis and fractures and decide whether, considering the limitations, it's worth it to you to have a bone-density test. And you can decide with your doctor what lifestyle changes you should undertake and whether you would be willing to take drugs. If you are not going to act on the test, it may not be worth taking. Most women aren't at risk, and the test is expensive.

I think the best policy is to change your diet and exercise program if need be when you hit fifty or so, but hold off on the bone-density test. Since the average age of a white American woman to have a hip fracture is eighty, it makes sense to wait to have a bone-density test until you are sixty-five. By then you will have declared yourself. Your body's propensity toward, or away from, osteoporosis will be clear. The women who have very low bone density will be obvious and can be treated to prevent later fractures. Those who are unlikely to have a problem will also be obvious and can be monitored periodically to see if the situation changes. If you have a normal bone density at sixty-five, you can repeat the test after three to five years. If you are osteopenic, then you might repeat it after two or three years. If you have osteoporosis and are started on treatment, you also should wait two years to repeat the test. Nothing in bone changes that fast, and the test is not that sensitive. Studies have shown that women will go on losing some bone over the first year on treatment and still have a benefit after two years.[38] In older women it is important to measure bone density in the hip, while measurements of the spine are appropriate for younger women because that is their major source of bone loss.

This is also the recommendation of the National Osteoporosis Foundation, which suggests that all women have a bone-density test at sixty-five, unless they have compelling risk factors suggesting a need earlier. This is a real shift from the first edition of the book when all women were being pushed to have bone-density tests at fifty. The reason for the change in approach is the fact that treating osteoporosis is more effective than we thought and prevention through drugs used to maintain bone density is not as valuable or necessary as we once believed.[39]

Estrogen: Is There Still a Role?

For many years the standard line has been that osteoporosis is caused by estrogen deficiency, and prevention is better than cure, so all women older than fifty should take HRT. Unfortunately, like the situation with heart disease, things are turning out to be much more complicated. It is true that as in heart disease, large long-term observational studies have demonstrated that women who took Premarin for more than seven years had 50 percent fewer fractures of the spine.[40] The Study of Osteoporotic Fractures (SOF) followed a cohort of 9,704 women over sixty-five for at least seven years. These researchers found that *current* users of estrogen had 60 percent fewer wrist fractures, 40 percent fewer hip fractures, and 35 percent fewer nonspinal fractures when compared with women who had never taken estrogen. Current users who started estrogen within five years of menopause showed an even larger effect: all nonspinal fractures decreased by 50 percent, and hip fractures went down 70 percent, as did wrist fractures, in comparison with women who had never been on estrogen. And women on estrogen and progestin showed the same effect. Notice the emphasis on "current users." Unfortunately, women who had taken estrogen and then stopped, even if they'd taken it for ten years, had no decrease in their risk of fractures. This was also true for those who started estrogen more than five years after menopause.

These data are quite consistent, and impressive, although they're from observational studies with all of the biases we outlined in Chapter 4. Moreover, this effect makes sense: animal and human studies have found that estrogen can halt the decrease in bone density and add 5 percent to total bone mass.[41] But don't get too excited—this figure of 5 percent is somewhat of an illusion. Estrogen appears to halt or slow bone resorption, rather than actually build bone: thus the 5 percent represents a filling in of resorption pits rather than a development of new bone. Returning to our metaphor of the "bone-house," it's as though estrogen finishes off the job of building new rooms that have already been started but doesn't help you build any more rooms after those. On the other hand, this beats having half-finished rooms. Also, estrogen may improve the microarchitecture of bone, making fracture less likely, and some studies have shown that estrogen increases your body's ability to absorb calcium from the intestine and increases calcitonin production from the thyroid. Progesterone and progestins have also been shown to decrease osteoporosis in animals, possibly through their androgenic effects. But the one randomized controlled study of natural progesterone cream showed no effect on bone density.[42] We are only now getting data on HRT and fractures. One randomized controlled trial of HRT has been reported that showed fracture reduction as the primary outcome.

Although it was initially presented as showing a 60 percent reduction in the risk of fractures, it actually showed no benefit when the number of women with new fractures was counted rather than the number of new fractures.[43] In the PEPI study, which was randomized but studied the effect of HRT on cholesterol levels, there was no reduction in fractures. The women were young (forty-five to sixty-five), however, and not at increased risk.[44] Finally the HERS study (see Chapter 6), which randomized women with heart disease to take Prempro or placebo, showed no difference in the number of fractures in either group. In addition, there was no difference in the loss of height in the two groups after five years. It should be noted that most of the women in HERS did not fit the definition of osteoporosis and were overweight. This would make it less likely that they would see an effect.[45] Sally E. M. Bell-Syer and David Torgerson tried to put together all of the randomized data on fractures and HRT to get a hint of an effect. Most of the studies were designed to look at something else and just happened to collect data on fractures. They found a small (27 percent) reduction in the risk of nonvertebral fractures that was statistically significant. Interestingly, they noted that the effect might be attenuated among older women. This is interesting because these are the women at most risk.[46] One of the results of the Women's Health Initiative that has gotten lost in the surprise about the breast cancer and heart risk is the benefit to the bone. It is the first randomized controlled study done on the effect of Prempro on fractures. It showed that there was a decrease in hip and vertebral fractures of about one third. It is worth noting that the overall rates of fracture were low in the entire study with ten per ten thousand in the HRT group and fifteen per ten thousand in the placebo group. This would be good news if HRT had other benefits, but the fact that there are alternative drugs (see Chapter 14) makes it less significant. I eagerly await the data from the WHI study, due in 2006, examining vitamin D and calcium supplementation as a strategy for fracture prevention.[47]

What Should You Do to Prevent Fractures?

At fifty you should look at your lifestyle. Make sure you are getting adequate levels of vitamin D and calcium, and start an exercise program, if you don't have one already, that includes weight training and aerobics. If you are at a very high risk of osteoporosis, you can consider a bone-density test. If not, wait until you are sixty-five to be screened.[48] This is based on the recent findings that women with small amounts of their own estrogen may not have an increase in fractures, that bone loss at menopause is less accelerated than had been previously believed, and that the period of high loss is briefer than had been feared.[49] And when a woman is sixty-five, we can more precisely estimate her risk of hip fracture and target her treatment more accurately. It's beginning to appear that, at sites other than the spine, bone loss continues unabated into very old age and probably accelerates at the hip—the most important region for predicting hip fractures.[50] Recent studies indicate that a low dose of estrogen (.3 or even .15 milligram of Premarin) can be used for this purpose, or you could take any of the other drugs that have been proven to prevent fractures.

Prevention or Treatment?

The usual line is that prevention is better than treatment, and this has certainly driven the use of HRT in postmenopausal women. This may not actually be the case, however.

New studies of other drugs such as Fosamax (see Chapter 14) suggest that women who had already suffered at least one spinal fracture and were treated with Fosamax reduced their risk of breaking a hip by 51 percent and of breaking a wrist by 44 percent.[51] Fractures of the spine were 46 percent lower for women who took this drug than for those who took only calcium. The women on Fosamax also lost less height than women who didn't take it. Fosamax had much less benefit in women who had osteopenia than in women who had osteoporosis. Raloxifene or Evista (see Chapter 7) has also been shown to be quite beneficial in women in their sixties who have been diagnosed with osteoporosis already. And new drugs such as parathormone will actually build new bone in women who are found to have osteoporosis in their later years.

This suggests that there's an alternative to thirty years on estrogen.[52] Have a bone-density study at age fifty if you are high risk for fracture (family history). If it's very low (more than 2.5 standard deviations below that of a thirty-five-year-old), consider lifestyle changes and possibly drugs (see Chapter 14). If your bone density is moderately low (1 to 2.5 standard deviations below that of a thirty-five-year-old), you could take dietary calcium and vitamin D, change your diet, begin an exercise program (see page 242), and then repeat the test in five years. If your bone density is high or normal, wait and have another test at age sixty-five, when you can better estimate the risk of hip fracture, since by that time the process of loss is starting to be visible. If you are not at high risk, hold off having a bone-density test until you are at least sixty-five. If the bone scan at sixty-five reveals high bone loss, you can start drugs then and still reduce the number of possible of fractures.

Managing Osteopenia

Because the bisphosphonates and raloxifene are so effective in reducing bone loss in women with osteoporosis, it's easy to assume that they should be prescribed to women with osteopenia as well. But that isn't the case. In fact, osteopenia does not need to be treated with any drugs at all.

At first, this may sound like it doesn't make sense. But the research has shown that these drugs do not significantly reduce fracture risk in women with osteopenia. Why? Because women with osteopenia have had so little bone loss and have such a low risk for fracture that there is very little for the drug to do. "There is no evidence," says Dr. Cummings, at the San Francisco School of Medicine, "that any of the drugs decrease the risk of hip, wrist, or rib fractures, broken ankles, or anything that would cause you to go to a doctor in women with osteopenia."[53]

So why are women with osteopenia being prescribed medication? According to Cummings, it is "because doctors have come to believe that osteopenia is a problem and no one is disseminating information about the benefits or risks or worthwhileness of taking treatment if you have osteopenia." Doctors and their patients hear the word *osteopenia,* he continues, "and they get worried and think that they should do something. What I've told women is that in this particular case, the drugs are principally anti-anxiety, not anti-fracture drugs because you don't have much of a risk to start with and there is no reason to take a drug." All you would be doing, he explains, "is hoping that taking the drug now would mean that you would have a lower risk of fracture ten to fifteen years from now—and that is completely unproven."

(There are some unusual circumstances in which a woman with osteopenia should take drugs, but they are few and far between, Cummings says. "It may be worthwhile for a woman who is just starting to take corticosteroid pills and has a T score of −2 to be treated for osteopenia," he says, "because that is a situation where you know the drugs will lead her bone density to go down in a hurry and a lot, and you know her risk of fractures will go up in a hurry and a lot. But that's very unusual.")

Further, when it comes to osteopenia, time really is on a woman's side. "A woman who has osteopenia is likely to lose maybe seven percent of her bone density every ten years," explains Ettinger. "So ten years later she will still have osteopenia, but twenty years later she will have osteoporosis. And if she does develop osteoporosis, he continues, "we already have drugs that can put back six to eight percent of bone density and there are drugs coming that can put back eight to fifteen percent." Further, in five or ten years, there will probably be even better drugs, "which means all the more reason to not do anything now."

Aromatase Inhibitors, Osteopenia, and Osteoporosis

Some women are now receiving drugs called aromatase inhibitors, instead of tamoxifen, as hormonal treatment for breast cancer. These drugs—like anastrozole (Arimidex) and letrozole (Femara)—work by blocking aromatase, the enzyme that converts androgens into estrogen. Initial clinical trials have shown the aromatase inhibitors to be effective, but they have also been found to increase bone fracture risk. For women who have osteoporosis and are on aromatase inhibitors, bisphosphonates should help reduce fracture risk. For women with osteopenia, though, it still makes more sense to wait until osteopenia has advanced to osteoporosis to begin taking these drugs. "I don't think that osteopenia by itself is a reason to take drugs during breast cancer treatment," says Cummings. "If you are really close to −2.5 in the hip or spine and starting on an aromatase inhibitor, then it may be wise to take something else, like a bisphosphonate. We're not sure of that, but it seems wise."[54]

NEW TREATMENTS FOR OSTEOPOROSIS: IS PREVENTION NECESSARY?

Finally, it's important to remember that the study of osteoporosis is continuing. There's a lot of research going on about how osteoporosis happens. In addition, new drugs are being developed all the time. We may soon be able to test for microarchitecture as well as bone density, and to determine genetically who is actually going to be a fast loser or a slower one. We're likely to have drugs that will allow us not only to prevent bone resorption but actually to build bone. There is a great deal of research on new ways to grow bone, and such different approaches as novel matrices (latticework for bone to grow on), bone morphogenic proteins, gene therapy, and stem cells are all showing promise. It's naive to think that the way we approach osteoporosis today is the way we'll approach it twenty or even ten years from now. My guess is that this disease, which has been such a hot topic in recent years, will become less important as new treatments make drugs that promise a shaky sort of "prevention" unnecessary and obsolete.

SIX

HEART DISEASE: WHAT'S YOUR REAL RISK?

The image of heart disease has undergone a transformation in recent years. Once perceived as an almost exclusively male concern, it's now recognized as a major problem for women as well. We're assaulted with the fact that almost half of all women in the United States die from cardiovascular disease—disease of the heart and blood vessels.

This can sound alarming, and was used in the past to frighten women into taking hormones as a preventive. However, there are problems with this approach. One problem is that we now know that hormones won't prevent heart disease. A second problem is that the death rates aren't as dire as they sound. Ultimately, everyone dies of "heart failure": your heart ceases to beat, and you die. Many deaths from heart disease occur in elderly people whose bodies have been weakened by other diseases. Death certificates rarely record "old age" as the official cause of death. So to some extent the dire statistics simply mean that you have to die of something, and your risk of cardiovascular disease increases with age. (Premature heart disease is another matter and deserves some attention, although it has never been associated with hormones.) Interestingly, discussions of this issue usually ignore the fact that deaths from heart disease are decreasing in this country. This is probably due to the fact that we are eating better, smoking less, and treating heart attacks more effectively.

The basis for the hypothesis that estrogen protects women from heart disease comes in part from the fact that men have more heart disease than women. Since we all know that the "only" difference between men and women is that we have more estrogen, this is assumed to be the cause of the difference. As with many of the observations we have used to base our theories on, this one is not quite true. If you look at the rates of heart disease in women and men starting in the 1950s, there is a large discrepancy. If, however, you widen your view and track the differences since the beginning of the nineteenth century, you uncover a different picture. Although there has always been a difference in heart disease rates between women and men in some countries (such as the United Kingdom, the United States, and Australia), this difference was relatively small until the 1920s, when a dramatic increase in heart disease in men, but not women, suddenly appeared.[1] This increase persisted until the later parts of the century, when it started to decrease.

Although the cause of this increase has not yet been determined, there are several theories. Some have attributed it to men's increased smoking, some to their intake of dietary fat, and others to their increased alcohol consumption. All suggest it's not that women's estrogen had been protective, but that men developed these "bad habits." This is underscored by the fact that the epidemic in male heart disease of the early nineteenth century never happened in Japan and only slightly in France.

This reevaluation of the epidemiologic data is just another example of what happens when you look at data with preconceived ideas and as a result find just the evidence you were looking for. First we had women artificially living too long (see Chapter 1), and now we have estrogen getting undeserved credit for their decrease in heart disease.

Heart disease has never been a "symptom" of menopause. Heart disease is heart disease. It's more common in postmenopausal women than in premenopausal women, but that's because postmenopausal women are older than premenopausal women. It's like gray hair: you're more likely to have gray hair after menopause than before it, but menopause doesn't cause gray hair—rather, they both tend to happen in later life. But the increase of heart disease with age has been seen to confirm the misconception that women are protected from heart disease as long as their bodies make estrogen, and then after menopause they lose that protection and the rates of heart disease for men and women become equal. But, in fact, the rates *never* become equal. In this country, women in their sixties and seventies have 45 percent less heart disease than men in the same age bracket. Women develop heart disease much later than men—seven or eight years later. Women's risk rises continuously as they get older, but there's no sudden increase with menopause.[2] We never catch up.

WHAT IS HEART DISEASE?

Heart Disease and Cardiovascular Disease

I should clarify what I mean by *heart disease.* I'm not talking here about congenital heart disease, which you're born with, or the kind caused by rheumatic fever. No one has ever claimed that these are connected to estrogen or to menopause. In fact, these fairly rare conditions can even hit very young adults, like the athletes who have been in the news in recent years. The kind of heart problems at issue here are the kind caused by atherosclerosis, the narrowing of the arteries that feed the heart.

Cardiovascular disease is a broader term, which usually includes both heart disease and stroke. Stroke, like heart disease, is a vascular disease: a disease of blood vessels. In both cases, the blood vessels become narrow, either through spasm or through atherosclerosis, and not enough blood gets to a critical place: to the heart in the case of heart disease, and to the brain in the case of stroke. Cardiovascular disease also encompasses high blood pressure and coronary artery disease.

Arteries and Cholesterol

We're really only beginning to understand some of the mechanisms of atherosclerosis and arterial blockage (see Figure 6.1). Judith Berliner and her group at UCLA stated in 1995 that "atherosclerosis is a chronic inflammatory condition that's converted to an acute clinical event by the induction of plaque rupture, which in turn leads to thrombosis."[3] But what does that mean in English?

I've been trying to figure out a good analogy for this process. Since I live in Los Angeles, a freeway came to mind. In Chapter 5, I talked about the "bone-house," so for this chapter let's move outdoors. Imagine a three-lane freeway that has a chronic problem of litter thrown into the ditch on the side of the road (see Figure 6.2). That's similar to chronic inflammation and plaque formation. (A plaque is a thickened area in the lining of the artery.)

The first step involves a buildup of cholesterol. Cholesterol is a type of fat made by the liver. People often think of "fat" as either the stuff in your food or the body fat that shows up in your hips and tummy. But there are numerous kinds of fat in your body. Just as fat you eat can take the form of butter, lard, or olive oil, fat in your body can take the form of cholesterol and triglycerides, as well as the fatty tissue that makes you appear

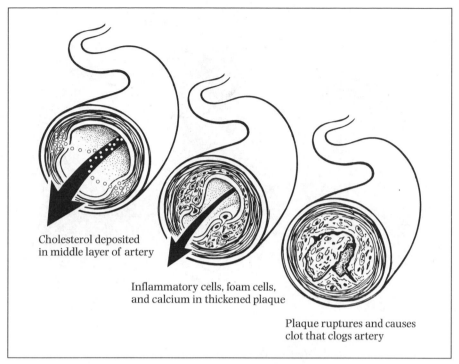

Cholesterol deposited
in middle layer of artery

Inflammatory cells, foam cells,
and calcium in thickened plaque

Plaque ruptures and causes
clot that clogs artery

Figure 6.1. The atherosclerotic process.

chubby. You always have cholesterol circulating in your blood. It's a building block for many of the hormones the body makes. Estrogen, vitamin D, and testosterone all start out as cholesterol.

Our bodies make lots of cholesterol—nearly all that we require. So we really don't need to eat any. Unfortunately, though, we do eat it. Meat and dairy products, which figure strongly in the American diet, are full of cholesterol.

It used to be thought that there was just one kind of cholesterol, but then scientists discovered that it's broken down into two types: "good" HDL (high-density lipoprotein) and "bad" LDL (low-density lipoprotein). What makes these "good" and "bad" is what happens within the blood vessels.

An artery has three layers. The smooth inner lining (the endothelium) is like the highway. The middle layer, which is a latticework (the media), is like the drainage ditch on the side of the road, and the outer layer (the adventitia) is like the outer wall that blocks access to the highway. LDL can pass through the lining of the artery and sit in the middle layer. Let's

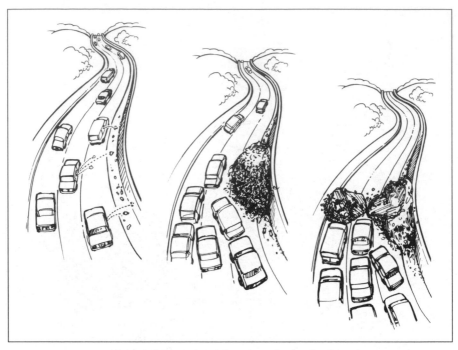

Figure 6.2. A metaphor for atherosclerosis.

say the LDL is represented by the garbage that's being thrown out of the cars into the drainage ditch. The more LDL there is in your blood, the more of it gets into the middle layer of the blood vessels. After a while, the cells in the artery secrete materials that can oxidize LDL—chemically change it into a more dangerous form (the garbage becomes rotten). This process ends up creating cholesterol-loaded cells that form a fatty streak in the artery wall. These can actually be seen in the lining of the arteries. HDL (good cholesterol) has been found to protect against LDL oxidation (like a street sweeper who cleans up garbage before it has time to rot).

The next step toward atherosclerosis is an inflammatory reaction. Certain white blood cells, part of the body's immune system, are attracted to the arteries that have been damaged by LDL and get trapped there, forming a plaque. The reaction feeds on itself, like rats attracted to the garbage piling up in the ditch; finally, the pile gets so big that it starts to encroach on the slow lane of the highway, causing traffic (blood flow) to start slowing down.

The inflammatory plaque then causes calcium to be formed, and this in turn causes the arteries to harden—and to constrict. (The pile of rotten, rat-infested garbage is by now blocking the slow lane and narrowing the middle lane.) Then the heart gets less and less blood to feed its own muscle. When the heart is deprived of too much of its blood supply, there is severe pain. This pain, *angina,* frequently follows strenuous activity that increases your need for blood. Often it gets better when you rest. (This is like a rush-hour traffic jam; the narrowing of the highway will make it hellish at rush hour, but the flow of traffic is better during the rest of the day.)

Angina is always a serious warning signal. If the underlying problem isn't taken care of, eventually the soft inflammatory plaque ruptures into the vessel, forming a clot that blocks the blood vessel and stops the blood flow. The heart muscle fed by that artery dies. This is a heart attack. (The pile of garbage spills into the middle lane, blocking traffic completely.)

I've gone into this much detail because it's important to understand that there are different things you can do at each step along the way to help minimize the likelihood of getting a heart attack. The earlier you start, the better your chances: get that litter off the road the first time it shows up. I'll talk about that more in Chapters 12 to 14.

WHAT PUTS YOU AT RISK OF A HEART ATTACK?

Family History

As with almost every other disease, family history is important in coronary artery disease. It can indicate whether you've inherited genes that make you more susceptible to the atherosclerotic process, whether you're more likely to have high LDL, and whether you're more likely to oxidize LDL or to develop an inflammatory reaction. Research is now going on to determine the precise ways in which genetic factors contribute to coronary artery disease.

Lipid Levels

The fats and fatty substances in your body, *lipids,* include HDL, LDL, cholesterol, and triglycerides. Your lipid "profile" can determine your risk for a heart attack. In general, you want high HDL and low LDL, cholesterol, and triglycerides (see Table 6.1, page 124).

Many factors influence the levels of triglycerides, LDL, and HDL. Insulin, diet, exercise, obesity, age, and hormones all affect the way fat is metabolized.

TABLE 6.1
Cholesterol Levels

	Total Cholesterol	HDL	LDL	Triglycerides
Good	<200	>70	<130	50–250
Borderline	200–240	35–70	130–159	250–500
Bad	>240	<35	>160	>500

Key: < = less than; > = greater than

One factor that's clearly controlled by genes is how you metabolize dietary fat (see Chapter 12 for a discussion of dietary fat). This can be partly measured by testing your blood cholesterol. Across cultures, men with high cholesterol have a higher death rate from coronary heart disease than men with low cholesterol. Women are also affected by cholesterol, but it turns out that we're less affected than men are. Don't get too cheery, though: women are more susceptible to problems that result from a bad ratio of LDL to HDL. Remember, overall cholesterol isn't all that matters. You really need to know your LDL and HDL as well, and you need to have your triglycerides measured after an overnight fast.

In women, the level of HDL is usually higher than it is in men. An increase in HDL cholesterol of 1 milligram per deciliter (mg/dl), the units in which cholesterol is usually measured in the United States, is associated with a 3.2 percent decrease in the risk of heart disease in women (compared with 1.9 to 2.35 percent in men). In fact, HDL trumps total cholesterol. Most of these levels are a result of a combination of genes and diet. Some lucky people can eat a whole cheesecake and still have low cholesterol, while others just look at a cheesecake through the bakery window and their cholesterol shoots up to 400. The lucky ones have genes that make it easier to metabolize cholesterol.

Other factors affect lipid levels as well. As you age, your good HDLs fall and your bad LDLs rise. Some of that change may be related to menopause. After menopause, particularly if you gain weight, your LDL increases. Exercise increases HDL and lowers cholesterol levels. Moderate alcohol intake raises HDL levels. (Remember, that's moderate alcohol;

too many three-martini lunches are likely to give you a heart attack, not prevent one.)

It is important to realize that there is no absolute number for cholesterol (or HDL and LDL, for that matter) that is bad or good. It is a continuum—the higher your LDL, the higher your risk. This means that lowering your cholesterol, whatever it is, will lower your risk of heart disease. The key is that at lower and lower rates of heart disease, the benefit is extremely small. In 2002 new guidelines for cholesterol came out recommending treatment at a lower level. This is just like setting the level of bone density that needs treatment in osteoporosis (see Chapter 5): the lower you set the threshold, the more drugs you will sell to prevent disease. But at each lower level the number of women at risk is also lower, while the number being treated and getting no benefit is greater. It is important that we find out exactly what the risk of heart disease is and what the absolute benefit is in each case so that we can properly decide the best therapy.

Homocysteine

Since the first edition of this book, increasing attention has been paid to high homocysteine levels as a risk factor for heart disease. Homocysteine, a product resulting from the metabolism of the amino acid methionine, is thought to damage the inner lining of arteries, triggering an increase in smooth-muscle cells. In the Physicians' Health Study (on men), the likelihood of having a heart attack increased 3.4-fold among doctors with the highest blood levels of homocysteine—putting this amino acid by-product on a par with smoking and high blood cholesterol as a risk factor for heart disease. It has been estimated that every 10 percent rise in homocysteine is matched by almost the same increase in coronary artery disease.[4] In July 1997 a research group from the University of Washington School of Public Health found a twofold increased risk of heart attack among women with higher than normal blood levels of the protein homocysteine and lower than normal blood levels of the vitamin folate.[5]

The exciting part of this story is the fact that it appears to be very easy to lower homocysteine levels. Studies have shown that B vitamin supplements, especially folate, reduce the levels of homocysteine. The missing piece of the puzzle came in February 1998, when an important report from the Nurses' Health Study found that women with the highest intake of folic acid had 47 percent less heart disease than women with the lowest intake. And a high intake of vitamin B_6 reduced heart disease by 51 percent. The authors found, however, that the current recommended daily allowances of these B vitamins were insufficient. You need at least 3 milligrams of B_6 and 400 micrograms of folate to benefit. Another interesting finding was that women who consumed alcohol had the biggest benefit. The largest contributors to intake of folate were multivitamin supplements, beef, cold cereal, lettuce, eggs, broccoli, and spinach. The B_6 came from multivitamin supplements, beef, cold cereal, potatoes, bananas, chicken, milk, and tuna fish.[6] So what should you do right now? Well, this is yet another reason to eat five servings of fruits and vegetables a day. You could also take a standard multivitamin/mineral supplement containing at least 3 milligrams of vitamin B_6 and 400 micrograms of folate. And stay tuned.

C Reactive Protein

Another measure that has been added to the list of blood tests predicting heart disease is C reactive protein. This one is a bit easier to understand since it goes up with inflammation. Women who have high levels of C reactive protein double their risk of heart disease. This is independent of their cholestorol level.[7] Interestingly, estrogen increases C reactive protein.

Personality Type

There are other factors related to cholesterol levels that are less well publicized (maybe because they don't fit our biases). For example, there is some relationship between personality, the mind, and cholesterol levels. We've all heard of the type-A personality. Recent research by Redford Williams has found that the factors that really increase heart disease are self-involvement, hostility, and cynicism.[8] A researcher from the University of California in San Francisco who taped conversations found that the more frequently people referred to themselves, the greater the likelihood that they would develop heart disease and die from it.[9] There are also many studies supporting the concept that social isolation is an important risk factor for heart disease; but although this is an important finding, it's less relevant to women, who by and large tend to be more social. Problems with women come more when they lose control over their lives.

Some fascinating observational studies of monkeys demonstrate biologically how that works. In a group of female monkeys, one is dominant; the others are subordinate. When monkeys were fed a high-fat diet, the HDL levels of the subordinate ones went down and their lipids changed, far more than was the case with the dominant monkeys. The subordinate monkeys had a risk of heart disease three times greater than the dominant ones.[10]

Recent studies on humans parallel this. One study noted that working women had more risk factors for heart disease than housewives—they were more likely to smoke, less likely to exercise, and more likely to drink alcohol and coffee.[11] Nonetheless they still had higher HDL levels than the housewives. If they quit working and became housewives, their HDL levels went down. A similar study hypothesized that women with high-powered jobs would have the most heart disease because they were under the most stress.[12] What they actually found was that the career women had less heart disease. It turned out that the more control a woman had over her life, the less likely she was to have heart disease. So cholesterol levels may relate to being in a role where you perceive that you have less control over your life—like a housewife who spends twenty-four hours a day at the beck and call of her children and spouse. It shows an interesting mind-body connection.

I'm not necessarily advising that you lower your cholesterol by getting a job—a particular woman may in fact have more control over her life as a housewife than she would in an outside job. What is much more significant about these studies is that they demonstrate that diet is not the only factor determining your cholesterol level.

Diabetes

Diabetes is a disease of sugar metabolism. There are two kinds of diabetes. The first, which usually occurs in childhood, is *insulin-dependent* (formerly *juvenile*) diabetes. It's caused by the body's failure to produce enough insulin, the hormone that regulates sugar metabolism. People with this form of diabetes take daily insulin injections to compensate. The second, more common, form of the disease is *adult-onset, non-insulin-dependent,* diabetes. This occurs when the body makes insulin but for some reason is unable to use it. Adult-onset diabetes is most likely to develop in people who are obese, come from families with diabetes, and have high blood pressure. It can often be controlled by diet, weight loss, and exercise.

Uncontrolled diabetes of either type has a treacherous effect on the very small arteries throughout the body. Diabetes doubles a woman's risk of coronary heart disease. When you've got diabetes on top of high blood pressure, obesity, high cholesterol, and high triglycerides, it quadruples the risk of heart disease. In fact, 80 percent of diabetics die of heart attacks. This is a particular problem for women. When a diabetic woman has a heart attack, she's more likely to die from it than either a diabetic man or a nondiabetic woman.

Smoking

Smoking at least triples the risk of coronary heart disease, probably chiefly because it increases the oxidation of LDL and secondarily because it increases vessel spasm—and spastic vessels don't transport blood very well. The more you smoke, the more effect smoking has. Further, it increases the risk of adult-onset diabetes—which, as we've just seen, is a risk factor for heart disease. It doesn't take much smoking to increase the risk. Women who smoke as little as half a pack a day may have a 50 percent increased risk of heart disease compared to women who have never smoked, while women smoking a pack or more a day (twenty cigarettes) may have a 100 percent increased risk.[13]

Overweight

Obesity—defined as being more than 20 percent over the target weight for your height—is a strong risk factor for coronary heart disease in women. Forty percent of coronary heart disease found among all women is related to excess weight. Even women of average weight have about a 30 percent higher risk than thin women. And here is where the famous apple/pear shapes come in. Women who have a high ratio of waist to hip (the apples) have a greater risk of heart disease than those who carry their fat in their hips (the pears).

High Blood Pressure

High blood pressure, like cholesterol, can lead to heart attacks. It increases the stress on the blood vessels and thus increases the chance of artery narrowing and plaque rupture.

In part, obese people tend to have high blood pressure because they have more blood vessels, which the body creates to bring blood to all that fat. Weight loss is more likely to control high blood pressure (hypertension) in women than in men. However, women get less benefit from antihypertensive drugs. All women over forty should have their blood pressure checked regularly. Doctors call it the "silent killer" because it's asymptomatic.

Blood Clots

If your blood clots easily, you're more prone to heart disease. There's a balance between factors in your blood that make clots and factors that break them up. If you have more of the factors that make clots and fewer of those that break them up, you're at a greater risk for a heart attack. This is why doctors advise many men to take an aspirin a day: aspirin thins blood so that it won't clot as much. Once the doctors started studying women and heart disease, they discovered that we need less aspirin than men do—half a tablet a day. If you think you're at risk of heart disease, though, don't just start popping aspirin. Get a medical workup from your doctor. Aspirin is a drug, and like all drugs it has side effects, so don't take it regularly without checking with your doctor.

THE NATURAL HISTORY OF HEART DISEASE

Heart disease in women doesn't usually occur until their seventies or eighties. A fifty-year-old white American woman has a 46 percent lifetime probability of developing heart disease and a 31 percent probability of dying of it. The median age at which a heart attack occurs is seventy-four years.[14] Smokers have three times as much heart disease as nonsmokers and account for most of the early deaths from heart disease.

Some women will experience angina (chest pain) as a symptom of heart disease before they have a heart attack, but about a third of women with heart disease never have any warning symptoms—they have a sudden, massive heart attack and die instantly. (Although this is often described in the medical literature as a terrible event, it may actually be a better way to die than a lingering, painful illness—particularly if you're at an advanced age in which death in the near future is inevitable.)

What is it like to have a heart attack? A heart attack is usually accompanied by crushing chest pain. (Any new chest pain should be evaluated by your doctor.) However, women often have other patterns of pain—such as pain in the arm, neck, jaw, teeth, or back—usually associated with physical exertion or emotional stress and lasting longer than two minutes. You may also feel dizzy, faint, sweaty, nauseated, short of breath, or weak. If you think you're having a heart attack, stop what you're doing and lie down immediately. Get help: call 911 to get an ambulance or have someone take you to a hospital. If you can get to a hospital within four to six hours after the first hint of a problem, emergency treatment may be able to dissolve the clot that caused the attack or use angioplasty to open up the artery that is blocked.

After the initial treatment, you'll go to a coronary care unit (CCU) where the rhythm of your heart can be monitored. Once the acute event is over, you'll be moved to an intermediate care unit and rehabilitation will begin. This usually means evaluating your risk factors and lifestyle and starting you on a low-fat diet and an exercise program. Six weeks later you'll undergo further studies to see whether you need surgery or angioplasty (a method to open up narrowed arteries). You may need to take drugs such as beta-blockers, aspirin, and ACE inhibitors (see Chapter 14) to decrease the chance of another attack.

Women have a higher probability of dying in the year following heart attacks than men do (45 percent of women compared with 10 percent of men); and 40 percent of women, compared with 13 percent of men, have a second heart attack within that year.[15] Some of this is due to the fact that, by and large, women who have had heart attacks are older, have more high blood pressure and diabetes, and have more severe or unstable angina than their male counterparts. Women are more likely than men to suffer psychological consequences of a heart attack. They're less likely to return to work, and if they do return, they tend to return later than men do. They have more frequent depression and are less likely to return to their previous activities. This may be in part because they are more likely to be older and widowed. However, with good rehabilitation, psychological and social support, and lifestyle changes, women can recover from heart attacks and resume their lives.

ESTROGEN AND HEART DISEASE

By now you have some inkling of where the assumed connection between estrogen and heart disease came from. In addition to the epidemiologic data on the differences between women and men that we have already mentioned, there have been further observations fueling the hypothesis. The first mention of estrogen therapy to prevent heart disease was by Michael Oliver in 1959. He had noted that women who had had their ovaries out had a higher risk of heart disease and suggested that "a case could even be made out for administering small doses of oestrogens for a number of years to all menopausal women."[16]

These observations led to a search for a biological explanation for the presumed effect. As is often the fact, scientists quickly accepted the data that supported their theory—i.e., that estrogen reduced cholesterol— and downplayed the effects that did not fit, such as the increase in triglycerides seen with estrogen therapy.

Natural Estrogen: Not a Factor?

The claims that estrogen therapy could prevent heart disease were always interesting but problematical. For one thing, levels of women's own natural estrogen seemed to have little or no effect on their rate of heart disease. There's something mysterious in this. In osteoporosis, breast cancer, and endometrial cancer, factors associated with the body's own estrogens correlate with the risk of the disease. For example, the larger your lifetime supply of estrogen—whether because you started menstruating early, took certain medications, or drank alcohol—the greater your risk of breast cancer and the lower your risk of osteoporosis. After menopause, women who are obese and have more of their own estrogen have less osteoporosis and more breast and endometrial cancer. Estrogen, whether it's your own or you get it from medication, has a consistent effect on risk for these conditions. But there's no clear relationship between heart disease and your body's own estrogen. The amount of estrogen your body makes over your lifetime doesn't appear to have any effect on your risk of heart disease. Onset of menstruation doesn't seem to affect risk; nor does anorexia or amenorrhea (lack of periods).

In 1995, Elizabeth Barrett-Connor did studies to see if levels of hormones in the blood affected heart disease.[17] She measured testosterone, estrone, and androstenedione. She found no relationship between the blood levels of these sex hormones and heart disease in postmenopausal women, or in men. Nor did she find any relationship between blood levels of estrogen and cholesterol levels, LDH, and triglycerides. Other studies have confirmed this finding. Although obesity increases blood levels of estrogen, it certainly doesn't decrease heart disease in the way it decreases osteoporosis. On the contrary, as we all know, obesity is one of the greatest contributors to heart disease.

Obviously the argument that hormones could prevent heart disease was always on shaky ground.

Estrogen Therapy and Heart Disease

As we mentioned in Chapter 1, the first clinical study on estrogen and heart disease took place with men and showed that giving them estrogen increased their risk of heart attack.[18] Later observational studies suggested that giving estrogen to postmenopausal women seemed to decrease their risk of heart disease.[19] In 1991, Meir Stampfer and Graham Colditz did a review of all of the observational studies that had looked at the connection between estrogen therapy and heart disease. They found that women on estrogen therapy alone had a 50 percent lower risk of heart disease than women who weren't on estrogen.[20] In a second review they found that women on both estrogen and progestin had a similar decrease in their risk of heart disease.[21]

There have been many observational studies on this issue and although most of them have been consistent, the fact that they are observational means that the question remains whether estrogen lessens the risk of heart disease, or whether women with generally good health were more likely to be on estrogen in the first place.[22] This is where all the biases we mentioned in Chapter 4 come in. None of these were large, randomized, controlled blinded studies. In all of them, the women who took estrogen were of higher socioeconomic status, better educated, thinner, more likely to be nonsmokers, and more likely to have had a hysterectomy (60 to 80 percent).[23] These women were more likely to go to doctors (that's how they got their hormones in the first place) and therefore more likely to have had overall preventative care, such as having their blood pressure checked and their cholesterol monitored. Finally, the women who stayed on hormones were more likely to be compliant (see Chapter 4).[24]

Remember that all of these other factors can themselves affect vulnerability to heart attack. Cardiovascular disease in people over sixty-five is 80 percent higher among those who are least educated than among those who are college-educated—and in people under sixty-five, it's at least twice as high. Also, the least educated people have twice the risk of people with a high school education.[25] Since better-educated people tend to get better-paying jobs, the fact that women who take hormones have a higher socioeconomic status and more education is really significant. Remember the monkeys—the dominant ones had higher HDL levels.

The compliance mentioned above is also an issue. Only one fourth of all women who are prescribed estrogen take it for an extended period of time, as their doctors recommend. The other three fourths decide for themselves at some point not to take it or to stop taking it.[26] As you'll recall from Chapter 4, there is some evidence that compliant patients in general, regardless of what they're complying with, have a significantly reduced risk of heart disease.

Even taking all this into account, though, there are still possible biological explanations for at least some of the apparent effect of estrogen on heart disease. The first to be identified was the effect of estrogen on cholesterol. Estrogen increases HDL and decreases LDL. This can have a marked effect on subsequent heart disease. The first randomized controlled study to investigate estrogen and progesterone therapy and its effects on lipids in women was the three-year PEPI study.[27] They compared placebo to Premarin alone, Premarin plus micronized (natural) progesterone, and Premarin plus Provera on two different schedules. The results were reported in 1995 showing that the average increase in HDL was similar for Premarin alone and Premarin plus micronized progesterone.[28] In both of the groups of Premarin and Provera the increase in HDL was significantly lower. Triglyceride levels increased in every group except the one that received the placebo.

In addition to the lipid-lowering effects confirmed in the PEPI study, there were many experiments in animals showing other direct benefits of estrogen on blood vessels. Still all we had was a large body of circumstantial evidence suggesting that estrogen therapy could prevent heart disease. As I suggested in the first edition of this book, that is not enough to prove cause and effect.

HERS and WHI, The Surprising Answer

In an attempt to provide the final piece of proof, the HERS trial was launched of women who already had heart disease, randomizing 3,000 women to take Prempro or placebo.[29] The company that makes Premarin was so confident of the result that they funded the study. The results after four years were a surprise to everyone. Overall there was no effect of the HRT on fatal or nonfatal heart attacks, even though cholesterol was indeed lowered. Even more surprising, in the first year of the study there was a 50 percent increase in heart attacks in the women on HRT. The HRT advocates were quick to come up with explanations. Perhaps the Provera (a form of progestin given to prevent cancer of the uterus) blocked the benefit as it had in PEPI. This theory was quickly disproven when the results of the ERA study were reported.[30] In this study using angiography (an X ray in which dye is injected into the arteries to see if there is narrowing) women who had heart disease were randomized to Premarin alone, Premarin and Provera (if the woman still had a uterus), or placebo. The angiogram was repeated after 3.2 years, and there was no benefit shown from either the Premarin or the Prempro.

The observations in HERS of an increase in heart attack deaths in the first year led many to claim that if you didn't die first, HRT could be preventive (a bit crazy, but they were thinking about all the women who were already taking HRT and hadn't died). In fact, there was a slight trend in that direction, but it was not significant. The HERS investigators followed the women who stayed on their original drugs for an additional 2.7 years unblinded (everyone knew what they were taking). They found that at the end of 6.8 years the lower rates of heart disease in the hormone group did not persist and overall there was no decrease in heart disease.[31] After the HERS study the question remained as to whether estrogen and progestin could prevent heart disease in healthy women. Luckily the Women's Health Initiative was already underway, and, as we have already seen, the randomized study of estrogen and progestin answered that question quite clearly. In the group that received HRT, the rate of women experiencing heart disease was increased by 29 percent over that of the women receiving placebo. Most of the increase was in nonfatal heart attacks. This was not a huge increase, as the risks in this group were low: out of ten thousand women on HRT, there would be seven more cardiac events a year.[32] Nonetheless, this is a significant number and confirms the HERS study. Another trial being done in Europe (WISDOM) was stopped prematurely in October 2002 for scientific and practical reasons. Since the data from HERS and WHI have come out, there have been several new meta-analyses looking at the heart and HRT connection and lending more support to the conclusion that there is no connection.[33] This is truly a reminder that you can't prove cause and effect with observational data.

There is no substitute for randomized, controlled studies. Unfortunately it took us fifty years to get around to doing them.

Effects of Other Hormone Additives

Needless to say, if we're unsure about the effects of progestin in coronary heart disease protection, we're completely in the dark regarding other hormonal additives such as testosterone. One small study on women showed no difference in lipid levels in the women taking androgens along with estrogen. No direct effects on blood vessels were studied.[34] One study in monkeys showed that their lipid profiles did not deteriorate when testosterone was added. This does not, however, shed any light on possible long-term effects. I think it's naive not to recognize that estrogen can have so many varied effects while maintaining that male hormones like testosterone will affect only libido. Although there are as yet no long-term studies, the fact that heart disease is so much more common in men than women is enough to give one pause.

Directions for Further Research

Almost all the studies done in the United States on estrogen and heart disease have used Premarin, which is taken by mouth and broken down by the liver. In this process it affects the production of the lipids that pose such a risk factor for heart disease. Other estrogens—especially those that are absorbed through the skin, by injection, or vaginally—may not have the same effect on lipids, although their direct effect on the blood vessels should be the same. But again, we can't be certain until further studies are done, using these other forms.

What You Really Want to Know: Should You Take Estrogen to Prevent or Treat Heart Disease?

Meanwhile, should you take estrogen—with or without other hormones—to prevent heart disease or to treat existing heart disease? The American Heart Association gave us some direction with their Science Advisory Statement on the topic in July 2001.[35] They recommended that women with heart disease should *not* be given HRT in an effort to prevent further disease. Women who are already on HRT and have heart disease should continue only if there is a good reason other than heart disease to do it. They stated that the data are not strong enough at this time to suggest that healthy women start HRT to prevent heart disease. With the additional information from the WHI about the increased risk of breast cancer in the women on HRT, most experts are now recommending that women who have been on HRT for more than five years consider stopping. Hormones are not the way to prevent heart disease. Luckily there are other ways to prevent heart disease that are better proven, from lifestyle changes to drugs that can lower cholesterol and high blood pressure (see Chapter 14).

SEVEN

BREAST CANCER: EVERY WOMAN'S FEAR?

Until the recent past, we heard much about all the wonderful benefits of HRT, while the potential risk of breast cancer was downplayed. Now, with the first report out of the Women's Health Initiative showing that estrogen and progestins increase the risk of breast cancer after only four years, it is harder to dismiss this concern.[1]

HOW BREAST CANCER BEGINS

In order to understand the relationship between estrogen and breast cancer, we need first to understand what is known about how and why breast cancer develops (see Figure 7.1). Breast cancer starts in the lining of the milk ducts. First, extra cells begin to form in this lining—a condition called hyperplasia (hyper means "too many," and plasia means "cells"). These cells then become odd looking (atypical hyperplasia) and start filling the duct. Most of the time, neither hyperplasia nor atypical hyperplasia leads to cancer. When the cells start to look bizarre, like cancer cells, and are filling the duct but are still totally contained within it, they are called ductal carcinoma in situ, DCIS. DCIS is also called precancer. About 30 percent of the time, the cells develop the ability to break out of the duct into the surrounding fat—this is called invasion—and at that stage, you have cancer. These same cells can then gain access to a blood vessel and head out to the rest of the body. This process is termed metastasis. And it is metastasis that eventually kills you.

What starts this process? Cell growth, division, and invasion are all programmed by our genes. Cancers are started by faulty genes. You can inherit a faulty gene from your father or mother (or both), or you can inherit normal genes but something in the environment can come along and damage one of them. Actually, even an inherited gene needs some-

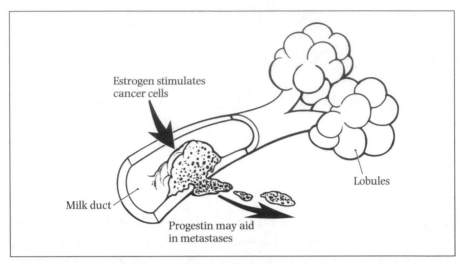

Figure 7.1. Hormones and breast cancer.

thing in the environment to cause the final mutation needed to lead to breast cancer—so breast cancer, like other cancers, is caused by a combination of abnormal genes and carcinogens in the environment.

Over the past several years, many discoveries have been made about breast cancer genes. For example, BRCA 1 (which stands for "breast cancer" 1) is a gene prevalent in families that have a lot of breast and ovarian cancer; BRCA 2 is a gene prevalent in families with a lot of male and female breast cancer. However, BRCA 1 and BRCA 2, important as they are, explain only 5 to 10 percent of breast cancer; they are not responsible for the vast number of cases.

More important for the average woman are the factors in her life that can cause a mutation in a normal breast gene or cause a mutated gene to grow and propagate. In this regard, the most common culprits are estrogen and progesterone.

RISK FACTORS IN BREAST CANCER: ESTROGEN AND PROGESTERONE

Are estrogen and progesterone a deadly duo? Estrogen was once thought to be the only hormone involved in starting and causing the progression of breast cancer. This idea came about because researchers believed that the breast responded to hormones in the same way as the uterus. In the uterus, estrogen causes cancer and progesterone protects against it. But the breast isn't the uterus; the breast responds to hormones quite differently.

Most hormones work through receptors on the outside surface of a cell. A receptor is like a lock that a specific hormone fits into, allowing the hormone to enter a cell or at least cause something to happen in a cell. Researchers initially assumed that all of the locks were the same; if progesterone blocked the effects of estrogen in one place, it would block them everywhere. We are now finding that this isn't entirely true. The researcher Katherine Horwitz has shown that the progesterone receptor in the uterus is completely different from the progesterone receptor in the breast.[2] For example, in the uterus, the drug RU 486 will block progesterone (that's how it causes a miscarriage); in the breast, it will act like progesterone and stimulate tissue to grow. This has been a source of confusion. In addition, as with the heart, we can't assume that progesterone and progestins have the same effect in the breast.

Malcolm Pike, a researcher from the University of Southern California, has theorized that unlike cancer of the uterus, which is caused by estrogen alone, breast cancer is caused by estrogen and progesterone together.[3] Examining the risk factors for breast cancer provides some evidence that gives weight to Pike's hypothesis. Recently we found out that even estrogen receptors are not as simple as we thought; a second estrogen receptor has been identified. This beta receptor is present in some of the same organs as the classical alpha receptor, as well as in some different organs. It has some of the same effects as well as some different effects.[4] With the premature termination of the estrogen and progestin arm of the Women's Health Initiative because of the increase in breast cancer, Pike stands on firmer ground. It is important to point out that this does not mean that estrogen alone is home free—simply that the combination is more carcinogenic. At the time of this writing, some of these effects are just being sorted out, but expect to hear more about this issue. This demonstrates yet again that the issue of hormone therapy is a work in progress and that we never really understand it all.

Your Own Estrogen and Progesterone as Risk Factors

One of the first studies done on the connection between hormones and breast cancer looked at 6,908 women who had had hysterectomies between 1920 and 1940 and compared them with 1,479 women who had gone through natural menopause.[5] Women who had had both the uterus and the ovaries removed before age forty had a remarkably lower incidence of breast cancer—75 percent lower. But there was no such decrease among the women who had kept their ovaries. This was the first study to suggest that early surgical menopause protected women from breast cancer, and that hormones had something to do with the disease.

Since then, many other risk factors point to the effect of your own estrogen and progesterone on the risk of breast cancer. We know, for example, that the younger you are when you start your period and the older you are when you enter menopause, the higher your risk of getting breast cancer will be. In other words, the more exposure you have to your own hormones, the more you are at risk. If you become pregnant before age thirty, you decrease your risk of breast cancer; and if you have no children, your risk increases. If you exercise more than three times a week in the years before menopause, your risk of breast cancer decreases, presumably because you've altered the length of your cycle and decreased your levels of estrogen and progesterone. Postmenopausal obesity increases the risk of breast cancer, presumably because it raises the level of estrogen. Alcohol consumption also raises estrogen levels and increases the risk of breast cancer.

There are other signs of high estrogen that predict for a higher risk of breast cancer. Women with a high bone density have an increased risk of getting breast cancer, as do women with dense mammograms.[6]

Of course, there are also risk factors for breast cancer that aren't hormonally related. But having more than one risk factor can compound the risk—and this often involves an interaction between hormonal and non-hormonal factors.

Radiation, for example, especially at an early age, appears to increase the risk of breast cancer. In the 1950s, doctors were radiating people for a variety of problems, believing that radiation was completely safe. As a result, a large number of women who were treated for various conditions with radiation as girls and young adults in the 1950s have developed breast cancer.[7] Researchers theorize that breast tissue doesn't develop fully until you've gone through a full-term pregnancy and are capable of making milk, and immature breast tissue is thought to be more sensitive than mature breast tissue to carcinogens such as radiation. Because of this, radiation in younger women is more dangerous than the same radiation later on. On the other hand, some things may serve to mature breast tissue early and therefore decrease risk. In the 1950s, HCG (human choriogonadotrophic hormone)—the hormone that rises during pregnancy, inhibiting estrogen and progesterone—decreased the risk of breast cancer when it was given to women for weight loss.[8] Perhaps this caused the breast tissue to be more mature.

Many other external environmental pollutants are carcinogenic because they mimic estrogen. The pesticide DDT is metabolized into DDE, which is a form of estrogen. Some researchers believe that such environmental pesticides are contributing to the increased incidence of breast cancer.[9] Although studies have not been able to show a direct link between environmental carcinogens and breast cancer, this does not rule out an effect.[10] It may depend on when the exposure occurs. Or there may be combinations of effects—birth control pills and environmental estrogens, for example. Some studies have shown that the average sperm count has declined in men; this is also thought to be related to higher environmental estrogens.

At the same time, plant compounds (phyto-SERMs), such as those found in soy, seem to protect against breast cancer in the test tube.[11] (This last is important, since test-tube results aren't always the same as the effects on actual human beings.) Substances in soy appear to block estrogen in the breast while acting like estrogen in other organs, such as the bones (see Chapter 12). One hypothesis about how soy protects against breast cancer is that a diet high in soy protein given to girls during puberty may cause early breast tissue differentiation much as early pregnancy does, making it less susceptible to carcinogens. Whether this is true, or even whether soy can prevent breast cancer in women, remains to be studied.

What you eat may affect the amount of endogenous estrogens you have. For example, vegetarians have lower levels of estrogen in their urine than meat eaters. Several studies have even shown that women who develop breast cancer have higher blood levels of estrogen and testosterone.[12] And the breast itself may make estrogen from testosterone. Studies of breast duct fluid show that it has forty times the level of estrogen in the blood.[13]

Hormones as Drugs and the Risk of Breast Cancer

Since your body's own hormones can cause breast cancer, it makes sense to conclude that hormones taken as drugs will also increase your risk.

DES, a form of estrogen that was given to pregnant women to prevent miscarriages in the 1950s, increased their risk of breast cancer.[14] Birth control pills taken for more than ten years increase the risk of breast cancer in those women still taking them.[15] (We don't know about the current low-dose pills, as they haven't been used long enough.)

Although many people were surprised when the Women's Health Initiative showed a 26 percent increase in breast cancer risk in women on estrogen and progestin postmenopausally, this result had been predicted by the observational studies.[16] More information will be coming from the Women's Health Initiative; meanwhile, examining the previous studies can give us some insight into the risk.

A study by Catherine Schairer looked at women in the Breast Cancer Detection Demonstration Project (BCDDP), a nonrandomized screening program.[17] It compared women on estrogen and progestins with those who weren't and found that women on estrogen and progestins had a slightly increased (20 percent higher) risk of breast cancer. Ron Ross confirmed this, showing that women on estrogen alone increased their risk by 1 percent per year, while women on both estrogen and progestin increased their risk of breast cancer by 8 percent per year.[18] One of the biggest studies we have to date, the Nurses' Health Study, which we discussed in Chapter 6, showed in June 1995 that adding progestin to estrogen not only failed to reduce women's incidence of breast cancer, but actually increased it—as Malcolm Pike's model (discussed earlier) would suggest. This wasn't a huge increase, but it's an effect nonetheless. Women taking estrogen alone had a 36 percent increase in their risk of breast cancer; those on estrogen plus progestin had a 50 percent increase; those on progestins alone had a 240 percent increase. However, the number of women on progestins alone was small, so it is important to look at a larger number of women before we give that finding too much credence. This study also looked at women who were taking estrogen and testosterone, which had been added to their regimen in the hope that it would restore libido. These women's risk of breast cancer was increased by 78 percent.[19]

Another important finding of the Nurses' Health Study had to do with the effects of age and duration of use. Women who at the time of the study had been taking estrogen and progesterone for five to ten years had a 46 percent increase in their risk of breast cancer. Also, the older a woman was, the higher her risk. Women between ages sixty and sixty-four who had been taking hormones for five years or more had an increase in risk of 71 percent.

Some experts have argued that since the estrogen–alone study of the WHI (in women who have had hysterectomies) has not been stopped prematurely, it must be safe. They are blaming the whole risk on progestins. This is unlikely. As we have seen, the risk from estrogen alone is lower than that for estrogen plus progestin, but not zero. It will take a little longer for the WHI results to show up but it is likely that, when the study is finished in 2006, we will also find that the risk benefit does not work.

The explanation for the difference in risk when progestins are added may not be due to the progestin per se but rather the type of woman who takes it. First, as we discussed in Chapter 4, the women on estrogen alone have usually had a hysterectomy and had their ovaries out. This surgery is done most commonly premenopausally for bleeding. We know that women who have their ovaries out prior to menopause have a lower risk of breast cancer than women undergoing a natural menopause.

In addition, it is the studies that have looked at the duration of use of estrogen that show the biggest risk. The WHI estrogen–alone study has been going for less than five years at the time of this writing. Bruce Ettinger of Kaiser Permanente looked at a series of women who had used estrogen for at least seventeen years. The study found a doubling of the risk of breast cancer.[20]

The WHI estrogen plus progestin study has been criticized because it studied synthetic and not the bioidentical hormones that are closer to what our own bodies make. The implication is that natural progesterone and estradiol will be safer for the breast. There is no data to support that hypothesis at this time. In fact, in the PEPI study progesterone increased mammographic density to the same degree as Provera did, suggesting that its effect on the breast is the same.[21] Other studies have looked at bioidential hormones, especially studies done in Europe, where Premarin was not as widely used, and they also show an increased risk of breast cancer.[22] In fact, in October 1997 the Collaborative Group on Hormonal Factors in Breast Cancer brought together and reanalyzed about 90 percent of the worldwide epidemiological evidence on the relation between the risk of breast cancer and the use of hormone replacement therapy of all types. Individual data on 52,050 women with breast cancer and 108,411 women without breast cancer from fifty-one studies in twenty-one countries were collected, checked, and analyzed centrally. The study found an increased risk of breast cancer of 35 percent after five years of use and a 53 percent increase for more than five years. Five years after stopping hormones, this increased risk completely disappeared.[23]

To me the conclusion is clear: there's an increased risk of breast cancer for women who take hormones postmenopausally for five or more years. It is not a huge increase, however. In the WHI study there were eight more cases of invasive cancer per ten thousand women per year. After five years this would be four out of one thousand women. After thirty years it would be twenty-four women out of one thousand. And the risk was across all groups of women, not just in women who had a family history of breast cancer. In fact the big surprise to me from the WHI is that the risk is not higher. Nonetheless, this risk does give one pause. When we still thought that HRT would decrease heart disease, there was a reasonable argument that that was more important. Now that the studies are not showing a benefit in heart disease, I have to ask whether it makes sense to use a drug for prevention when there is even the slightest risk that it could cause harm, especially when there are safe alternatives such as lifestyle changes.[24]

One crucial question is whether cancers caused by postmenopausal hormone therapy are the same as cancers that occur on their own. There's a continuing tendency to extrapolate from what we know about the uterus, and so some researchers have theorized that hormonally promoted cancers might be less aggressive. The endometrial cancers caused by estrogen tend to be fairly unaggressive and treatable, as you'll read in Chapter 8. This led some early researchers to assume that the same would be true of breast cancer: if you got breast cancer from taking hormones too long, perhaps it would be easier to cure because it would be less aggressive than other breast cancers.

Two studies have seemed to confirm this, as did data from my own research at UCLA.[25] The percentage was not large, but there was a slightly higher proportion of low-grade cancers among women on hormones. We can't be sure why this is. One possible explanation, though, is that women on hormones, as we've noted before, tend to be people who get better medical care than others, so they're more likely to get regular mammograms—and the kind of breast cancers that mammograms are best at finding are precisely those cancers that respond best to "early detection." At least four recent studies have shown an increase in lobular cancers in women on HRT.[26] This makes some sense, since lobular cancers are almost always sensitive to estrogen. However, they are harder to feel or see on a mammogram and are often diagnosed at a later stage.

Still, these aren't the only findings that have come up. The Nurses' Health Study showed a 45 percent increase in the risk of death from breast cancer in women who took hormones for more than five years. So it isn't just relatively harmless in situ cancers that women get from hormones.[27]

If You're Already at Risk

Some studies have looked at whether women already at risk for breast cancer will compound their risk if they use estrogen. This question is not clear-cut, because risk factors don't always add up: it's somewhat like a prisoner who's committed two crimes getting concurrent sentences rather than consecutive sentences. In the WHI the increased risk in breast cancer was the same in all groups, regardless of risk factors or lack thereof. Women who are at low risk for breast cancer are not safe,[28] and women who are at high risk are probably increasing their risk, at least to some extent.

Recently, there have been disturbing studies about still another possible effect of hormone therapy on the risk of breast cancer. This has to do with detection of breast cancer. Young women have dense breast tissue. Usually, breast tissue in postmenopausal women is less dense and thus doesn't hide cancers as well. But taking hormones can stimulate breast tissue, causing it to become denser. Cancer and breast tissue are the same density, so the effect on a mammogram is like looking for a polar bear in the snow.

This problem of detection appears to be worse when women take combined estrogen and progestins. One study reported that 30 percent of women on estrogen and progestins will show an increase in dense tissue.[29] A report from the *Journal of the National Cancer Institute* said that the mammograms of women on hormone therapy were more difficult to read.[30] I used to see this in my own breast-surgery practice all the time: I'd look at a patient's mammogram and think, "She must have started hormones," because suddenly her breast tissue was dense, which it hadn't been in previous mammograms. Then, if the woman stopped her hormones, within six months her mammogram would be back to normal.

Retrospective studies have demonstrated that women with dense breasts in general have more breast cancer.[31] Density may represent hormones stimulating the tissue, which in turn could cause more cancer. These two implications create a frightening double jeopardy: you're more likely to get breast cancer, and less likely to catch it in time to save your life—yet another reason that long-term use of HRT is just not worth it.

BREAST CANCER AND YOU

Early Detection

The recent questions about mammography and breast self-examination should make you leary of dismissing concerns about the increased risk of breast cancer on the assumption that if you're diligent about your health care, your cancer can be detected early and cured. I wish this were true, but as I've seen so often and so tragically in my practice, it's not something you can count on. Even apart from the obscuring effect hormones have on breast tissue, mammography at its best is far from a guarantee that breast cancer will be caught at an early, curable stage. A mammogram isn't the equivalent of a Pap smear, and the concept of "early detection" is somewhat misleading. It works only about 30 percent of the time. Women can still get small cancers that have already spread by the time they're diagnosed.

In fact it was my frustration with the limitations of our means of detecting cancers that led me to develop ductal lavage. This new technique is based on the fact that all breast cancer starts in the lining of the milk ducts. If we had a way to sample the cells from the milk-duct lining, we could find not only cancers, but cells that are just thinking of becoming cancer some day when they grow up. Then we could do something to prevent that from happening, such as take tamoxifen. The procedure requires a tiny catheter that the doctor can thread into a milk-duct opening through the nipple for a short distance, then squirt in salt water and suck it back out, collecting hundreds of cells to look at under the microscope. If you have atypical cells on lavage, you have a higher risk of subsequent breast cancer, and if you have a family history of breast cancer along with the atypical cells, the risk is even higher. Right now this procedure is available only to high-risk women, but as we do more research, I think it will become more helpful to women who are trying to make decisions about HRT.

Prevention of Breast Cancer

The good news is that we have some options for preventing breast cancer, and, not surprisingly, most of them work by blocking estrogen. Tamoxifen, which blocks the estrogen receptor in the breast when given to women who are at increased risk of breast cancer for four years, will reduce the risk by 50 percent. As you would expect, it prevents the cancers that are sensitive to estrogen and not the ones that are estrogen receptor negative. Raloxifene, a designer estrogen, was studied in women with osteoporosis to see if it would decrease fractures and was noted to significantly decrease breast cancer risk. There is currently an ongoing study (STAR) comparing raloxifene to tamoxifen in high-risk women to find out whether one is better than the other. The other, more drastic way to decrease breast cancer is to remove the breasts preventatively. This measure is usually reserved for women who carry the gene for breast cancer.

What You Really Want to Know: What Is It Like to Have Breast Cancer?

Breast cancer often takes a woman by surprise. Seventy to eighty percent of women with breast cancer have no risk factors. No one in their family has ever had it, and they did everything right. The first sign is usually a lump you find while showering, rolling over in bed, or making love, or an abnormal routine mammogram.

When a biopsy reveals cancer, you'll need to have the tumor removed by either a lumpectomy or a mastectomy. During the surgery, a few lymph nodes will be removed from under your arm and examined for cancer cells. If there is cancer in the nodes or if there's another reason to believe that there might be microscopic cancer cells elsewhere in the body, you'll receive chemotherapy for four to six months, tamoxifen (an estrogen blocker) for five years, or both. (Which of these systemic treatments is best depends on a number of factors.) If the nodes are negative and there's no reason to believe that there are cancer cells elsewhere in the body, you'll probably have only local treatment: lumpectomy and six weeks or so of radiation therapy; or mastectomy, with the option of breast reconstruction.

The median age for breast cancer is sixty-nine. Approximately one-third of the women diagnosed with breast cancer will die of it. A fifty-year-old woman has a 10 percent lifetime probability of getting breast cancer and a 3 percent chance of dying of the disease.[32] Most women who develop breast cancer tolerate their therapy while continuing their normal lives. Neither the treatment nor the disease is physically disabling unless the disease spreads. Once this spread (metastasis) develops, the course is usually fairly rapid, with most women dead within two to three and a half years.

What You Really Want to Know: When You've Already Had Breast Cancer

We have long felt that women who have already had breast cancer would increase their risk of a recurrence of the original cancer or of a second breast cancer if they took hormones. This made sense since part of the treatment of breast cancer is blocking estrogen either by tamoxifen or now by one of the aromatase inhibitors. Yet the solution is not so clear. Several small, nonrandomized studies of the use of hormones for postmenopausal women with breast cancer show no increase in recurrence.[33] The follow-up, however, has been short, and the studies were of women who were already at low risk of recurrence, so they're hard to evaluate. Until we have a lot more evidence that it's safe, I feel that preventive hormone therapy for women who have had breast cancer is a bad idea. One worrisome, albeit small, study followed four women who were taking both estrogen and progesterone after treatment for breast cancer.[34] They all developed metastasis. When they were taken off their hormones, however, the metastasis temporarily disappeared. This suggests that the hormones were fueling the metastases. Limited as this study is, it does give one pause.

Finally, it's important to realize that a woman who's had cancer in one breast already has an increased risk of developing cancer in the other breast. The risk to any woman with breast cancer is a recurrence or a second cancer. This overwhelms any possible benefit of hormone therapy in preventing osteoporosi .[35]

Once in a while, I've had a breast-cancer patient who, knowing the risks, still wants to be on short-term hormone therapy to relieve menopausal symptoms. A study of women with breast cancer done at Johns Hopkins showed that 49 percent of women experienced a physical or emotional problem related to menopause after the diagnosis of breast cancer. Half of these women felt they were in need of treatment.[36] Obviously, we need to develop appropriate treatments for this group of women. In Europe they sometimes combine estrogen and tamoxifen in their prevention trials, with no obvious harm. The Milan group is starting a study to look at this option for women with breast cancer on tamoxifen with severe symptoms. Meanwhile, though, if a woman has severe symptoms that are interfering with the quality of her life, I think she would be wise to investigate many of the alternative methods for relieving symptoms before settling on hormone therapy. (We discuss some of these in Chapter 11.) At the very least, if she feels she must take hormones, she should take the lowest dose for the shortest possible time.

As I've said before, there's no free lunch.

EIGHT

ENDOMETRIAL CANCER: THE FIRST PROBLEM WITH ESTROGEN

The one danger from long-term estrogen therapy that isn't disputed is its link with cancer of the endometrium—the lining of the uterus. (Because cancer of the actual uterine wall is very uncommon, the term uterine cancer almost always refers to endometrial cancer.) I described in Chapter 1 the complicated hormonal dance that occurs monthly in your body between puberty and menopause. As part of that dance, the endometrium is first built, then sloughed off with your period, and then rebuilt.

UNDERSTANDING ENDOMETRIAL CANCER

The endometrial lining is meant to be replaced monthly unless it's needed to support a pregnancy. If it's not shed regularly, it can become cancerous. Endometrial cancer is genetic, just as breast cancer is. It starts with flawed genes that are either inherited or acquired through exposure to carcinogens. Estrogen may cause some mutations, but we believe that its main role in endometrial cancer is to increase cell division, giving any mutations already there the opportunity to multiply. Progesterone can block this process if it causes the lining of the uterus to shed (see Figure 8.1). All the mutated cells, even the cancerous ones, flow out during your period. Because of this, endometrial cancer is unusual in a woman who is menstruating normally, since she's regularly shedding her endometrium.

After menopause, unless you've had a hysterectomy, you still have an endometrium. Usually, if your own levels of estrogen production aren't too high, this lining atrophies or becomes inactive. So even if precancerous cells are present, they lie dormant. If for some reason the cells are stimulated to divide, however, the precancerous or cancerous mutations

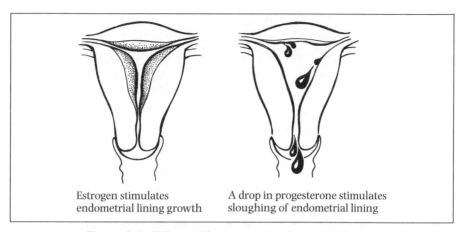

Estrogen stimulates
endometrial lining growth

A drop in progesterone stimulates
sloughing of endometrial lining

Figure 8.1. Effects of hormones on the uterine lining.

will have a chance to increase, and they won't be automatically shed at the end of the month in a period. This is how women get endometrial cancer.

Once endometrial cancer develops, it can invade the blood vessels (just as breast cancer can) and spread to other organs. So, like any cancer, it can kill you.

But unlike breast cancer, endometrial cancer gives you early warning signs. As the uterine lining builds up, it causes spotting or bleeding. Spontaneous bleeding in a woman who hasn't had a period in a year always needs to be checked out. So does persistent heavy menstrual bleeding. (As we said in Chapter 3, the problem isn't always cancer; there are a number of more likely possibilities.) Fortunately, the uterine lining is readily accessible and can be easily biopsied in a doctor's office.

Sometimes the biopsy will find signs that the endometrium is precancerous. Though precancer is a frightening idea, it's a far cry from cancer itself, especially when it's in the short-lived endometrium rather than a permanent, critical organ. Still, you want to be careful with it.

The first indication that there may be a problem is if the biopsy finds an increased number of cells. This is called simple or adenomatous hyperplasia (*adenomatous* means in a gland-forming organ; *hyper,* as we saw in Chapter 7, means "too many"; *plasia* means "cells"). Hyperplasia is often a cause of irregular or heavy bleeding in perimenopausal women (see Chapter 3). This is thought to arise because some women have cycles in which they don't ovulate and therefore don't produce progesterone to help them shed the endometrium. You may have several such cycles and then, when you do ovulate, end up with a period in which the blood just seems to gush—"your basic flooder," as one of my friends calls it. If you have such cells and they're abnormal looking, they're called atypical (see Figure 8.2). Atypical hyperplasia can be simple or complex, depending on whether the increased cells are also interfering with the normal architecture of the uterine lining. Complex hyperplasia is more ominous than simple hyperplasia.

The next step after atypia is thought to be cancer. But this is far from an inevitable progression. In 1985, the researcher Robert Kurman showed that only 1 percent of women with untreated simple hyperplasia went on to develop uterine cancer; and even with complex atypical hyperplasia, only 29 percent of women developed cancer.[1]

Hyperplasia can be treated with a progestin. It's given for twelve days to balance the estrogen, and then when it's stopped, it causes the lining of the uterus to slough off, thereby eliminating any precancerous cells that may be there.

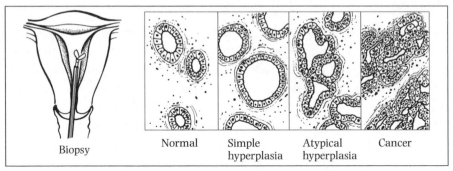

| Biopsy | Normal | Simple hyperplasia | Atypical hyperplasia | Cancer |

Figure 8.2. Uterine cancer development.

What Is It Like to Have Endometrial Cancer?

Actual endometrial cancer is usually a disease of older women, the median age being sixty-eight years. This cancer is very curable.

If the problem is precancer, as just noted, it can be treated with progestin. But if the problem is cancer, a hysterectomy is usually needed. (See Chapter 11 for a description of what to expect with a hysterectomy.) When endometrial cancers are detected at an early stage—as most are—

this is all the treatment necessary. Women with more advanced disease usually need radiation therapy as well. Although early-stage endometrial cancer is 93 percent curable, there are still some women who are diagnosed at a later stage, and women do die of this disease.

RISK FACTORS IN ENDOMETRIAL CANCER

All of the risk factors for endometrial cancer have to do with increased estrogen that isn't balanced by progesterone—so-called unopposed estrogen. So women who take estrogen are obviously at risk.

Weight is also a major risk factor because, as I said earlier, fat has an enzyme called aromatase that produces estrogen in postmenopausal women. Postmenopausal women who are between twenty and fifty pounds overweight have three times the normal risk of endometrial cancer; if you're more than fifty pounds overweight, you have nineteen times the risk of endometrial cancer. In fact, the best way to prevent endometrial cancer is to keep your weight down with exercise and a healthy diet.

Diabetes triples your risk of endometrial cancer. So does high blood pressure. It's not clear, however, whether these are independent risk factors or are related to being overweight. (Both adult-onset diabetes and high blood pressure are often associated with obesity.)

The breast cancer drug tamoxifen, since it blocks estrogen in the breast but acts like estrogen in the uterus, has also been shown to cause endometrial cancer.

At the same time, there are some factors that *decrease* the risk of endometrial cancer. Premenopausal women who take birth control pills have a lower incidence of endometrial cancer, and the protection lasts for at least fifteen years after they've stopped taking the pills. This is probably because the balanced estrogen and progesterone in the pill prevent abnormal buildups in the lining of the uterus. Regular exercise decreases the risk of endometrial cancer by lengthening your menstrual cycle and thus lessening the amount of both hormones you're exposed to in your lifetime. Eating a diet high in soy protein will have a similar effect. Smoking, which does so much harm in other ways, decreases the risk of endometrial cancer because it reduces the amount of estrogen you have naturally. (I need hardly add that I don't advise taking up smoking as a preventive measure—lung cancer is a ghastly alternative to endometrial cancer.)

Estrogen as a Risk Factor

It isn't surprising that estrogen given alone (unopposed by progesterone) to postmenopausal women increases their risk of endometrial cancer significantly. The researcher Deborah Grady published a meta-analysis of endometrial cancer in 1995.[2] (A meta-analysis takes a large group of studies and combines their results.) Women who had used estrogen at any point in their lives, whether for one year or thirty years, had 2.3 times the normal risk of endometrial cancer. Those who took it for less than a year had 1.4 times the normal risk. Those who took it for more than ten years had almost 10 times the normal risk. Those who took it for twenty years had 20 times the risk.

Interestingly, women who took Premarin had a greater risk than those who took synthetic estrogens. Users of Premarin were 2.5 times more likely to get endometrial cancer than nonusers, while women who used synthetic estrogens like Estrace were only 1.3 times more likely to get it than nonusers.

Women who used unopposed estrogen were four times more likely to get an early-stage cancer than a late-stage one. Women on estrogen had six times as many noninvasive cancers (precancers) and four times as many invasive cancers as nonusers. This finding has been interpreted to mean that estrogen is much more likely to stimulate an in situ or noninvasive cancer and is said to support the theory that the kind of endometrial cancer caused by unopposed estrogen is a "better"—or at least slower-growing—kind of cancer. As with all the diseases we've been discussing, though, we have to consider the "healthy woman" effect. These women were going to the doctor to get their hormones and were thus more likely than women who were not on hormones to have their cancer detected at an early stage. But even at that, these women weren't completely out of the woods. Their death rate from endometrial cancer was almost three times that of women who had never taken hormones. If you take estrogen, your risk of endometrial cancer is worse if you smoke cigarettes or are thin. Obese women have a lot of their own estrogen, and one would think that would make their risk of endometrial cancer worse. But it seems to be the opposite. It's the women who don't have that much of their own estrogen and who then supplement it who are more at risk.

It's important to remember that for a fifty-year-old woman the lifetime risk of developing endometrial cancer is 3 percent. So doubling your risk by taking estrogen would raise it to 6 percent.[3] As we've pointed out before, an increase in risk can be less important if a disease is less common but more important if a disease is more common. It may or may not be worth it to you to take that increased risk.

Progestins as a Risk Factor

You'll remember from Chapter 7 that the first wave of postmenopausal women who took hormone therapy in the United States received only estrogen. When the reports came out about increased rates of both endometrial hyperplasia and endometrial cancers in women who had taken unopposed Premarin, the drug companies and doctors had to do something. The risk was related to the fact that with estrogen the lining of the uterus built up continuously and unnaturally, without being shed. So doctors began adding progestin to the estrogen regimen for a few days in each cycle. When the progestin was stopped, the uterine lining would shed and eliminate the risk. This combined hormone therapy caused a prompt decrease in the incidence of both hyperplasia and cancer of the endometrium in women taking it (and a prompt increase in sales of tampons and sanitary napkins, since they all started bleeding again).

However, there are still no good long-term studies of progestin and how it affects cancer. Some cancers take many years to develop, so we can't tell to what extent the combined therapy really results in fewer cancers and to what extent late-developing cancers will prove the benefits illusory. In addition, since many postmenopausal women are encouraged to take hormones all their lives, we need long-term studies to see the effect of twenty or thirty years of hormone use.

There are other unanswered questions about progestins. It isn't clear how much progestin is necessary to prevent uterine cancer. In one study, women who took estrogen with progestin for ten days of the cycle had a 50 percent increased risk of uterine cancer, while those who took the added progestin for twelve days had no increase in uterine cancer.[4] Some doctors are doing research to see whether taking progesterone only every three or four months to shed any uterine buildup might not be enough to protect against endometrial cancer. Intrauterine progesterone, which is inserted by a doctor like an IUD, is also being studied. In the PEPI study, discussed in Chapter 6, 200 milligrams of micronized progesterone daily for twelve days appeared to be enough to protect the uterus without counteracting the positive effects of estrogen on lipid levels.[5] Another approach, suggested by Bruce Ettinger at Kaiser, is using lower doses of estrogen and giving progestin every six months.[6]

Many of the symptoms of perimenopause and menopause actually become worse when you take progestins and progesterone (see Chapter 15); women complain especially of bloating and depression. The biggest problem, however, is that you start bleeding again. Women who are menopausal will get periods again, and those who are perimenopausal may have heavy, irregular bleeding. Needless to say, this hasn't pleased women. In fact, it's the reason most women stop taking postmenopausal hormone therapy.

In an effort to prevent this bleeding, doctors began giving the progestins in a different way: continuously. The idea was that taking a smaller dose every day might counteract the stimulating effect of the estrogen and allow the uterus to become inactive. If you take progestins this way, you'll still bleed at first, but after six months to a year, the bleeding will peter out. (Of course, you may need a few biopsies along the way to make sure that there's no cancer—see Chapter 4.) This solves the bleeding problem, but once again, it's changed the picture. We can't simply extrapolate the data from cyclical estrogen and progestin therapy to continuous therapy. As we discussed in Chapter 6, continuous progestins have a different effect on the heart from cyclical progestins, which means that they might have different effects in many other areas. I'm amazed that doctors continue to prescribe drugs and combinations of drugs for which we have no actual data on long-term safety, and no proof that they're effective for anything but short-term symptoms.

The real question is the effect that these approaches will have on the breast cancer risk. Now that the WHI has confirmed that estrogen plus progestin increases breast cancer risk, researchers will need to study whether variations in the progestins, doses, or schedules make a difference. The real risk from the WHI data at this writing is that women will go back to taking unopposed estrogen and trade breast cancer for uterine cancer. I don't think that is wise when there are other risks such as stroke and blood clots from estrogen even when given alone.

A Cautionary Tale

The story of endometrial cancer and the long-term use of estrogen is a cautionary tale indeed. As we've discussed in Chapter 2, Robert Wilson's book *Feminine Forever* set off a mania for long-term estrogen therapy for every woman. At the time, there were no studies documenting the alleged beneficial effects; nor were there studies on the safety of this approach. That, of course, didn't stop anyone. Here was the fountain of youth, and both women and their doctors enthusiastically ran toward it. It made sense, after all, according to the dogma of postmenopausal "ovarian failure" and "estrogen deficiency." And women had estrogen in their bodies naturally before menopause, so how could it be dangerous?

As we now know, nothing is that simple. The uterus is controlled by a bevy of hormones, not just estrogen, and supplementing only one of them throws off the choreography of the hormonal dance. Women have died from endometrial cancer caused by the estrogen they were taking to keep them young. Yet we did it again. We gave women progestins to protect their uterus without any studies on its effects on any other organs. But we plunged ahead with widespread use because "it made sense." The WHI study confirmed that the risk of breast cancer was significant, repeating the scenario. I hope we can finally learn our lesson and demand adequate data about safety and firm evidence of benefit before we jump onto a bandwagon that may again sacrifice women's lives to the pharmaceutical fad of the day.

NINE

FOR BETTER OR WORSE: HORMONE THERAPY AND OTHER DISEASES

In chapters 5, 6, and 7 we discussed the diseases most commonly linked with hormone therapy. The newspapers are also chock-full of other potential associations—some positive, some negative. In this chapter I'll review the data we have for them. We'll start with the disorders that hormones are thought to help; these include Alzheimer's disease, colon cancer, and osteoarthritis. We'll then go on to areas of potential harm: stroke, ovarian cancer, gallbladder disease, thromboembolic disease, fibroids, endometriosis, and a few others.

THE GOOD NEWS?

Alzheimer's Disease

As we mention later, there are some data suggesting that estrogen might affect thinking and memory (see Chapter 11). Because of this possibility, some people have wondered whether estrogen might also protect against Alzheimer's disease, the best-known form of dementia—and a form that's more common in women than men.

Risk Factors for Alzheimer's Disease
We know that Alzheimer's disease runs in families and therefore is caused in part by genetic defects, but we don't yet know what its other causes are. Women have 1.5 to 3 times more risk of getting Alzheimer's disease than men. This may, in part, be simply because women live longer. But there's also a greater risk if you're thin or if you've had a heart attack—and both of these factors, as you've seen, are related to estrogen levels.

Natural History of Alzheimer's Disease

Although many of us fear dementia more than most other diseases, Alzheimer's actually isn't all that common. Also, it's most likely to happen when you're very old. It's fourteen times more common in people over age eighty-five than in those between sixty and sixty-five. A 1995 study of a community in Boston found that the probability of getting Alzheimer's disease is 0.6 percent in people between sixty-five and sixty-nine, 1 percent in those between seventy and seventy-four, 2 percent in those between seventy-five and seventy-nine, 3.3 percent in those between eighty and eighty-four, and 8.4 percent in people eighty-five and older.[1] Senile dementia, which includes Alzheimer's as well as other dementias, levels off at 40 percent at age ninety-five. Few of us live to be ninety-five, however.

What Is It Like to Have Alzheimer's Disease?

The earliest symptom of Alzheimer's disease is an inability to learn or recall new information. Patients have trouble finding words, become disoriented, or have a tendency to get lost. They may have behavioral problems such as depression, irritability, suspiciousness, or delusions. Deterioration continues inexorably over a period of up to a decade or longer. Eventually, many patients lose the ability to communicate or even to recognize their closest relatives. Although there's some difference in the symptoms in men and women, the course of the disease and its severity are the same.

Estrogen and Alzheimer's Disease

Unfortunately the studies on Alzheimer's and estrogen are all observational and subject to the same biases that we have been talking about regarding heart disease.[2] (The biggest predictor of Alzheimer's disease is level of education, and there is no question that the women who chose to take ERT/HRT tend to be better educated than the women who don't.) Because of this we need much better studies to answer the question.

In terms of Alzheimer's, most of the reports are based on observational data at this point. The data we do have, however, are not promising. A randomized controlled study of women with mild to moderate Alzheimer's disease who had had a hysterectomy demonstrated no benefit from one year of estrogen.[3] The FDA has approved the first drug designed to address the cognitive deficits of Alzheimer's disease. Tacrine increases the levels of acetylcholine, a neurotransmitter in the brain. Unfortunately, its benefits are modest at best, and many people experience side effects. Although it wasn't directly studied, there's some evidence that women on estrogen as well as Tacrine had a better effect than either drug alone or placebo.[4] Recent studies have also shown that nonsteroidal anti-inflammatory agents (ibuprofen) reduce the incidence of Alzheimer's disease by 55 percent.

Estrogen and Thinking

Interestingly, the first study to look at levels of estrogen in the blood and cognitive function showed that women with high endogenous estrone levels performed significantly more poorly on two of three cognitive-function tests than women who had lower levels of estrone and that estradiol levels were unrelated to change in test performance.[5] (Although there have been several studies showing direct effects of estrogen on the growth of new neurons, synapse connectivity, and increases in neurotransmitters, as with heart disease these findings do not necessarily translate to a benefit to women's health.[6] A review of all the observational data available indicated that estrogen might have some benefit in women with symptoms of menopause but had no benefit for asymptomatic women.[7] Could this be a result of sleeping better?)

There are data showing that giving estrogen to women right after hysterectomy improves their thinking. But we don't know if it is the symptom relief or the estrogen itself that is allowing them to think better. Studies will need to look at women at different ages and different formulations of HRT to even begin to answer this question. Luckily there are several very large randomized controlled studies (such as the Women's Health Initiative Memory Study and the Women's International Study of Cognitive Aging) looking at cognitive function in relation to estrogen and menopause directly, and their findings will be reported in the next few years.

Meanwhile we have hints from randomized studies investigating other problems that included cognition in the data evaluation. The HERS study found no benefit in older women, and the MORE study of raloxifene also showed no cognitive benefit.[8] The large randomized studies will finally give us some answers, but until then it is probably not worth taking ERT/HRT as a means of improving your thinking or memory.

Colon Cancer

Colon cancer is the second most common cancer in women (after breast cancer). Some observational data suggest that women on hormone therapy have lower rates of fatal colon cancer.[9]

Colon cancer begins in the lining of the large intestine and grows to a size that can bleed or obstruct the large bowel. Most colon cancers are thought to arise in adenomatous polyps—outgrowths of the lining of the colon. These polyps occur in 30 percent of men and women, without any symptoms. Only about 1 percent or less of these polyps ever turn cancerous, however.

Risk Factors for Colon Cancer

Polyps are one risk factor. The biggest risk factor is a family history of the disease, which increases your risk by 50 percent. There is an inherited disease called familial polyposis coli in which the colon is studded with polyps, many of which turn into cancer when you're young. This cancer also occurs more often in people who have had ulcerative colitis, a chronic bowel disease characterized by bloody diarrhea.

If you eat a meat-based diet, you have twice as high a chance of getting colon cancer than if you eat meat less than once a month. Obesity increases the risk of colon cancer by 30 percent. Finally, constipation increases the rate of colon cancer. A diet high in fiber and fruits and vegetables decreases the risk of colon cancer. So does an aspirin a day.[10] (Don't take aspirin for this purpose without checking with your doctor.)

In retrospective studies, colon cancer appears to be more common among women who have had breast, ovarian, or endometrial cancer.[11] This implies a genetic or hormonal link.

Some characteristics of colon cancer suggest that hormones may have an influence. For example, the fact that pregnancy affects bile salt metabolism, which has long been believed to be a factor in the development of colon cancer, has led some researchers to investigate whether pregnancy protects against colon cancer. To date, these studies have been contradictory. Some studies have suggested that the more children a woman has and the earlier she has them, the lower her risk, but others have shown no connection.[12] One study found that both men and women with many children had a lower rate of colon cancer than those with few or none—which suggests that if there is a connection, it's related more to lifestyle than to biology.[13] So the link between hormones and colon cancer is neither consistent nor simple.

Estrogen and Colon Cancer

Observational studies in recent years have found an almost 50 percent lower risk of colon cancer among women on estrogen therapy.[14] The Women's Health Initiative estrogen and progestin study confirmed this connection, demonstrating a 37 percent reduction in cases of colorectal cancer or six fewer cases per ten thousand women per year. While this was good news, it was overwhelmed by the risks of heart disease, stroke, and breast cancer.[15]

Osteoarthritis

Preliminary studies suggest that estrogen therapy may lower the risk of osteoarthritis, a form of arthritis that affects sixteen million Americans, mostly women over age forty-five. A large observational study of 4,366 white women age sixty-five and older showed that women taking estrogen had the lowest incidence of osteoarthritis.[16] More studies need to be done to see if ERT can actually prevent osteoarthritis, but this finding is promising.

THE BAD NEWS

Of course, for every preliminary study of the good that estrogen therapy might do, there's another story about potential harm. The potential damages are an increase in your risk of stroke, ovarian cancer, gallbladder problems, and thromboembolic disease (disease caused by blood clots), and possibly other disorders.

Stroke

Two contradictory factors have led researchers to look at a possible connection between stroke and hormone therapy. The first is that the early formulations of birth control pills increased the rate of stroke in women over thirty who took them. These pills had higher doses of hormones, and some of the risk showed up only in smokers, who are already at risk for stroke. Nonetheless, we do know that high-dose estrogen increases blood clots, so there's been a concern that hormone therapy would increase strokes.

What Is a Stroke?

There are several types of strokes. The most common, the thrombotic stroke, occurs when a clot forms in a narrowed artery and blocks the flow of blood. This is similar to the way a heart attack occurs. An embolic stroke occurs when a clot travels from another area (usually the heart) or a particle of plaque breaks off from a hardened artery (usually the carotid) and is carried through the bloodstream into a narrow vessel, which it blocks. There's a third type of stroke called a hemorrhagic stroke, which happens when a blood vessel breaks and bleeds into the brain. This type has no relationship to estrogen.

Stroke is really a word for any condition in which blood is kept from flowing into an area of the brain normally served by a suddenly blocked or damaged blood vessel. That section of the brain dies, and the area of the body that it controls becomes nonfunctional. If you're lucky, the surrounding areas of the brain compensate for the dead part, and you'll recover some function. But if the area is too big, the stroke can cause significant disability, or even death.

Risk Factors for Stroke

Strokes are more common in older people. They occur in men more frequently than women, and in African Americans more frequently than Caucasians. A family history of stroke increases your risk, as do high blood pressure, heart disease, smoking, obesity, and high levels of red blood cells. A diet high in salt or a sedentary lifestyle can also increase your risk of stroke, by increasing your risk of high blood pressure.

Hormones and Stroke

What does all of this have to do with estrogen? In fact, none of these risk factors appears to have any relationship to estrogen or progesterone. Not surprisingly, the studies that have looked at the risk of stroke in women who have taken hormones postmenopausally have shown mixed results. Some have found a small decrease in the rate of stroke, while others find no effect.[17] A meta-analysis of all of the studies revealed no effect of estrogen on stroke.[18] In 1997, further study showed no decrease in the incidence of stroke in women on estrogen alone or combined with a progestin.[19]

Indeed the HERS study, which randomized women with heart disease to take Premarin and Provera or a placebo, showed no effect.[20] A second randomized controlled study looked at women who had just had a stroke. They were randomized to take estrogen or placebo. After about three years, there was no decrease in either the chance of a second stroke or death from the original stroke; in fact the women randomized to take estrogen had a higher risk of fatal stroke, and their nonfatal strokes were associated with slightly worse neurologic and functional deficits.[21] The Women's Health Initiative finally gave us data based on a large group of healthy women. In this study the women who were randomized to estrogen and progestin had a 41 percent higher risk of stroke than the women on placebo. This translated into eight more strokes per ten thousand women per year.[22]

Ovarian Cancer

Ovarian cancer isn't very common, but it's deadly and therefore very frightening. Ever since the comedian Gilda Radner died from ovarian cancer, women have been especially aware of this potential killer. One in fifty-seven women (1.7 percent) will develop ovarian cancer. Like breast cancer, ovarian cancer is more common among older people. The median age of a woman getting ovarian cancer is fifty-nine.

The major problem with ovarian cancer is that we don't have a good way to detect it early. Because the ovaries are hidden deep in the abdomen, ovarian cancer is often far advanced by the time it's detected. Thus the treatments aren't very effective; only 38 percent of women with the disease live for five years after it's been diagnosed.

It's not clear what causes ovarian cancer, but as you might expect with an organ whose job is to create hormones, there seems to be a hormonal link.

Risk Factors for Ovarian Cancer

Ovarian cancer is most common in women whose families have a history of it. The lifetime probability of ovarian cancer increases from about 1.6 percent in a thirty-five-year-old woman who has no family history of ovarian cancer to about 5 percent if she has one first-degree relative (a mother, sister, or daughter) with it and 7 percent if she has two affected first-degree relatives. Women who have the BRCA 1 gene (see Chapter 7) have a 50 percent risk of ovarian cancer over a lifetime.[23]

The risk for ovarian cancer increases the more you ovulate. So the younger you are when you get your first period and the older you are when you reach menopause, the higher your risk. There have been several observational studies of a possible link between fertility drugs (which increase ovulation) and ovarian cancer. Although there seems to be an increased risk, these studies were too small to allow certainty. Several large studies are now looking into the issue.[24]

Birth control pills, on the other hand, decrease the risk of ovarian cancer, probably because they decrease ovulation. The thirty-five-year-old with two relatives who have ovarian cancer could reduce her risk to about between 3 and 4 percent by taking birth control pills for five to nine years.

One retrospective observational study found that women who had hysterectomies reduced their chances of getting ovarian cancer by about 30 percent.[25] But this study is a bit shaky because among the women who had hysterectomies, it wasn't always clear how many still had one or both ovaries. In some cases, the surgeons had taken out one ovary and left the other. In some cases, part of an ovary was removed. In others, the ovaries were left intact. That could well account for some of the apparent reduction of risk. Some critics of the study have also pointed out that the surgeon doing the hysterectomy had a chance to look at the ovaries and was likely to leave them in only if they looked healthy.

Estrogen and Ovarian Cancer

Large observational studies have suggested that estrogen therapy may actually increase the chance of getting ovarian cancer. One study found that women on estrogen replacement therapy had higher death rates from ovarian cancer.[26] Between 1982 and 1989, the researchers observed 240,073 peri- and postmenopausal women who hadn't had either a hysterectomy or ovarian surgery. In those seven years, 436 women died of ovarian cancer. The incidence was higher in women who took hormones postmenopausally for more than six years; their risk increased by 72 percent. The women who took hormones for a time and then stopped had a 48 percent increase in risk. Another observational study noted that women who took estrogen alone for ten or more years had a 60 percent increased risk of ovarian cancer.[27]

A meta-analysis of all of the studies looking at HRT and ovarian cancer published in 1998 suggested that use of HRT for more than ten years was associated with a 27 percent increased risk in ovarian cancer.[28] Of more concern was a large prospective study of U.S. women which demonstrated that estrogen replacement therapy for more than ten years was associated with an increased risk of ovarian cancer mortality that persisted up to twenty-nine years after cessation of use.[29]

All of these studies are worrisome but do not prove a connection. Again we need randomized controlled data. So far there were no data on this topic in the first report of the Women's Health Initiative, but ovarian cancer is such a comparatively rare disease, it is unlikely that we will have enough women diagnosed with it to answer the question once and for all.

Gallbladder Disease

Estrogen affects the way bile is metabolized, and thus it can lead to gallstones. Because of this, gallbladder disease is more common in women than in men. Observational studies have demonstrated that women on Premarin have two and a half times as many gallbladder operations as other women.[30] The risk is higher if you're currently taking hormones, and it decreases five years after you stop. In the HERS randomized controlled study there was a 38 percent increase in the relative risk for biliary tract surgery in those women on HRT than in those on placebo.[31] Gallbladder removal can now often be done with a laparoscope and so entails less time in the hospital; still, it's an operation and it's not a lot of fun.

Risk factors for gallbladder disease include being overweight, eating a high-fat diet, having a family history of the disease, and high fertility. Generally it's a disease of middle-aged women. When I was in medical school, the teachers said that the risks for gallbladder disease were being female, fat, fertile, and forty.

Thromboembolic Disease

The term *thromboembolic disease* refers to conditions in which the body is more likely to form blood clots. It includes thrombophlebitis (clots in the veins), pulmonary embolus (blood clots that have traveled to the lungs), and clots that form in arteries in the legs. Strokes and heart attacks can also be considered thromboembolic if they're caused by a clot traveling to and then blocking an already narrowed artery.

There are experimental data showing that estrogen increases clotting factors. This appears to be related to dose: the higher the dose of estrogen, the higher the risk of clotting. If you smoke, the risk is even higher. In one study of oral contraceptives, smokers on the pill had 4 times more clotting episodes than women who weren't on the pill, while nonsmokers had only 1.7 times the risk of women who weren't on the pill.[32] Another study of postmenopausal women on estrogen, however, found no effect.[33]

But in October 1996, three studies increased the concern about thromboembolic disease caused by hormone therapy. Each of the three studies showed a two- to fourfold increase in phlebitis in the veins of the legs, whether the women took estrogen alone or combined with a progestin.[34] In addition, there was a doubling of the risk of pulmonary embolus, a potentially fatal condition that occurs when one of the clots travels to the lungs. The increase in phlebitis occurred soon after the women started hormone therapy, which means that if you're prone to phlebitis, you should be careful about taking hormones even for a short time to relieve your symptoms.

One recent finding is that some women have inherited a factor that makes them more prone to clotting, Factor V Leiden mutation. This mutation is found in 4 to 6 percent of the American population and increases the risk for thromboembolic disease by three- to sixfold. It may well be that the women with this propensity comprise a percentage of the ones who get into trouble with clot-promoting drugs such as estrogen.[35] It is certainly reasonable to stay away from estrogen if you have a family history of clotting problems or phlebitis.

In the HERS trial there was a 2.7 times increase in thromboembolic disease in the women with heart disease taking HRT. Another way to put it is that one of every 256 women on HRT had a problem with clots. This was worse in the situations that tend to increase clotting anyway, such as surgery, lower extremity fractures, and cancer. It was also better in women on aspirin or statins, which thin blood and tend to decrease clotting.[36] The Women's Health Initiative also demonstrated an increase in thrombosis with a bit more than doubling, or a 213 percent increase, in pulmonary emboli in the women on estrogen and progestin. This translates into eight more pulmonary emboli per ten thousand women per year. Since these can often be fatal, this is a significant risk. In addition there was a doubling, or a 200 percent increase, in deep-vein thrombosis.[37]

Some clinicians feel that if you have any history of clotting problems such as thrombophlebitis, you shouldn't be on estrogen therapy. Others feel that only repeated episodes of clotting represent a contraindication.

Since this risk occurs immediately, it could be significant in women at risk for thrombosis who want to take short-term HRT for symptom relief.

Fibroids

As we mention in Chapter 3, fibroids tend to shrink with menopause. This would lead you to believe that fibroids will bloom again if you start hormone therapy. And you are probably right. One study showed that much of the bleeding problems of postmenopausal women on estrogen came from submucosal fibroids that were reactivated by the hormones.[38] Another study found an increase in size of fibroids in women using the patch and a progestin, but not in those taking estrogen and a progestin by mouth.[39]

Endometriosis

Endometriosis is a condition in which some of the lining of the uterus travels to other areas, usually in the abdomen. Patches of uterine tissue can end up on the bladder, the large intestine, or the lining of the abdomen. This wouldn't be a problem except for the fact that these patches can respond to your cyclical hormones and bleed or swell, causing pain. The treatment is often with hormone blockers such as Lupron. If that doesn't work, you might need a total hysterectomy and removal of both ovaries. If you are then started on estrogen therapy and there are any patches left over somewhere, you may still have problems.[40] This may be one reason to either forgo hormones or add a progestin to estrogen even though you have had a hysterectomy.

Lupus

Lupus is an autoimmune disease that attacks almost every organ of the body. It can be fatal. It's more common in African-American women than in white women. The Nurses' Health Study has found that women on hormone therapy double their risk of lupus.[41] Other retrospective studies have suggested that the risk of flare is not increased with hormone therapy. However, as we mentioned above, hormones do increase clotting, which can be a problem in women with lupus. A prospective study, SELENA, designed to help clarify whether taking estrogens causes severe flares in lupus, was halted after the WHI showed more risk than benefit of taking HRT.[42]

Other Diseases

Small observational studies have linked estrogen therapy with an increase in risk for several other diseases. One is *asthma,* but the data are so preliminary it's hard to know how to interpret them.[43] Some studies suggest that estrogen therapy can increase the risk of *melanoma,* a severe kind of skin cancer that's often fatal if not caught early. Melanomas are known to be sensitive to hormones, and any woman with a history of melanoma should be cautious about hormone therapy.[44]

In the spring of 1996, a report came out showing that women have a higher death rate from lung cancer than men and have more lung cancers even when they don't smoke.[45] This preliminary study suggested that estrogen therapy could increase the risk of lung cancer, but the finding was not confirmed by the WHI.[46]

None of this means that you shouldn't consider taking hormones to relieve short-term symptoms. But combined with our previous discussions of the risks of heart disease and breast cancer, it should discourage you from long-term use.

TEN

APPROACHES TO SYMPTOM RELIEF

So far we've been talking about what causes perimenopausal and menopausal symptoms, what diseases you're more vulnerable to as you get older, and how hormones affect them. And you've probably been sitting there thinking, "Well, yes—but what am I supposed to do right now?" Preventing life-threatening diseases is ultimately more important to your health than dealing with current symptoms, but it's also less immediate. You can decide next month, next year, or later than that if you want to take steps to prevent osteoporosis or heart disease. But if you're experiencing unpleasant symptoms right now, even next month can be a long time away. You want to know how to get a good night's sleep tonight. You need your hot flashes gone by next week when you have to speak at a convention. You need a solution for vaginal dryness before your two-week vacation in Hawaii.

In chapters 12 to 15 we'll talk in more detail about lifestyle changes, alternative approaches, drugs, and surgery as they relate to a healthy life and to prevention of disease. Chapter 16 will offer suggestions about how you can incorporate all the information in the book into a personalized formula to help you determine what, if anything, you want to do about menopause. But in this chapter and the next, I want to focus on different options for what you're feeling right now. If you're one of the lucky 10 percent of women who have no perimenopausal or menopausal symptoms, you can just skip ahead.

The first step is to let you know that *there are different options*. This is something that is only now being acknowledged. With all the controversy about hormones it is lucky that there are other options and other drugs that work as well or better. And you should know about all of them before you decide what to do—or what not to do.

The second step is to remind you that you may not want, or need, to do anything. I'm always struck by the absurdity of a doctor telling a symptom-free woman with a spry ninety-year-old mother that she must do something to "treat" her menopause or dire things will happen. Your symptoms may be so mild that you'd rather just put up with them for a while and not change your habits or risk your health to control them. For many women, the best way to "manage menopause" is to just go about your life and let it happen.

My goal here is not to give you a prescription but rather to present a menu from which you can choose what seems most reasonable to you. What you choose to do may depend on how much your symptoms are bothering you or how fast you feel you need to relieve them—or on a number of other factors, which we'll discuss in depth in Chapter 16.

Since nothing exists in a vacuum, you'll soon see that some of the options for addressing short-term symptoms also help prevent disease. The exercise you do to help you deal with hot flashes and insomnia may have the "side effect" of adding years to your life. The estrogen you use for vaginal dryness may help prevent osteoporosis. Therefore, you'll probably want to read all of chapters 11 to 16 before you decide on a course of action.

OPTIONS FOR TREATING SYMPTOMS: THREE LEVELS OF APPROACHES

The strategy I'm always most comfortable with is one that starts with the least risky approaches and goes on to riskier approaches only if necessary. Unless you're in an emergency situation, I always think it's worth trying the lowest-level, safest approach first, and moving up to the next level or levels only if that fails. And I find it useful to categorize the levels as (1) lifestyle approaches, (2) alternative approaches, and (3) drugs and surgical approaches.

The first level, lifestyle approaches, makes changes in the way you eat, exercise, or otherwise go about your life. Level 1 involves little or no risk. Some of the interventions at this level are simply common sense: if you have hot flashes, dress in layers. Some are less familiar: eat more tofu to decrease hot flashes. Unlike the lifestyle options, the second-level alternative approaches require you to buy something (such as herbs or supplements) or to go to a practitioner (such as an acupuncturist). But they're still approaches that, if embarked on carefully, involve little or no risk. Interventions at level 3 involve the highest risk and often the highest cost.

Some approaches, or treatments, are specific for a particular symptom, while others are good for many symptoms. I'll discuss each approach in general first, in this chapter, and then discuss their applications for specific symptoms in Chapter 11.

LEVEL 1: LIFESTYLE APPROACHES

Surprisingly, there has been less research on how changing your lifestyle can affect symptoms of perimenopause and menopause than on how it can help prevent disease. Nonetheless, a healthy diet, exercise, and stress reduction are important tools for combating many of the symptoms you may have. Becoming more fit, as we discuss in Chapter 12, will help you feel better in general, and that certainly will affect your short-term symptoms. What you eat is important; as we have discussed in Chapter 2, Japanese women have few menopausal symptoms and no word for hot flashes. This has been attributed to their lifestyle, including a diet that is high in soy, which has estrogenic and antiestrogenic effects. And techniques for reducing stress can lessen or even eliminate some symptoms.

LEVEL 2: ALTERNATIVE APPROACHES

Alternative medicine, including herbal remedies and acupuncture, has been getting increasing attention as we begin to realize that Western medicine may not have all the answers. Still, the United States is behind most of the world in accepting them. Only one third of Americans are now seeking complementary therapies, compared with 50 percent of Europeans and 80 percent of the world's population as a whole.[1] Also, unfortunately, alternative methods can sometimes be more expensive than hormone therapy and other Western medicine, because most insurance plans won't cover them. This is changing, however, and some managed-care plans do cover alternative practitioners.

What you most want to know, of course, is how effective alternative approaches are. Ideally, we should have many solid, long-term scientific studies to turn to. Sadly, we don't. Some alternative remedies have been tested scientifically and some haven't. (Of course, as we have seen, we don't have many scientific studies on hormone therapy, either.) Many Western scientists, with their proprietary attachment to our own allopathic, or traditional Western medical, approach, have ridiculed or ignored alternative approaches. American researchers in this country are starting to remedy this, however. Growing interest in this area has given rise to the recently created Office of Alternative Medicine at the National Institutes of Health. A study done by the North American Menopause Society in 1998 reported that 8 to 10 percent of menopausal women were using some form of dietary supplement. They found that soy protein was the most common (10 percent) followed by herbs (9 percent) and "natural hormones" (8 percent).[2] (In a survey of San Franciscan women who attended a health conference, 48 percent of the women used some form of dietary supplement. But then it was San Francisco....) Soy products were the most popular, along with gingko and black cohosh. Many women combined HRT and dietary supplements.[3] (It is hard to know whether the increase in use of alternatives is due to the different women being surveyed or the fact that their use has become more common over the intervening five years.)

And over the last five years, as with hormone therapy, we have started to replace observational studies with randomized controlled data. Still, as with hormone therapy, we still have lots of questions to answer and lots of areas without data. This doesn't mean that you might not want to try something, even if it isn't proven—you just should know that it isn't. Committed as I am to vigorous scientific research, I don't believe that the comparative lack of studies on most of these alternatives should keep you from considering them, any more than it should keep you from considering hormone therapy. Most of these approaches come out of centuries-old traditions and have worked for millions of people.

Unfortunately, in the eternal quest for easy answers, some people now deify alternative methods as they once deified Western medicine. But just as we're learning to insist on proof that what the M.D.s tell us is really accurate, we need to demand as much proof as possible for every alternative mode. In the same way that we can't say with certainty that the combination of estrogen and progesterone is effective and safe for long-term use, we can't say with certainty that homeopathy or Chinese herbs are effective or safe. People tend to be in one of two camps: either they feel that since these methods haven't been studied for years in a Western laboratory setting, they must be quackery; or they believe that since these methods don't involve drugs in the commonly used sense of the word, they're safe and natural. Neither belief is wholly accurate. As with Western drugs, we need to look at each alternative therapy to see what is known about its long-term safety or efficacy, and how that knowledge has been acquired. In both situations you have to consider all the information available and make your own choices. When you've acquired enough information, or at least understood the limits of the information you have, then you can decide which approach or combination of approaches is best for you.

Indeed, a combination of approaches is often the most useful route to take. An either/or mentality toward conventional and alternative approaches can deprive you of the best solutions for your health issues. My coauthor, who has had severe chronic asthma for many years and was taking large amounts of medication daily, has been working with an acupuncturist since 1995. Now she sees the acupuncturist about once a month and continues to take her medications. But she takes a quarter of the medication she used to take, and her asthma is far better controlled than it was by the drugs alone.

Just as you should shop around until you find a gynecologist or primary care physician whose skill you trust and who you feel shares your philosophy of health and life, you need to find an alternative practitioner who meets your standards. Some forms of medicine (such as Chinese medicine) are associated with philosophical or religious points of view. They are based on a belief that spiritual, emotional, and physical harmony or balance is the key to health. Other traditions, such as homeopathy, have a different theory of treatment. Some disciplines, such as naturopathy, include several differing schools of thought, some of which you may feel more comfortable with than others.

I think we need to approach every practitioner and practice the same way—with a critical and questioning mind. Throughout this book, I've been asking you to question the standard Western approach to menopause as a disease that requires drug treatment, and we need to be equally questioning of, for example, the Chinese theory that menopause is a diminishing of jing energy. By "questioning," I don't mean "dismissing." As you question, you come up with answers, and they aren't always the answers you might have expected before you started asking your questions. The theory behind any practice is important, but it isn't the only thing that matters. You may not believe that menopause is a disease, but you can still get relief from your hot flashes with hormones. Nor do you have to believe in jing energy to get relief from acupuncture or Chinese herbs.

Some practitioners, such as those who practice acupuncture, are licensed by the state. Others, such as herbalists, are not. In Appendix 1, I list various governing or licensing bodies for some of the different disciplines and ways to find an appropriate practitioner. Even if they're not actually licensed, however, all reputable practitioners have some kind of training, and it's worth your while to find out what that training is when you're thinking of working with any health care practitioner. (Like M.D.s, most alternative practitioners are likely to display their accreditation certificates on their walls, so if you're too shy to ask, you can start from there.)

As with Western doctors, making sure practitioners have the appropriate credentials or training is only a first step. You also have to make sure you're comfortable with and confident about their approach to your problem. The relationship between practitioner and patient is one of the most important aspects of any healing tradition. Practitioners of alternative healing are as varied in their personalities and approaches to patients as are medical doctors.

Some of the more relevant alternative approaches for perimenopausal and menopausal symptoms—herbs, biofeedback, acupuncture, and homeopathy—are worth reviewing generally before we get specific.

Herbs

An *herb,* as I'm using the term here, is basically a plant used for a medicinal purpose. In this country, their use is now considered alternative, though in France and Germany 30 to 40 percent of medical doctors use herbal remedies as their primary approach. Many drugs currently used in the United States are based on herbs, but because a plant can't be patented, American pharmaceutical companies sometimes isolate the active ingredient of an herb and then patent that as a drug. In addition, the FDA requires that any herb marketed for a medical purpose must meet the same standards as a drug—an expensive and time-consuming process that many manufacturers don't want to undertake. As a result, most herbs are sold as food supplements rather than as medications. Many Americans thus have the impression that herbal preparations are weak and ineffective. This has been a double-edged sword. People often either dismiss the healing properties of herbs or underrate the potential dangers. (I read a report of digitalis poisoning that occurred because an inexperienced consumer mistakenly used foxglove to make tea.)[4]

In Europe, herbal products can be marketed as drugs only if they have been proven safe and effective. In countries such as Japan and Germany, herbs are better-regulated, dispensed only by licensed pharmacists, and covered by insurance when a doctor has prescribed them. Because all this is lacking in the United States, there is no regulation of herbs, and thus there's a great variation in quality. There have been recent reports of "ginseng tea" with no ginseng. And, as we discuss in Chapter 13, there have been rare but serious problems with contaminated traditional Chinese herbal formulas.

Many factors go into making an herb effective. The plant must be properly identified, and it has to be harvested at the right time of year, when it's most potent. The best way to ensure the quality of any herb you use is to collect and process it yourself. This, of course, requires a certain degree of expertise—not to mention time and energy. If you pick the wrong herb, you may harm instead of help yourself. For those of you who are interested, I recommend Susun Weed's books, which show pictures and give recipes for processing.[5]

If you don't want to grow or collect your own herbs, you can order them by mail or buy them in a local health food store, a Chinese pharmacy, or sometimes even in a local grocery. I suggest that you carefully read the label on any herb you buy; it should include the amount of the active ingredient in each capsule. If you're getting herbs off the shelf rather than through a qualified practitioner, you might be wise to get a recognized brand. Identify the herb you're buying by its botanical name, to avoid confusion.

Another concern is always whether herbs are safe. It's one thing to make sure an herb has the right active ingredient—but can that ingredient do any harm? The increased use of herbs has highlighted some of the potential harm. Kava Kava has recently been shown to cause liver problems and has been withdrawn from the European market. And keep in mind that *natural* does not mean *safe*. You can walk into your local health food store and easily buy herbs capable of causing miscarriage, heavy menstrual bleeding, or worse. Recently a supplement called ephedra was banned in several states when reports surfaced linking it with several fatalities.

This makes it very important for you to know the source of your medications. Not all herbs are equal. As with drugs, some can counteract others. You need to read up on the subject and work with a reliable practitioner who can guide you. I suggest that you seek the advice of an herbalist, a traditional Chinese doctor, or a naturopath—just as you would consult with your doctor before taking a new medication. This is also the best way to ensure that if you take an herbal pill, it will be effective and safe. Further, working with a qualified practitioner gives you the benefit of someone who will take your whole medical history into consideration, just as a principled M.D. will do. And always tell your primary care doctor if you're taking any herbs. Both of your practitioners can help you determine if the herbs could interfere with any other medications you're on or could aggravate any medical condition. For example, some herbs can be dangerous for people with high blood pressure. Other herbs that are relatively safe have been shown to interact with anesthesia. Marie Cargill, an herbalist and acupuncturist from Boston, notes that many Americans have very disturbed, dysfunctional digestive systems, resulting from the birth control pill, antibiotics, or various and sundry other drugs. "This changes the whole flora of your stomach and gastrointestinal tract," she says, adding that since many herbs need to be digested, this change in flora can affect their absorption and make you ill.[6]

Herbs can be taken in a number of forms. Sometimes you prepare them as a tea. This is usually a small amount of herb brewed in hot water for a short time. It's a good way to deliver some herbs but is relatively weak. A very strong tea—a lot of herbs brewed for a long time—is called an infusion. Tinctures or fluid extracts are made by soaking the herb in alcohol. Tinctures are generally the most effective method of taking herbs. Pills are a grab bag—many are good, but others contain so little active herb that they're virtually worthless. Nonetheless, pills are the most popular for Americans—we're accustomed to taking our medications in pill form rather than taking the time to brew or soak them. And we tend to dislike the taste of many herbs, though some, like chamomile, have become fairly popular. If you're taking an herb in capsule form and it appears to be having no effect, consider trying a tincture or tea before abandoning it entirely.

Everyone has an individual reaction to herbs, just as to foods and drugs—and this includes allergic reactions. I suggest that you stick to one herb at a time, or wait until you have used one herb for a period of time before adding a second. Side effects from herbs are usually milder than those from drugs, but they can happen. If you find that an herb is affecting your digestion, stick with it for a few days to see if your body is simply adjusting to it. An herb that really doesn't agree with you may cause nausea, dizziness, stomach pains, diarrhea, headache, or blurred vision, and these effects generally come on quite quickly. If you experience any of these reactions, stop taking the herb immediately—or decrease the dose drastically—and report the reaction to your practitioner or doctor. Trust your body. If something makes you feel worse, don't take it. And never assume that if a little is good, more is better—any more than with Western medication. One aspirin will make your headache go away; twenty will land you in the hospital.

Herbs used specifically for menopausal symptoms are those that appear to have plant hormones or hormone precursors in them, or those that stimulate the formation of these hormones. These herbs are selective estrogen-receptor modulators or SERMs. They have weak estrogenic properties that cause them to act like estrogen in some organs and block estrogen in others. They have the interesting ability to raise a low level of estrogen but to lower a high level (by replacing a strong estrogen with a weaker one). Because of this, they're often known as "balancers." In a premenopausal woman, they decrease estrogen; in a postmenopausal woman, they increase it.

Women who have had breast cancer are often concerned about using herbs that have been termed phytoestrogens. Or better said, phyto-SERMs. Will such herbs cause a recurrence, or a new breast cancer? The answers are really not in yet. The level of estrogenic effect from these plants is very low; their activity is at most only 2 percent as strong as estradiol.[7] All this depends in part on dose, however. The current ubiquitousness of soy isoflavones in many foods may be giving us much higher levels than those found in the average Japanese diet. These high levels may not be as safe as eating one serving of tofu a day. In addition, some of the phyto-SERMs, such as the genestein in soy (see Chapter 12), block tyrosine kinase, an important enzyme for cancer growth, and also block the development of new blood vessels in tumors. These antitumor effects may outweigh any slight estrogenic stimulation they might have. There is also a theory that some phyto-SERMs might act like tamoxifen (a SERM used to treat women with breast cancer), blocking estrogen in the breast and acting like it in other organs. But we're not certain of this. The recent discovery of a second estrogen receptor may bring us better understanding. Until then, I think it is better to use these substances in food in moderation and under the supervision of a trained practitioner.

Biofeedback

Biofeedback uses physical measurements to help you to learn to regulate certain bodily functions. This technique can be helpful for people who have trouble being aware of their bodies. It's also useful in influencing or controlling other symptoms such as headaches, chronic pain, asthma, and muscle disorders. Biofeedback has been effectively used to treat urinary incontinence, which is discussed in Chapter 11.

Acupuncture

In the fall of 1997, the NIH came to the conclusion that acupuncture is an acceptable treatment. This statement must have brought a smile to the faces of the Chinese, who have believed in acupuncture for centuries. Acupuncture, which is the form of Chinese medicine most familiar to Americans, has been used for many of the symptoms of menopause. It's based on the premise that acupuncture needles can be placed in the body so as to affect *ch'i*, the life force energy, which travels through paths known as meridians. Along the meridian are many points. Each meridian and each point are involved in a number of problems—or imbalances. For example, point 6 in the spleen meridian is considered the origin of many menstrual problems, and an acupuncturist treating heavy bleeding would include this point in the needling process. Fibroids, uterine cysts, and migraines also belong in part to this point. The kidney meridian is also involved in most of these type problems.[8]

An acupuncture treatment targets several points along one or more meridians. Today the needles are usually disposable, since patients fear AIDS. Some practitioners prefer to use nondisposable needles, which they sterilize, but you can always insist on disposable needles. Sometimes a needle can sting very slightly, but usually you don't even feel it going in.

Many acupuncturists prefer to work with a combination of acupuncture and Chinese herbs, both of which are components of traditional Chinese medicine. Not all acupuncturists are practitioners of Chinese herbal medicine, but almost all practitioners of Chinese herbal medicine are also acupuncturists. So if you're interested in combining the two—which may be the most effective use of Chinese medicine—it's important to ask if an acupuncturist has studied Chinese herbal medicine when you're seeking out a practitioner.

There are more than thirty American schools and colleges of acupuncture and Chinese medicine. In addition, there is an Accreditation Commission for Acupuncture and Oriental Medicine which approves the schools that train and educate, and the National Commission for the Certification of Acupuncturists, which helps to ensure competence. There are also national associations. To date, acupuncture has been legalized as a form of health care in more than twenty states; several other states are in the process of legalizing it. Some insurers will even pay for acupuncture for certain conditions. In states where acupuncture is licensed and regulated, you can find the names of practitioners by contacting the state department of health or department of licensing. In other states, make sure that an acupuncturist is board certified. This usually means that "Dipl. Ac."—for "diplomate of acupuncture"—appears after the practitioner's name.

Homeopathy

Homeopathy claims that its roots go back to Hippocrates. It was formally organized by Samuel Hahneman in the 1790s. He proposed the law of similars, or "Like cures like." This means that a substance that can produce a set of symptoms in a healthy person can be used in greatly diluted portions to treat someone who suffers from those symptoms. This isn't as odd as it might first sound. It's similar to what we do with vaccines, in which we use a small, modified virus to enable the body to develop immunity to the disease caused by the virus. It's also similar to desensitization methods used in treating allergies.

Underlying this principle is the concept of vital energy, which is similar to *ch'i* in traditional Chinese medicine. When you're healthy, the theory goes, you're in a state of balance and harmony. When the balance is destroyed, symptoms are the body's way of trying to restore it. Therefore you should never simply suppress symptoms. Allopathic (traditional Western) medicine tries to help the body get well by destroying the pathogens that cause a disease, while Chinese medicine seeks to strengthen the body's ability to deal with disease. Homeopathy tries to provoke the body in order to strengthen its vital force so that it can heal itself. Homeopathic practitioners feel that the pharmaceutical approach of Western medicine doesn't strengthen the body but may actually weaken and disrupt it further. There are homeopathic remedies intended for acute and chronic symptoms, as well as some intended to strengthen the constitution so that the symptoms won't recur. A homeopathic practitioner carefully studies the symptoms and then chooses the remedy that will most closely mimic them.

Homeopathy can be helpful with many of the symptoms of menopause, since it's an individualized approach and each woman's symptoms manifest themselves differently. The exact match of remedy and symptom is important for the success of homeopathy. (Since homeopathy focuses on symptoms, it isn't used for prevention.)

There have been some studies and clinical trials of homeopathy, including double-blind prospective studies, and they've found that it often has an effect. (Unfortunately, though, none of the studies looked at the treatment of menopausal symptoms.) Some researchers feel that results achieved with homeopathy are simply the placebo effect—that the amount of the active ingredient is too small to have any real effect. Many doctors are uncomfortable about encouraging homeopathy because they can't explain how it works. I find this prejudice rather ludicrous; there's much in Western medicine that we still don't fully understand but that we use anyway because we know it works—aspirin, for example.

There is currently no licensing in homeopathy. Most practitioners are licensed providers from another discipline, and they include practitioners of other healing arts. Many are M.D.s, chiropractors, naturopaths, acupuncturists, nurses, nurse practitioners, physician's assistants, pharmacists, or dentists. You should ask about the training of any practitioner you're considering working with. Several organizations have tried to establish a certifying exam, but the exams are relatively new, so lack of certification doesn't necessarily mean that a practitioner is no good. (A list of training institutions and certifying groups is given in Appendix 1.)

You'll see many over-the-counter homeopathic remedies at health stores and even supermarkets, but because of the highly individualized nature of the practice, they're probably a waste of money. The one you pick off the shelf may or may not match your symptoms well enough to benefit you. I suggest consulting a trained homeopath first, to direct you to the right remedy. Nevertheless, for your information, we'll point out some of the most commonly used remedies for menopausal symptoms in Chapter 11.

LEVEL 3: DRUGS AND SURGICAL APPROACHES

We can talk all day about the benefits of a healthy lifestyle and the advantages of herbs and other alternative approaches, but there will always be women who need or want to go to the third level of treatment, which includes drugs (hormones and others) and surgical procedures, both major and minor. Side effects are inevitable with this approach, and they run the gamut from mildly irritating to devastating. Often, however, the side effects are well worth the relief or the protection that this approach provides. The risk may well be worthwhile in your individual case, but you need to know exactly what you are risking. I'll discuss all the combinations and permutations of hormonal drugs in Chapter 15.

Remember that these three levels of approaches aren't mutually exclusive. You can use different approaches at different times or combine several at the same time. There are all kinds of possibilities, depending on what you need at any given moment.

ELEVEN

FROM FLASHES TO FUZZY THINKING: WHAT YOU CAN DO RIGHT NOW

Let's look now at the most common short-term perimenopausal symptoms and the ways they can be treated. I'll tell you where we have data and where we don't. If you have a symptom not covered here, you may still want to try one of these approaches by seeing a practitioner who can fashion a treatment just for you.

HOT FLASHES AND NIGHT SWEATS

Hot flashes and night sweats can be extremely variable. You can get them every day for two weeks, and then they're gone for a month or two. This can make it difficult to know whether a treatment is having an effect. It seems to work, you breathe a sigh of relief— and a few weeks later you're flashing again. With hot flashes, you really need a lot of patience. Try something, see what happens, and if it works, stick with it for a while. Then, after a few months or a year, stop what you're doing and see if the flashes are gone for good. In the following lists, the treatments that have been proven in randomized, controlled studies are in **boldface.**

APPROACHES FOR HOT FLASHES

LIFESTYLE: dress in layers, avoid caffeine and alcohol, exercise, eat a diet with soy proteins (one or two servings a day); try meditation, stress reduction, visualization, affirmations

SUPPLEMENTS: vitamin E (800 mg/day); B vitamins; bioflavinoids (250 mg 5 or 6 times a day); herbs such as **black cohosh** or **RemiFemin,** dong quai, fennel, anise, sarsaparilla, wild yam root, motherwort

TREATMENTS: acupuncture, paced respiration, homeopathy

DRUGS: clonidine, Effexor, Paxil, natural progesterone cream, Megace, estrogen therapy or hormone therapy

Lifestyle Changes

Keep It Cool

The first steps in dealing with hot flashes are the obvious ones. Dress in layers so that you can adapt your attire to your temperature at any given time. Keep the temperature of the room cooler. Although this may sound too simple, there's actually scientific evidence that it works. One study found that women who stayed in a cool room (68 degrees F, or 19 degrees C) had significantly fewer and less intense hot flashes than women in a warmer room (86 degrees F, or 31 degrees C).[1] The researcher in this study reported that a woman whose drenching hot flashes woke her up hourly at home slept through the night when she stayed in the cooler laboratory as part of the study.[2] Sleeping in a cooler room has certainly helped me decrease my night sweats.

Exercise

Only two studies, both observational, have looked at whether exercise can affect hot flashes. In one, women who belonged to a fitness club reported less severe hot flashes than those who did not.[3] Unfortunately, this study didn't examine how much physical activity the women performed. The second study found that only 6 percent of physically active women have hot flashes, compared with 25 percent of women who don't exercise regularly.[4] Many woman have suggested that they "walked their way through menopause," and I'd certainly recommend trying exercise—it's got so many benefits to offer and little downside (see Chapter 12). I have taken up running and am sure it helps, but then again maybe I am sweating so much from my running that I don't notice the hot flashes as much.

Pinpoint Your Triggers

Some women can pinpoint what will trigger their flashes—a hot cup of tea, for instance, or a stressful family battle. Some triggers are more avoidable than others. You can forgo tea, but unless your teenager transforms herself into Mother Teresa, family battles may be inescapable.

Nonetheless, you might find it helpful to keep a "hot flash diary" for a few days to help identify your triggers, which you can then avoid. Even if you can't circumvent triggers completely, just knowing ahead of time that a certain situation is likely to cause a flash will help you feel more prepared for it. (Not all flashes have identifiable triggers, unfortunately.) Many women find that eliminating spicy foods, caffeine, and alcohol can reduce their flashes. Drinking lots of cool water can help as well.

Eat Soy Protein

A diet high in soy protein has been suggested as a good way to treat hot flashes. Initially this was based on the observational data suggesting that women in Japan had fewer hot flashes than women in the United States. In addition, it was found that soy contained isoflavones, compounds that can act like estrogens in some organs and block estrogen in others. Since then there have been several randomized controlled studies of soy protein, isoflavones in pill form, and other variations to try and demonstrate a decrease in hot flashes. In fact the data are mixed. A recent randomized controlled double-blind study of an isoflavone supplement was representative of the type of data that are being reported. Both the placebo and the soy group experienced a statistically significant reduction in the number and severity of hot flashes and night sweats. The soy supplement had a more rapid effect, but after twelve weeks the difference between the two groups was not quite statistically significant.[5] Part of the reason that it is so hard to demonstrate a difference for soy over placebo is the fact that placebo works very well for hot flashes. Some of this may be the natural variation in hot flashes that women experience from day to day and week to week and some may just be that placebo works.

The real question about using soy protein for menopausal symptom relief is the question of its safety especially in terms of breast cancer risk. Again the data are mixed. We have test tube data, animal data, and very little women data. Eating soy as food is probably safe as long as it is in moderation (one or two servings a day).[6] On the other hand, we really do not have data on the safety of isoflavone supplements, so I would be careful of their use. It is also important to be aware of all the extra soy isoflavone supplementation that is occurring in other foods, such as cheese and even hot dogs—you may be eating more than you're aware of. (In Chapter 12, I'll discuss more about soy and different ways to add it to your diet.)

Reduce Your Stress

Most women with hot flashes say that stress exacerbates them. It should therefore come as no surprise that reducing stress and using certain behavioral techniques can have an effect on hot flashes.

The best study on this randomly divided women with hot flashes into three groups.[7] The first group received training in paced respiration, the second received training in progressive muscular relaxation, and the third group—the control group—received training in biofeedback. The "paced respiration" group had 40 percent fewer hot flashes over twenty-four hours, compared with the other two groups. Paced respiration is quite easy. You breathe from deep inside your abdomen, slowing down to six times a minute (the normal rate is about ten to fifteen breaths a minute). Try breathing in for five seconds and then breathing out for five seconds, and you'll have the right timing. To get the right feel, put one hand on your abdomen and the other on your chest, and let the hand on the abdomen rise and fall with your breath, making sure that the hand on the chest doesn't rise and fall. Practice this every day for fifteen minutes. Then whenever you feel a flash coming on, slow down your breathing.

In another study, women were randomly assigned to one of three tasks: (1) perform the relaxation response (see Chapter 12) daily for seven weeks, (2) read a book every day for seven weeks, or (3) do nothing. The women practicing relaxation reported a 28 percent drop in the intensity of their flashes and a smaller decrease in the number of flashes compared to the readers.[8] In another study, four women trained in several stress-reduction techniques reduced their hot flashes by 41 to 90 percent.

Though they haven't been studied in any formal way, meditation (see page 250), prayer, visualization, and affirmation (autosuggestion) have been used by many women to reduce symptoms. Visualization, which I'll discuss in more detail in Chapter 12, involves imagining that the changes you want to happen in your body (or in your life) are actually happening. For example, you might imagine that the hot flashes are leaving your body through your feet. Or you can imagine your discomfort metaphorically—as a fire, for example. Then, visualize your immune system as a force attacking it—a firefighter putting out the blaze. In affirmation, or autosuggestion, you use a verbal rather than a visual approach. You tell yourself, over and over, that you're in the state you wish to be in—for example, "My body is cool and comfortable." As we explain later, you shouldn't phrase this negatively; if you say, "I don't have hot flashes," you embed the idea of hot flashes even more in your mind. Also, you want to conceptualize in the present, not the future.

Alternative Approaches to Hot Flashes

Acupuncture

Acupuncture has also proven helpful in treating hot flashes in many women. A randomized controlled study in Sweden compared two groups of women.[9] One group received acupuncture with superficial needles at twelve points (this was as close to a placebo as the investigators could come), and the other received "classical acupuncture" at eight points and electroacupuncture (in which a very low electric current is applied to the needles) at four points. Both groups had less than half their usual number of hot flashes. In the placebo group, flashes increased again during the three months after treatment; in the electroacupuncture groups, the levels remained lower. This suggests that acupuncture may be a good, safe approach to hot flashes.

Vitamin E

Vitamin E has been suggested as a treatment for hot flashes in many popular books. Most of the clinical studies of vitamin E for hot flashes were actually done in the 1940s and were not placebo controlled, but they did find that vitamin E was helpful. The one double-blind placebo-controlled study I could find lumped hot flashes together with eleven other menopausal symptoms. This study compared vitamin E with estrogen and a placebo and found that vitamin E was no more effective than the placebo.[10] Although this study has been used to discredit vitamin E as a treatment for hot flashes, it's hard to draw that conclusion because the study didn't focus on this one symptom. A randomized controlled placebo-based crossover trial was done on vitamin E and placebo and was able to show a statistically significant decrease in hot flashes with vitamin E compared to placebo. The real question was whether it was clinically significant since it came down to one less hot flash a day and most women did not prefer the vitamin E to placebo.[11]

In a survey (not a study) of 438 women, 57 percent who had hot flashes reported taking vitamin E for them and 27 percent felt that it had helped.[12]

In the absence of data, those who suggest taking vitamin E advise that you start at 400 milligrams daily and increase the dose to 800 milligrams if necessary. You should not take more than 1,000 milligrams a day.

The use of vitamin E to treat hot flashes in women with breast cancer is more controversial. Several studies have compared the diets of women with breast cancer to those of women who do not have breast cancer. In the Iowa study of 1996, 34,387 women were followed prospectively, and the results showed no relationship between the consumption of anti-oxidant supplements (vitamins A, C, and E) and breast cancer.[13] The Netherlands Cohort Study 4 of 62,573 women was unable to show a statistically significant role for the intake of vitamins C and E, beta-carotene, retinol, dietary fiber, vegetables, fruit, and potatoes in the etiology of breast cancer.[14] The Nurses' Health Study, European Community Multicentre Study, and Canadian National Breast Cancer Screening Study also did not find any breast cancer protection from vitamin E intake; the Canadian study looked at both supplements and food sources.[15] The Boston group in another study[16] demonstrated that the risk of breast cancer was decreased in the women with the highest intake of vitamin E, but only when it was from food sources. This may well be part of the problem. As with beta-carotene, there may be more than vitamin E involved, and taking supplements may not have the same benefit as getting it from your food. Other studies have looked at the serum levels of vitamin E in women with breast cancer and controls. Most of the studies have found higher levels of serum vitamin E in women with breast cancer.[17] Two have shown decreased levels.[18] Studies have also looked at the levels of vitamin E in the fat (either any fat or breast fat specifically); they have shown lower levels of vitamin E in women with breast cancer.[19] In test tubes and petri dishes, vitamin E seems to have a cytotoxic effect on breast cancer tumor cells, that is, it poisons and kills the cells.[20] Most worrisome in the woman with breast cancer, however, are the data from Mariette Gerber and others that suggest there is some relationship between prognosis and vitamin E levels in the blood.[21] The women with more nodes and more metastatic disease had higher levels of vitamin E in their serum. The question that this study brings up is whether vitamin E acts differently in tumor tissue than in normal tissue. As is obvious from this overview, the data are inconsistent. Inconsistency in science means that our hypothesis may be wrong and that we need to find new explanations for the observations at hand. Until that happens, I feel that women with breast cancer need to know that there are some preliminary data that might suggest that vitamin E isn't totally safe. As is often the case, this means that these women now have to make a decision based on inadequate information. Each woman is going to have to decide for herself whether she wants to continue taking vitamin E until more definitive data are available or stop until we know for sure that it is safe.

Bioflavinoids

Bioflavinoids have an estrogenic effect about 1/50,000 that of estrogen. They've been used to treat hot flashes as well as vaginal dryness, bladder problems, and water retention. The richest source of bioflavinoids is the inner peel of citrus fruits. They're also found in many other sources, from buckwheat greens to bourbon. (I learned about this in a delightful way: one of my patients from Kentucky brought me a bottle of bourbon labeled "Kentucky bioflavinoids.") They're often taken with vitamin C. The dosage is one 250-milligram capsule five or six times a day.

Other supplements, including B vitamins, have been suggested for hot flashes but have not been studied in any formal way.

Herbs

A number of native herbs are commonly recommended by naturopaths and herbalists to treat hot flashes. Each woman reacts individually to herbs, so you may need to try a few under the guidance of an herbalist. Susun Weed told me she found that hormone–rich herbs aggravated her hot flashes and sleeplessness and that the best herbs for her were "cooling" herbs, such as chickweed and elder, and "liver helpers," such as milk thistle and dandelion.[22] Other women I've talked to swear by black cohosh, vitex, or dong quai. One size doesn't fit all, so do your own research and find what works for you.

BLACK COHOSH (*CIMICIFUGA RACEMOSA*)
This plant is a member of the buttercup family and is also known as black snakeroot, bugbane (because its flowers repel insects), and squawroot. The root supplies estrogenic sterols (the building blocks for the steroid hormones such as estrogen, progesterone, and testosterone) and was used for menopausal symptoms by Native Americans and the colonists. It has been studied actively in Germany. In a randomized controlled double-blind study, eighty women were selected to take RemiFemin (a

capsule form of black cohosh), Premarin, or a placebo. After twelve weeks the women who took the herb reduced their menopausal symptoms as much as the women who took Premarin; both did better than the placebo group.[23] Another randomized controlled study compared RemiFemin, estriol, and Premarin plus progestin in women who had just had hysterectomies that included removal of the ovaries. This study found no difference in symptoms among the three groups.[24]

RemiFemin

One tablet contains 1 milligram of 27 deoxyacteine (the active ingredient), and you take two tablets twice a day. It's readily available in health food stores.

A study done at Columbia University looked at RemiFemin, a formulation of black cohosh, in women with breast cancer, many of whom were taking tamoxifen. Although it was not statistically different from placebo in the overall reduction in hot flashes, the severity of the flashes was better on black cohosh.[25] More importantly it showed no estrogenic effects. Since it has also been shown to reduce other menopausal symptoms such as mood swings, night sweats, and occasional sleeplessness, RemiFemin may be a good choice. A recent study reported in the *Journal of Women's Health and Gender-Based Medicine* confirmed that it does not affect hormone levels and so is safe in women with breast cancer.[26] It can be found in most pharmacies. It is important for women trying RemiFemin to realize that it can take as long as six weeks to kick in. So be patient.

Red Clover (Promensil)

Another commonly used herb, red clover contains the daidzein and genistein found in soy as well as formononetin and biochanin. It is marketed for hot flashes and menopausal symptoms. There have been two randomized controlled studies comparing it to placebo and showing no difference.[27] There is concern about its ability to stimulate breast cancer, but this has not been studied. In addition, the action of microorganisms on sweet clover produces dicumarol, which can block blood clotting. Whether this is significant in this product is unknown.

Dong Quai (Angelica sinensis)

This drug (also spelled *dang quai*) is used in the East to equalize high and low levels of estrogen. Dong quai may also have some beneficial cardiovascular effects, especially in dilating coronary blood vessels and preventing spasm in them.

It is probably not a good idea to use the products that combine many herbs. First of all, it is never clear whether combinations are good or harmful. Secondly, some of the ingredients may not be safe. Estroven, for example, a product for menopause, contains kava, about which there are safety concerns.

Other herbs are less well studied and include garden sage and motherwort. If you are interested in trying herbal remedies other than RemiFemin for hot flashes, I recommend that you see an herbalist who can guide you. An herbalist can help you design the right combination for your needs.

Although many Chinese herbs in addition to those listed above have been used for hot flashes, I couldn't find any specific recommendations for them and very little in the way of scientific study. Most traditional Chinese herbs are given in combinations or formulas that have been developed by trial and error over the centuries. They often include dong quai, *gan cao* (*Glycyrrhiza uralensis*, otherwise known as licorice), and *bai shao* and *chi shao* (*Paeonia lactiflora*, or peony). Both licorice and peony raise estrogen levels by increasing the aromatase enzyme that converts testosterone to estrogen.[28] Licorice can also raise levels of cortisol and other adrenal-gland hormones.[29] In large amounts (over 100 grams daily), it can cause low blood potassium and high blood pressure.[30] These effects appear to be exaggerated in women who are taking oral contraceptives.[31] Therefore, if you have heart problems or high blood pressure or are taking hormones, you should avoid licorice. Be sure to tell your doctor if you're trying licorice. (Fortunately, the herb has no relation to the candy, so you don't have to give up your Good & Plenty!)

Chinese herbal formulas used for hot flashes include *liu wei di huang wan* ("quiet contemplative"), which raises estrogen levels in menopausal women, and *xiao yao tang* ("relaxed wanderer"), which lowers the level of estrogen in women with benign breast disease and therefore may be safer if you've had breast cancer.[32]

I suggest that you see a traditional Chinese practitioner to help you sort through these various formulas, make up specific prescriptions for you, and suggest safe places to get other herbs.

Homeopathy

I could find no randomized controlled studies of homeopathic remedies, nor are there any reports of harm. Again, you'll do better to see a practitioner to help you identify the best remedy for you. As you read the following descriptions, you'll realize how individualized these remedies are. Some of the homeopathic remedies recommended for hot flashes are these:

- LACHESIS—especially for flashes that start from the top of your head, are worse just before sleep and immediately upon awakening, and are accompanied by sweating and headaches.

- PULSATILLA—especially for flashes that occur around the face and are accompanied by mood changes and tearfulness.

- AMYL NITRICUM—for burning heat and sweats that attack your whole body.

- BELLADONNA—useful when you experience waves of overwhelming heat, a flushed face, and throbbing.

Drugs for Hot Flashes

Nonhormonal Drugs

Since the last edition of this book there have been several new studies on nonhormonal drugs for hot flashes. These are especially important for women who have been treated for breast cancer and are experiencing chemotherapy-induced menopause. Such women often suffer from severe hot flashes, made even worse by the addition of tamoxifen, and shouldn't take estrogen. (See Chapter 14 for a discussion of the use of estrogen for women who have had breast cancer.) Before describing these drugs, I should point out that many of the studies of hot flashes and drugs (including estrogen as well as nonhormal drugs) have shown a significant placebo effect—in some studies up to a 40 percent reduction in rate and intensity of flashes. That's not to say that hot flashes are all in our heads, but that the mind-body component is real.[33]

The oldest drug used for hot flashes is Bellergal—a combination of belladonna alkaloids, ergotamine (which constricts blood vessels and is commonly used for migraines), and phenobarbital. It has never been quite clear to me whether Bellergal really stops hot flashes or the phenobarbital in it simply makes you stop caring about them. One double-blind study found that women on Bellergal had 60 percent fewer hot flashes than women on placebo.[34] It's still prescribed occasionally today, but the sedative effects of the phenobarbital limit its use somewhat. Bellergal may be worth a try if you're truly suffering over the short haul, but exercise caution: since it contains a barbiturate, it could become addictive.

More recently, researchers have been studying clonidine (Catapres) for hot flashes. This drug was originally used for high blood pressure because it affects the responsiveness of blood vessels (remember that hot flashes cause the blood vessels to dilate) and blocks norepinephrine (which goes up with hot flashes).[35] A double-blind crossover study found that clonidine reduced the number and frequency of hot flashes. (It also found that a placebo decreased hot flashes, although not as much.) Studies of women taking clonidine by mouth, vein, or patch have reported fewer hot flashes, although interestingly, their skin temperature and levels of leutinizing hormone were unchanged.[36] Whether clonidine changed the women's perception of these symptoms or this was a placebo effect was unclear. It was clear, though, that the women felt better.

The side effects of clonidine include dry mouth, nausea, fatigue, headaches, and dizziness. The usual dosage is 0.05 to 0.4 milligram. Unfortunately, you get both the best effect and the worst side effects with the highest dose.

Lofexidene is another nonhormonal drug used for hot flashes. In a double-blind placebo-controlled study, this drug decreased hot flashes by 74 percent with a dose of from 0.1 to 1.6 milligrams.[37] Since lofexidene is the same type of drug as clonidine, it has similar side effects: dry mouth, fatigue, and headaches.

Most interesting have been the recent studies of SSRIs (selective serotonin reuptake inhibitors), antidepressants. Several of these, including venlafaxine (Effexor), paroxetine (Paxil), and fluoxetine (Prozac), have been shown in randomized controlled studies to reduce hot flashes by 40 percent more than placebo. Venlafaxine was tested in women with breast cancer as well as men with hot flashes from treatment of prostate cancer.[38] And the doses needed are about half the dose used for depression.

On my website I am often asked whether SSRIs can cause breast cancer. This is based on one observational study that showed an increase in breast cancer in women who take Paxil.[39] Two other studies, however, showed no such increased risk.[40] These studies were all at the dose used for treating depression rather than the lower dose used over a short period of time to treat hot flashes. At this point, I am quite comfortable recommending them for women who have severe hot flashes and cannot or will not take estrogen. Women who try them need to be warned to talk to their doctors before stopping. These drugs should not be stopped cold turkey.

Hormones and Hot Flashes

Generally speaking, estrogen therapy in any form is good for eliminating or at least decreasing hot flashes and night sweats, as many studies have shown. If you need a reliable result rather quickly (in about two weeks), estrogen is probably your best choice. I think it's important for women who choose estrogen therapy for relief of hot flashes or night sweats not to feel that this is a bad choice. Although WHI indicates there is always a risk, it is very small for short-term use. (But in the case of women who have had or are at risk of breast cancer, we can't say it's safe, so it's wise to be cautious.) In Chapter 15, we discuss the various ways you can take estrogen therapy, any of which will work to quell hot flashes.

Adding progestin to the estrogen doesn't seem to change the response. In fact, estrogen and progestin have each been used individually to treat hot flashes. Megace (or megesterol) is a progestin that has been used to treat breast cancer that has spread. In an effort to find a reasonable alternative to estrogen therapy for women who've had breast cancer, a randomized controlled study was done to see if lower doses of Megace could be used to treat hot flashes.[41] The study, which included ninety-seven women who had had breast cancer and, interestingly, sixty-six men with prostate cancer who developed hot flashes from testosterone-blocking therapy, found that the hot flashes were reduced in frequency and intensity by 21 percent in the group receiving a placebo and by 85 percent in the group receiving megesterol. Although Megace at higher doses has been used to treat women with metastatic disease, its safety at this lower dose in not known.

It is becoming common for gynecologists to use birth control pills to treat hot flashes and menopausal symptoms in women who are still menstruating. Certainly the pill could help hot flashes by balancing out your hormone shifts, although I have been unable to find any studies on this approach. Smokers and women with high blood pressure should not take the pill because of the possible increased risk of stroke. My other concern is the risk of breast cancer. An analysis of the effect of birth control pills on the risk of breast cancer found no increased risk among women age twenty-four to thirty-nine but did find a risk for both younger and older women who were currently taking the pill.[42] Specifically, women age forty-six to fifty-four had just about double the risk of breast cancer. If they stopped the pill, the additional risk disappeared after three years. This would suggest that women should approach this therapy with the same caution as they would menopausal estrogen therapy.

Some of you may decide to take estrogen and stop there. Others may want to combine estrogen with some of the other approaches we've discussed here. One observational study looked at the use of black cohosh by women who were withdrawing from estrogen and testosterone given by injection. It found that women who took black cohosh were able to withdraw more easily with fewer additional shots of drugs.[43] You might want to start on estrogen while increasing the soy in your diet or beginning an exercise plan. Or you could start on estrogen and take it for a year or two and then try tapering off with the help of herbs. Hot flashes are often the reason women start on estrogen, but they shouldn't be the reason for long-term use. Generally, your hot flashes would naturally stop after three and a half years, and at that point you should be able to eliminate estrogen. (In Chapter 15, we'll discuss how to taper off.)

Heavy Bleeding

The symptom that sends many perimenopausal women to the doctor is bleeding. As I mentioned in Chapter 3, neither irregular bleeding nor heavy bleeding is uncommon. But both can be a real nuisance, and heavy bleeding can be frightening. The cause of most heavy bleeding is the decrease in progesterone compared to estrogen in anovulatory cycles. Thus it can happen for a month or two or can continue for longer. A second cause is fibroids, or benign tumors of the uterus. Most of the time, heavy bleeding is transient, a couple of months, and needs no treatment. But if it continues for more than a month or two, or if the bleeding is more than just slightly heavier than usual, you need to check it out (see page 57) as there is always the risk of endometrial cancer.

APPROACHES FOR BLEEDING AND FIBROIDS

LIFESTYLE: exercise

HOMEOPATHIC REMEDIES: lachesis, sepia

SUPPLEMENTS: Chinese herbs, bioflavinoids, flaxseed, vitex, wild yam root (the wild yam root is taken two weeks before you expect your period)

TREATMENTS: **D and C,** acupuncture

DRUGS: natural progesterone, **Provera, Lupron,** ibuprofen

SURGERY: **hysteroscopy, myomectomy, endometrial ablation, hysterectomy**

Lifestyle Changes for Heavy Bleeding

Getting enough iron is important, as is drinking a lot of fluid. This won't end the bleeding, but it will replace these nutrients, which are lost with the blood. Many practitioners support a low-fat diet high in fruits and vegetables; but while good diet is important for many reasons, I haven't found any evidence that it will specifically address bleeding.

Alternative Approaches for Heavy Bleeding

Acupuncture is said to be very effective for erratic bleeding or flooding, although I could find no specific studies in the literature supporting this claim.

I couldn't find any good randomized controlled studies of the use of herbs or homeopathy for bleeding problems, either. Nonetheless, certain herbal and homeopathic remedies are commonly recommended.

Herbs to Treat Heavy Bleeding

The herbs thought to be most helpful for heavy bleeding are those that act like or increase progesterone: vitex, lady's mantle, flaxseed, and wild yam root. As with all approaches, let your health care provider know what you are doing.

VITEX OR CHASTE TREE (*VITEX AGNUS-CASTII*)

I did find one randomized, controlled double-blind study of women with low progesterone levels caused by too much prolactin. Vitex was shown to normalize the cycles and raise levels of progesterone and estrogen.[44] It's therefore worth trying as a way to regulate your periods if you're bleeding too much or too frequently. This is especially helpful if you have high prolactin levels (sometimes manifested by a milky nipple discharge).[45]

Herbalists also consider it good for shrinking fibroids. It's a slow-acting tonic, so you might need to use it daily for two or three months before you feel its effects. Susun Weed recommends twenty drops of the tincture once or twice daily, three capsules of freshly powdered berries daily, or one cup of tea. In general, this should be an amount equivalent to 30 to 40 milligrams. The study cited above reported no side effects, but tell your doctor if you plan to try Vitex.

LADY'S MANTLE (ALCHEMILLA VULGARIS)
Lady's mantle is used in Germany to control bleeding. When taken for one to two weeks before your period, it will prevent flooding. The usual dosage is five to ten drops of the fresh plant tincture three times a day for up to two weeks out of the month. If you've already begun flooding, it can still help, though it will take three to five days to be effective. Let your doctor know.

FLAXSEED (LINUM USITATISSIMUM)
Flaxseed contains prostaglandins that are important for preventing flooding, but be careful—too many can cause cramping, so you'll want to keep your doctor informed. These prostaglandins are made from gamma-linoleic acid (GLA), which can be found in the oil of flaxseed. The oil is good only if it is fresh, so buy it in small quantities, store it in your refrigerator, and use it before it goes rancid. You can take one to three teaspoons of flaxseed oil in the morning or grind the seeds and sprinkle them on your cereal. Or you can soak the seeds overnight and drink the whole thing, seeds and all, for breakfast.

WILD YAM ROOT (DIOSCOREA VILLOSA)
Most commonly prescribed synthetic hormones are made from the wild yam, including all of the estrogens except Premarin, as well as progesterone, progestin, and testosterone. Wild yam contains diosgenin, which is the laboratory precursor of all of these drugs. Unfortunately, there's no evidence that the human body converts diosgenin to hormones. So wild yam or wild yam extract is not the same as natural progesterone, which we'll discuss in Chapter 15. It does, however, have some effects and has been suggested to help balance the cycle. A tincture of twenty to thirty drops taken daily for the two weeks before your period may help decrease bleeding from hormonal imbalance. Tell your doctor if you're thinking of trying this.

There are also herbs you should avoid if you're bleeding heavily or irregularly, such as black cohosh, dong quai, and motherwort, which, as we said earlier, can exacerbate such bleeding.

Homeopathic Remedies for Heavy Bleeding

As with hot flashes, none of these homeopathic remedies has been studied in randomized controlled studies.

Homeopaths recommend lachesis if your blood is dark and thick and if you're experiencing a lot of anger. Sepia is used for heavy, frequent, painful bleeding accompanied by backache or depression. Belladonna is used for flooding with clots; secale is used for flooding without clots. There are many other remedies. They should be tailored to your particular situation by a homeopathic practitioner.

Drugs for Heavy Bleeding

There are available now several approaches to bleeding. Low-dose oral contraceptives in women with no contraindication have been shown to decrease blood loss by 50 percent.[46] The progesterone-releasing IUD is an option in more severe cases of bleeding and may particularly be effective in women with fibroids.[47] Finally, some investigators have advocated the use of ibuprofen (800 milligrams, three times daily for at least five days), which has resulted in a 40 percent reduction of bleeding in women in controlled clinical trials, with or without the presence of uterine fibroids.[48]

Then there are hormones, which are given in an attempt to rebalance the hormonal shifts that often cause the bleeding. Sometimes they work, but at other times they simply intensify the problem, since creating the right balance in a hormonal environment characterized by constant change is extremely difficult.

The first step—after making sure you don't have a fibroid or a polyp—is to try a progestin. This will balance the estrogen and at the end of the cycle will cause your endometrium to slough so that you will get a period. You might be given Provera for three months in an attempt to stabilize the endometrium. Oral micronized progesterone could also be used for this purpose, although it has never been studied. "Natural" progesterone (see Chapter 15) might also be useful, although the amount found in the specially compounded skin creams is variable and there have been no studies on its efficacy.

If some type of progestin or progesterone doesn't seem to control bleeding, your doctor might prescribe Lupron. Lupron inhibits the hormones from the hypothalamus and puts you into a reversible menopause with all the attendant symptoms. It's sometimes used for two to three months to stave off bleeding until scheduled surgery. Although it will usually stop the bleeding, it doesn't work for everyone.

Surgery for Heavy Bleeding

Surgery is the ultimate "breaking and entering." As a surgeon, I know there's a time and a place for it. Nonetheless, the number of unnecessary operations that take place in this country is alarming. Hysterectomy is the most common major nonobstetrical surgical procedure in the United States. This is certainly the choice with the highest risk—not only short-term risk but also, often, long-term consequences. You can stop taking a drug if it turns out to be the wrong choice. You can't put your organs back in if you find you didn't need that hysterectomy.

Actually, however, surgery is more often the cause of menopause than a treatment for its symptoms. One third of the women in this country have had a surgical menopause before age sixty—a hysterectomy that includes removal of the ovaries. In Europe, the proportion is only one seventh. This is probably cultural as well as a reflection of the different medical systems. We don't put up with bleeding for very long in this country whereas in several European countries medicine is socialized and there is less of a profit motive.

Even if surgery is the best option for you, hysterectomy isn't the only possibility, and it may not be the best one. As we've mentioned in Chapter 3, there are several operations used to diagnose and deal with bleeding perimenopausally.

You can have a polyp or a fibroid removed without losing your uterus. A polyp can be removed by a hysteroscope. Fibroids can be removed by a myomectomy. There are two ways a myomectomy can be done. One is to go through the cervix into the uterus if the fibroids are in the inner lining of the uterus (this is more common with bleeding fibroids); the other is to surgically remove the fibroids through an abdominal incision.

Hormonal bleeding that doesn't respond to progestins can sometimes be treated by dilation and curettage (D and C), though this is less common now than it was in the past. As the lining of the uterus is scraped

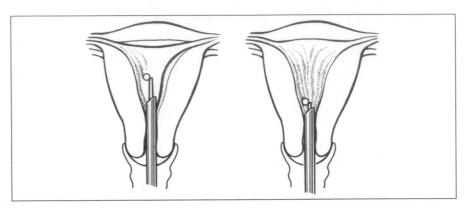

Figure 11.1. Uterine ablation.

away, it gets a chance to start anew. If your hormones are balanced, you won't bleed again.

If a D and C doesn't work and there's no sign of cancer, you can have an endometrial ablation (see Figure 11.1). Using an electrical cautery, the doctor burns and destroys the lining of the uterus. This is more thorough than a D and C, and the uterine lining scars as a result. Fifty percent of women who have this procedure will never have a period again. In 40 percent of women, a few lining cells will be left and they'll have a light period. Ten percent will have no relief. This procedure should be performed only if you don't want to have more children. The scarring and lack of adequate lining cells would make it hard to sustain a pregnancy. A recent prospective study from London followed 525 women for five years after endometrial ablation. For over 85 percent of the women, heavy bleeding was controlled by this simple office procedure; 79 to 87 percent were satisfied with the procedure. For 80 percent of these women, no further surgery was required. Only 9 percent needed a hysterectomy during the five years after the procedure.[49] Of course, no operation is without some complication. This study reported that 2 percent of the women had a perforation of the uterus, which was then sutured. Other problems included infection and bleeding. No one had to undergo an emergency hysterectomy, however.

A newer procedure is being tested in which a balloon is inserted into the uterus and then filled to compress the lining. An electric current is then applied to cauterize the endometrium. If it proves safe and effective, this procedure could be done in the health care provider's office. You may have to do a bit of research to find a practitioner who is trained in these new procedures, but it is well worth it.

Clearly, a hysterectomy should be your last resort for treating bleeding. If your gynecologist suggests it first, you need to get a second opinion. Nonetheless, many women with severe bleeding report that they are happy with having chosen surgery. I'm not antisurgery, after all. I'm just trying to counteract the current overuse of surgery and to encourage you to consider other options.

One survey of women who had had hysterectomies did find that they experienced marked improvement in a range of symptoms, including pelvic pain, urinary symptoms, fatigue, and sexual dysfunction.[50] One of my own patients called me while I was writing this book because she'd been having problems with bleeding. She'd had an endometrial biopsy and then a D and C and had some atypical hyperplasia, which can be a precursor to cancer. She wanted to talk about hormones after surgery. I had a long talk with her about whether she really wanted to have surgery. After exploring all of the options and discussing all of the risks, she told me: "I still think that a hysterectomy is right for me; when I had precancer of the breast I really didn't want a mastectomy and did fine with conservative surgery, but this time I feel that the right thing is to have my uterus out." (She did decide to keep her ovaries, however.) I was happy that she had made an informed decision.

A hysterectomy is major surgery, usually done in a hospital under general anesthesia. Depending on the reason for the hysterectomy, it can

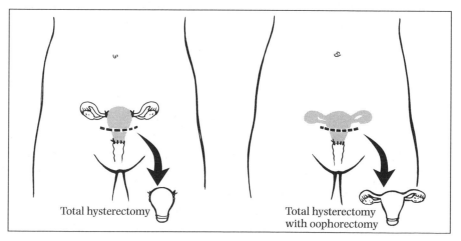

Figure 11.2. Hysterectomy.

sometimes be done through a long flexible tube called a laparoscope (so-called Band-Aid surgery). In a total hysterectomy, the uterus and part of the cervix are removed (see Figure 11.2). Sometimes this can be done through the vagina, a less invasive surgery that spares you an abdominal incision. In a total hysterectomy and bilateral oophorectomy, the uterus, cervix, both ovaries, and both fallopian tubes are removed. The vagina is retained. Sometimes the cervix is also retained, since some women feel that they have better orgasms when they have some cervical stimulation. (Sparing the cervix makes the operation easier from a surgical standpoint. Nonetheless, if you retain your cervix, some uterine tissue may be retained as well, and you should then consider adding a progestin to your estrogen therapy if you elect to take it.) You usually have a catheter in your bladder during surgery, and often postoperatively for a few days.

As I've mentioned, women who have hysterectomies and retain their ovaries typically go through menopause two years earlier than other women. But when the ovaries are removed, the effects are far more dramatic. Few women are clearly told that having their ovaries removed will plunge them into menopause. The effect is so immediate that some doctors put an estrogen patch on the patient while she's still in the operating room. Many women will have severe hot flashes within two hours after surgery. Unfortunately, estrogen therapy doesn't always compensate for the missing hormones. As I said in Chapter 1, the ovary makes more than just estrogen; when you lose your ovaries, you also lose progesterone and some of your testosterone and androstenedione—as well as any other hormone the uterus and ovary might make that we are as yet unaware of. The medical profession is becoming more conscious of this, and as a result we are reappraising the casual removal of ovaries in the course of a hysterectomy. A colleague of mine, the gynecologist Marcie Richardson, says that the only clear-cut reason for a woman to have her ovaries removed is if she has severe endometriosis. Endometriosis can spread to other organs, so you can still have it after your uterus has been removed. Reoperating to treat endometriosis after you have had a hysterectomy can be very difficult because of the scarring.

It's important to know that, contrary to popular belief, you still have some risk of ovarian cancer even if your ovaries are removed. There is ovarian tissue in the areas around the ovary, so that the danger of ovarian cancer, unlike that of uterine cancer, can never be completely eliminated. In one study, twenty-eight women in sixteen high-risk families all had their ovaries removed to prevent ovarian cancer. Three of these women subsequently developed the disease.[51]

Also, removal of the ovaries can produce its own set of problems. Women who undergo surgical menopause have worse symptoms of menopause, and, as I've mentioned, having your ovaries removed, whether or not you take hormone therapy, makes you far more vulnerable to osteoporosis and heart disease than women who experience natural menopause, probably because our bodies need more than just estrogen.

Furthermore, the idea that estrogen therapy can "replace" the work of the lost ovaries is misleading. Our new data on the other hormones produced by the ovary shows that it can't. Women who have their ovaries removed often don't feel normal when only estrogen is "replaced." This may relate to libido, orgasm, and just general well-being. Because of this complaint, the new fad is to add testosterone to the mix (see Chapter 15).

The earlier menopause caused by ordinary hysterectomy (removing only the uterus) suggests that there may be a connection we haven't yet discovered between the uterus and the ovaries—something akin to, or part of, the feedback loop of the brain, hypothalamus, pituitary, and ovary. The uterus may produce a hormone that responds to the ovary. Then, when the uterus is gone and the feedback ends, the ovary realizes it doesn't have any place to drop its eggs, so it stops trying.

The ovaries are highly sensitive to any change in the reproductive environment. One study reported that four out of seven women who had had tubal ligations produced less estrogen afterward. This could be because the operation disrupted the blood supply or because there's a hormonal connection we currently don't know about. This shouldn't be too surprising; as an environment, the body isn't all that different from the planet. If you cut down a rain forest, you affect more than just those trees; the whole ecology changes, causing the death of animals who would normally hide in the trees, the extinction of plants that flourish in the shade, and even damage to the ozone layer that will affect people on the other side of the earth. All environments consist of interwoven elements, and interfering with one affects the others.

As with all operations, complications can result from any form of hysterectomy. The most common is urinary tract infection. Bleeding is also common, and it can necessitate a return to the operating room for further surgery. You may have problems getting your digestive system working again. The wound can get infected. Because the organs are so close together, you may have damage to the bladder, rectum, or ureters (tubes that carry urine from the kidneys to the bladder).

There are also long-term effects. Thirty to 50 percent of women who have hysterectomies suffer from depression, although this is usually minor and short-lived, like postpartum depression. Other women complain of hot flashes, weight gain, and lack of interest in sex. Many women say that their orgasms change. This probably happens because the uterus produces prostacyclin, a hormone that may be involved in orgasm, and, often, because the cervix has been amputated. The cervix has many nerves, and pelvic thrusts, literally, have an impact on it. Finally, many women miss the rhythmic contractions of the uterus that often accompany orgasm.

Most women say it takes almost a year to recover, and some spend many more years tinkering with their hormones in an attempt to feel normal again.

So these operations aren't as benign as they may seem. You can't just pluck out an organ or disturb the body's balance without paying a price.

This isn't to say that no one should ever have a hysterectomy. It may be the only way to stop perimenopausal heavy bleeding or to deal with huge fibroids, after you've tried all the other options. But it's crucial that you know what you're getting into. Since at least one third of the hysterectomies done in this country are unnecessary, it's important that you get a second and even a third opinion before you proceed. There are very few conditions that require an emergency hysterectomy. Bleeding can be temporarily stopped with Lupron long enough for you to consider your options.

VAGINAL DRYNESS

Loss of vaginal lubrication is often described as an automatic result of menopause. As I've said, however, it certainly isn't universal; and it can be transient. Nonetheless, if you're suffering from vaginal dryness, it can have a major impact on your quality of life. Most often, this dryness sneaks up on you. Then on a particularly romantic night you attempt to have intercourse, and it hurts. This tends to make you less eager to try again. And so a cycle begins: less and less sex and more and more dryness. This leads to a significant change in your life; but don't despair—there are a variety of approaches you can use to get things back to normal.

APPROACHES FOR VAGINAL DRYNESS

LIFESTYLE: sexual exercise (masturbation and sexual activity with a partner as often as you like)

LUBRICANTS: Astroglide or others (be sure they're compatible with latex condoms if safe sex is a consideration)

SUPPLEMENTS: homeopathic remedies such as bryonia, lycopodium, and belladonna

TREATMENTS: **Replens**, vitamin E, Chinese herbs, acupuncture

DRUGS: **vaginal estrogen, Estring, Vagifem**

Lifestyle Changes for Vaginal Dryness

The vagina is one organ where use makes a difference. Sexual exercise— either alone or with a partner—will increase your natural lubrication.

Drinking lots of water—eight eight-ounce glasses a day—can help your whole body, including your vagina, stay hydrated. You can drink your water in the form of fruit or vegetable juices or herbal teas. Coffee and alcohol, on the other hand, will dehydrate you. There are some reports that women with vaginal dryness have more urinary tract infections. Of course, infections can occur for other reasons, too. But in any case drinking lots of water can help both problems at once.

There's one study on the use of dietary remedies for vaginal dryness.[52] Women supplemented their usual diet with 45 grams of soy flour (about six tablespoons) and twenty-five grams of flaxseed (about two tablespoons) daily. Researchers monitored the estrogenic effects on vaginal mucus. After six weeks the women had quantifiable estrogenic changes. Their vaginal moisture remained elevated for two weeks after they stopped their diet, but after eight weeks, the women were completely back to their prediet state.

There are lubricants that you can use at the time of intercourse that will make you more slippery. These include K-Y Jelly and Astroglide. One of my friends said that even though she didn't have vaginal dryness, she liked to keep a tube of Astroglide next to her bed because it made her feel so sexy. (Be careful of petroleum jelly, though, because it can break down the latex in a condom, increasing your vulnerability to HIV—the virus that causes AIDS—and other sexually transmitted diseases. Always check with your pharmacist to see whether a lubricant is compatible with latex.)

There are also products you use not specifically at the time of intercourse, but on a regular basis to eliminate vaginal dryness. These include Replens, which, applied vaginally, will cause your vagina to absorb water and become more supple. A randomized controlled study comparing Replens with vaginal estrogen found that they were equal in treating vaginal dryness.[53] You can also open vitamin E capsules and apply the oil daily inside your vagina, for a week or two at first and then once or twice a week.

Alternative Approaches for Vaginal Dryness

Herbalists suggest that taking motherwort tincture or dong quai in any form by mouth for three to seven days generally improves vaginal lubrication. Ginseng, which we'll discuss at length later, can also help.[54] Homeopathic remedies suggested include bryony, lycopodium, and belladonna, but I could find no good studies in support of these recommendations.

Drugs for Vaginal Dryness: Vaginal Estrogen

Vaginal estrogens can be very effective in treating dryness. There are a number of methods currently available for taking estrogen vaginally. In the United States, we have two forms of this, Premarin cream and Estrace (micronized estradiol). Both are very well absorbed and raise your blood levels of estrogen much the same as estrogen pills.

Estriol vaginal cream is available in other countries, but not in the United States. It's very well absorbed, producing blood levels that are about a quarter of those produced by the pill of the same dose.

Some women think that because you apply the cream only inside your vagina, none of it will get into the rest of your body. That isn't the case. Some of the estrogen will always be absorbed in your blood. How much is absorbed depends on which form of estrogen dominates the preparation and how much you use. Estradiol is absorbed very well and raises blood levels. Premarin, which is mostly estrone, isn't as well absorbed.

An example of how well vaginal estrogen can be absorbed was reported in a letter to the *New England Journal of Medicine*. A seventy-year-old man came to his doctor complaining of a lump in his left breast.

The lump was removed and found to be benign. But two months later he was back with a lump on the other side. This time the doctors checked his history before operating. It turned out that his wife had been using vaginal estrogen for eight years. She applied the cream twice a week for vaginal dryness and then two to three times a week as a lubricant right before intercourse—something, as we'll discuss shortly, that she shouldn't have been doing. The poor man had been absorbing this estrogen during intercourse. As soon as his wife stopped using it for lubrication, his breast lump disappeared.[55] Most women who use vaginal cream just want to get rid of vaginal dryness. This requires only a very low dose, which doesn't appear to have dangerous side effects. One study found that you can get effective relief from vaginal dryness with only 0.1 milligram of estrogen per use. For some reason (could it be that they want you to buy more?) the manufacturer's recommended dose is ten to thirty times that: 1.25 to 2.95 milligrams. But you're under no obligation to follow the manufacturer's recommendation. Remember what they used to say in the old Brylcreem commercial—"A little dab'll do ya." This is particularly important for women who have had breast cancer and don't want to risk a recurrence by using large amounts of estrogen. But it's also relevant to anyone who fears the increased risk of breast and endometrial cancer, whether or not she is at particularly high risk for these diseases.

When you start using vaginal cream, you apply a small dab just inside your vagina daily for three to four weeks. Then you can reduce it to once or twice a week. If you apply it daily for more than four to six weeks, it becomes less effective. It's important to remember that this is not a lubricant—use something else to lubricate your vagina right before intercourse (or you could end up with a partner with breast lumps).

Easier and less messy are the new sustained release products, Estring and Vagifem. Estring is a low-dose estrogen ring, marketed as Estring by Upjohn, that's placed in the vagina (much like a diaphragm) for three months at a time. It releases small amounts of estradiol over time. The estrogen dose is so low that it is not absorbed into the rest of the body. This makes it an alternative for women with breast cancer and severe vaginal dryness (atrophy). Newer products such as Vagifem involve using a tablet in the vagina rather than a ring. Both of these products have helped many women. In fact, one woman came up to me after a lecture recently and said, "You saved my marriage!" She had been suffering with vaginal dryness but was reluctant to take estrogen because of a breast cancer diagnosis. She heard me mention Estring and went right home and called her gynecologist to get a prescription. She was delighted with the results, as was her partner.

Estrogen pills or a patch will often help vaginal dryness. They don't always do so, however. At a recent medical meeting, one woman doctor said that I should tell my readers that in her case, Premarin alone was not enough to treat vaginal dryness—she needed the vaginal cream, too. If you're taking Premarin for hot flashes, it may help your dryness, but as my friend says, it may not, and you'll need to add one of the remedies we've discussed. But if you're using the pill or the patch just to address dryness, it's overkill. Most of it goes into your bloodstream and from there into other parts of your body. You're better off with a vaginal approach alone.

INSOMNIA

APPROACHES FOR INSOMNIA

LIFESTYLE: exercise, good sleep habits

SUPPLEMENTS: motherwort, valerian, chamomile, passion flower, **melatonin**

TREATMENTS: Chinese herbs, acupuncture

DRUGS: natural progesterone, **estrogen therapy, hormone therapy**

Lifestyle Changes to Help You Sleep

Insomnia can really mess up your life. As we mentioned in Chapter 3, some insomnia can be caused by night sweats; and when that's the case, you treat the insomnia by treating the night sweats. However, there is probably another component, unrelated to flashing.

Again, some of the lifestyle approaches are obvious. Cut down on caffeine and alcohol. It's ironic that people often use liquor to help them sleep, when it's far more likely to keep them awake or disturb the quality of their sleep. Don't eat a big meal right before bed. Keep your bedroom cool and dark, unless you're among the people who feel insecure in total darkness, in which case you might want to use a small nightlight. Use cotton sheets, which will cause less sweating.

Exercise is good for insomnia, for two reasons. First and most obvious, it makes you more tired. When you exercise, your natural blood levels of melatonin, a hormone that promotes sleep, decrease initially for a few hours. Perhaps this is the reason that exercise is invigorating. Later, your melatonin levels rebound and go up at night. This, in addition to the physical exhaustion, helps you fall asleep.

The relaxation response (see page 250) and meditation practiced regularly during the day have also been found to fight insomnia. And it wouldn't hurt to try visualization and affirmations. Visualize yourself sleeping soundly on your bed—you can even hear yourself snoring if that makes it more vivid. Say to yourself, "I choose to sleep soundly tonight."

Alternative Approaches for Insomnia

Herbalists recommend motherwort to help fight insomnia. Chamomile tea has become a popular treatment for sleeplessness—there's even a specific tea called Sleepytime, which combines chamomile with spearmint and other herbs. Oatstraw and nettle are also used. Valerian *(Valeriana officinalis)* has a reputation as a powerful plant sedative—practitioners recommend that you take twenty to thirty drops just before bedtime to help you sleep. Be careful, though, since valerian can be habit forming, as can any sleeping aid. I could find no studies on its use, but I know of many women who swear by it. Black cohosh (RemiFemin) has also been shown to be good for insomnia.

Drugs for Insomnia

Melatonin, a hormone available as a supplement, has received much attention lately as a "natural" way to combat insomnia. In fact, there are several good randomized studies of the use of melatonin in both men and women. It helped them sleep, it could be differentiated from a placebo, and it didn't cause a hangover.[56]

There are, of course, many soporific drugs and over-the-counter sleeping pills. Most of these are benzodiazepines, such as Valium, Xanax, Dalmane, Halcion, Restoril, and Ambien. They can be lifesavers at certain critical times in your life, but you should never use them for more than two to three weeks. They all have side effects, including loss of memory the next day, confusion, anxiety, and excitability. Use them only under a doctor's supervision.

Surprisingly, estrogen will improve insomnia almost immediately, not only by decreasing hot flashes but also by improving the quality of sleep itself. Micronized progesterone can also help—in fact, sleepiness is one of its side effects. Because of this, doctors recommend that you take it before bedtime.

MOOD SWINGS AND DECREASED LIBIDO

APPROACHES FOR MOOD SWINGS AND DECREASED LIBIDO

LIFESTYLE: exercise, diet, stress reduction, support group

SUPPLEMENTS: motherwort, black cohosh (RemiFemin), dong quai, Bach flower remedies

TREATMENTS: Chinese herbs, acupuncture

DRUGS: **estrogen therapy, hormone therapy, SSRIs such as Prozac, Paxil, Effexor** (these are good for moods and not libido)

Lifestyle Changes for Mood Swings

The lifestyle approach to mood swings really comes from reassessing your life. This is the time to look at how much alcohol and caffeine you consume, along with the rest of your diet. Eating a diet high in fruits and vegetables, incorporating exercise in your life, and reducing your stress can do wonders for smoothing out your moods.

Many women find a support group of perimenopausal women like themselves to be of enormous help. It's a place where you can share your feelings as well as remedies that have been helpful to you.

Meditation and the relaxation response have been shown to help enormously in evening out your moods. Randomized controlled studies have demonstrated the effectiveness of meditation on anxiety and premenstrual syndrome, even if it hasn't been specifically studied for perimenopausal mood swings. Try visualization and affirmations. You can imagine yourself smiling and calm, and you can develop affirmations like, "I am serene and comfortable with myself and my surroundings." As Rodgers and Hammerstein said, "Whistle a happy tune."

Yoga is especially good for women with mood swings.

Alternative Approaches for Mood Swings

Many herbalists recommend oatstraw as a safe herb that helps "nourish the nerves" (see Chapter 13). Garden sage, ginseng, black cohosh, and dong quai can all help with stress. Five to ten drops of motherwort is said to help when you feel your nerves starting to go. Dong quai is used for palpitations. Ginseng has a reputation for helping with libido. Regular use of vitex (chaste tree) for six to thirteen months is said to relieve all symptoms of PMS. These symptoms have not been very well studied, however, and I could find no scientific literature to support these recommendations.

One variant on Western herbs is specifically useful here. The Bach flower remedies are all compounded to soothe various emotional states. Their creator was a Harley Street physician in the 1930s who believed that the only way to really deal with illness was to treat underlying emotional causes. There are nearly forty of these remedies, each one designed for particular symptoms of depression.[57] To my knowledge there have been no studies on the remedies, but there is anecdotal evidence. Both my coauthor and my assistant have found Rescue Remedy, the most powerful of the flower remedies, extremely helpful. The remedies come in small bottles; you either put a drop directly on your tongue, or put four drops in a glass of water and sip it throughout the day. Aside from Rescue Remedy, the following are a few that practitioners suggest may help. The descriptions are quite evocative.

- Wild rose, larch, mustard, gorse, and gentian are said to help relieve apathy, resignation, despondency, self-doubt, and gloom.

- Cherry plum is used to help women who are filled with rage and feel that they are about to do something desperate. The usual dose is one to four drops taken frequently under the tongue.

- Mustard is for deep gloom.

- Aspen mimulus and red chestnut are for fear.

- Rock rose is for easing terror and panic.

- Walnut helps those who are too sensitive.

- Impatiens is good for impatience.

Because the essences are preserved in brandy, you'll get a minuscule amount of alcohol when you take them.

Homeopathic remedies are also used for specific mood problems. As I said earlier, it's much wiser to go to a practitioner and have a specific formula prescribed for you. Here are some common homeopathic remedies that have been suggested for mood problems.

- LACHESIS is used to even out moods.

- SEPIA is for when you want to be alone, have no libido, and are irritable with friends.

- ARUM METALLICUM is for when you're feeling unloved and joyless.

- "CALMS FORTE" is for depression with crying.

- MULIMEN and BELLADONNA are also used for mood problems.

Drugs for Mood Swings

Antidepressants such as Clonipin are often used for mood swings. They're strong drugs, however, and should be used only under the care of a psychopharmacologist, a doctor specializing in this type of drug. SSRIs such as Paxil, Prozac, and Effexor are all useful in getting you over the hump. Tranquilizers such as Valium and Xanax are also helpful. They're habit forming, so you should use them only for short times and only under medical supervision.

Studies have shown that estrogen therapy is not helpful for depression. In fact, estrogen therapy and hormone therapy with estrogen and progestin can actually cause depression. Provera especially has been found to cause depression in some women. If this is the case for you, the best thing to do is to stop taking these drugs. Testosterone has been suggested to treat women with decreased libido. There are no good studies on its efficacy or safety. In some women it will improve libido, and they will feel wonderful; in others, it can cause serious side effects (see Chapter 15).

Libido

APPROACHES FOR DECREASED LIBIDO

LIFESTYLE: exercise, sexual counseling

SUPPLEMENTS: **DHEA,** gingko, **arginine**

DRUGS: testosterone

Lifestyle Changes for Libido

Libido is a very difficult symptom to sort out because it is often the result of multiple factors. Nonetheless, there are definitely women who say: "I loved sex and had a healthy sexual appetite and after menopause it just disappeared and I feel as if that part of me is dead." This, more often than not, is a result of a hysterectomy where the ovaries have been removed. We are not good at replacing everything the ovary makes. It also may be the result of many psychological factors as well. It is helpful for women who are troubled by a severe decrease in libido to try seeing a sexual counselor who can give you exercises to increase the intimacy in your relationship.

Supplements for Libido
DHEA

(Dehydroepiandrostenedione) is a hormone made by the adrenal glands and converted into testosterone. It declines with age in both men and women. In one double-blind randomized study of 280 individuals (men and women between sixty and seventy-nine) over a year, the women over seventy but not the men or younger women reported an improvement in libido, and sexual satisfaction.[58] Side effects can include acne, greasy skin, and increased body hair. DHEA has also been reported to increase heart disease, and its safety regarding breast cancer is not known, though some reports are worrisome.[59]

ARGININE

As part of a proprietary combination therapy (ArginMax) arginine has been reported in a randomized double-blind study of seventy-seven women between the ages of twenty-two and seventy-one to show a 70.6 percent improvement in sexual desire compared to 41.9 percent in the placebo group. Frequency of intercourse and an improved sexual relationship were also reported with the supplement.[60] Although arginine is pretty safe, it should not be used by people with kidney disease.

TESTOSTERONE

This hormone has been suggested to treat women with decreased libido. There are no good studies on its efficacy or safety. In some women, it will improve libido, and they will feel wonderful; in others, it can cause serious side effects (see Chapter 15).

FUZZY THINKING

APPROACHES FOR FUZZY THINKING

LIFESTYLE: physical and mental exercise, diet

SUPPLEMENTS: sage, ginseng, gingko biloba

DRUGS: **estrogen therapy, hormone therapy**

Fuzzy thinking is probably the most disturbing symptom of perimeno-pause. It's known to be transient, but most women can't just stay home from work for a few months or years until their thinking clears up.

Lifestyle Changes to Help Your Thinking

As with the other symptoms, decreasing your use of alcohol and caffeine will help your thinking. So will a good diet high in vegetables and fruits. Increased physical activity seems to decrease the symptoms of aging; by increasing reaction time and blood flow to the brain, exercise may increase cognitive ability as well.

Exercising your brain will also help. My eighty-six-year-old Swiss grandmother decided that she'd memorize the capitals of all of the states as an exercise for her brain and a way to wow her grandchildren. Join a book club, go online, play bridge, or go back to school. As with your vagina, use it or lose it.

Alternative Approaches to Help Thinking: Herbs

According to Susun Weed, sage will help you "gain mental clarity, a strong memory and a calm 'craziness.'"[61] (This sounds like my usual state.)

Ginseng is also said to help memory. It comes in a number of forms: oriental ginseng *(Panax schinseng)*, American ginseng *(Panax quinque-folius)*, tienchi ginseng *(Panax pseudoginseng)*, and Siberian ginseng *(Eleutherococcus senticosus)*. Many of the beneficial effects of ginseng are notable during stress. It will not only help you cope but will also sharpen your mental abilities.

There are more studies in the scientific literature on ginseng than on any other herb I've researched. It's considered by the Chinese to be the king of herbs. It's been found, in good studies, to decrease anxiety in people and to improve a rat's performance under stress.[62]

Quality control can be a problem with ginseng, however. The majority of products in the marketplace contain only a trace of ginsenoside (its active ingredient), and some contain none at all.[63] Look for products that are standardized in terms of their ginsenoside content. According to Michael Murray, author of *The Healing Power of Herbs*, if you get a high-quality ginseng root extract containing 5 percent ginsenosides, your dose should be 200 milligrams.[64] It's best to start at a low dose and gradually increase it. Susun Weed prefers American ginseng, but you can experiment with different varieties. Weed finds that wild panax roots are the most effective. The kind of ginseng that's powdered in capsules or in foil wrappers is considered by most herbalists to be less effective.

Ginseng should not be taken with vitamin C, as it isn't as well absorbed with acid. But ginseng can be enhanced by taking it with vitamin E or flaxseed oil.

The dosage is five to forty drops of fresh root tincture thirteen times daily, or four to eight ounces of dried root infusion or tea daily. Usually, you'll notice an effect within two to three weeks. If you don't mind the taste, you can "chew a root as big as your little finger" daily for six to eight weeks.

One side effect of ginseng is a jittery, overstimulated feeling. It can also cause postmenopausal bleeding; if this happens, you should stop using it. Other side effects include high blood pressure, nervousness, insomnia, skin eruptions, and diarrhea. It can also exacerbate fever and cause euphoria (but that might not be so bad). Women taking panax ginseng may experience breast tenderness.

The Chinese herb ginkgo biloba is supposed to help memory. Although there has been much publicity surrounding this herb, I could find only three studies. One was a randomized controlled study of 48 patients who did find some effect on age-associated memory impairment.[65] A second randomized controlled study of ginkgo for memory enhancement looked at 203 participants who underwent standardized neuropsychological tests and then took ginkgo or placebo for six weeks. The study showed no improvement in performance on standard neuropsychological tests of learning, memory, attention, and concentration.[66] A third randomized controlled study of 309 patients with mild to severe dementia (including Alzheimer's disease) was conducted using Egb 761. This extract of ginkgo biloba is one of the most popular herbal remedies used in Europe to alleviate symptoms associated with a range of thinking disorders and has recently been approved in Germany for the treatment of dementia. In this study it was found to be safe and capable of stabilizing and, in a substantial number of cases, actually improving the cognitive performance and the social function of demented patients for six months to one year. Although modest, the changes induced by ginkgo biloba were objectively measured and were of sufficient magnitude to be recognized by the patients' caregivers.[67]

Drugs to Help Thinking

As we reviewed in Chapter 3, estrogen therapy probably does not sharpen your thinking permanently but may help in times of hormonal fluctuation. However, you don't have to take it forever. I suggest that you take it for two to four years and then taper off and see how your thinking is doing. It may be that your hormones have largely balanced out by that time.

URINARY INCONTINENCE

APPROACHES FOR INCONTINENCE

LIFESTYLE: **Kegel exercises, tampon,** pessary, Femsoft

SUPPLEMENTS: **biofeedback**

TREATMENTS: surgery

DRUGS: **oxybutynin (Ditropan)**

Lifestyle Changes to Deal with Incontinence

The biggest cause of incontinence is surgical; that is, having a hysterectomy.[68] Yet another reason for us to keep all our parts!

Treatment of urinary incontinence depends in part on the problem. If the problem is urgency (always feeling as if you have to go but then producing only a little urine), there are behavioral modifications you can make, such as slowly training yourself to wait longer before emptying your bladder—one hour, then two hours, and then three.

If the problem is stress incontinence (losing urine when you laugh or sneeze), you should first try Kegel exercises to strengthen your bladder. This involves exercising your pubococcygeal (PC—no, that does not mean it's politically correct) muscle. (I told you exercise was good for everything.) To find the muscle, simply stop your flow while urinating: it's the PC muscle that contracts to do this. Practice a few times to get used to the feeling of the muscle. Stop and start your flow at will. Try some stronger and weaker contractions until you can contract the muscle when you're not urinating. You can do your Kegel exercises anytime you wish, while waiting for the bus or walking down the street, sitting at your computer or sitting in traffic. There are several different exercises. One is to contract your PC muscle for three seconds and then release it for three seconds; repeat this six times three times a day; then go to twelve times a day. Second, you can contract your PC muscle strongly for one second and then release it for one second; repeat this twenty times, three times a day. Speed up the contractions until you have a fluttery feeling. Another exercise is to contract the PC muscle for ten full seconds, working at holding the contraction. Repeat this five times three times a day. Once you have your PC toned and can do all of these exercises well, you can do them just once a day. You can also use vaginal weights called Femina cones to enhance Kegels. As with most exercises, it helps to have a routine. Lest you think I am making this up, there are actually randomized controlled studies showing that these exercises can help incontinence.

Studies have shown that drinking one or two eight-ounce glasses of cranberry juice a day can help stave off urinary tract problems.

Alternative Approaches for Incontinence

If you're having trouble actually finding and feeling the PC muscle, you can use biofeedback to help you. (You'll need to go to a specialist for this.) Biofeedback is really the first step for any problems of urinary incontinence, in my opinion.

A pessary is a plastic ring you insert just inside your vagina, above the bone, to help keep the organs in proper alignment and decrease leakage. It's especially helpful if the problem is weak pelvic muscles, which can result after many pregnancies.

There's actually an even simpler tool you can use—one that you probably already have in your medicine chest. One study looked at three groups of women with stress incontinence.[69] One group used pessaries, the second used normal menstrual tampons, and the third used nothing. The women drank three glasses of water and then did aerobics. In this situation, the tampon worked best. You might consider using a tampon to help prevent stress incontinence. (If you do use a tampon, remember to change it every four to six hours to prevent toxic shock syndrome.) A new product called FemSoft takes advantage of this finding. It is a small single-use liquid and silicone device a woman inserts into her urethra before exercise and removes afterward. It has been shown to reduce the leakage of urine 87 percent.[70]

Black cohosh (RemiFemin) is also used for incontinence.

Drugs and Surgery for Incontinence

Although it has been commonly believed that HRT and even local estrogen were good for incontinence and frequent urinary tract infections, observational studies have certainly not borne this out in older women.[71] (In fact, in the HERS trial there was an increase in incontinence and urinary tract infections in the women on HRT versus those who were not.[72]) Finally, surgery is sometimes done for incontinence. In certain specific situations it may be helpful, but I'd use it as a last resort.

OTHER SYMPTOMS

Obviously, we have touched on only the most common symptoms. If you have symptoms I haven't discussed, you should research them in a similar manner. What are the lifestyle approaches to this symptom? What are the alternative approaches? See an herbalist, homeopath, naturopath, or traditional Chinese doctor and get a recommendation. And consider drugs or surgery as well. Be aware of all of the options open to you. Sometimes one practitioner may have a solution that another is not aware of.

Ellen Brown and Lynn Walker, in their book *Breezing Through the Change*, tell the story of a woman who said that her tongue was burning hot.[73] Her doctor said that she'd just have to live with it. She saw an herbalist who suggested a Chinese herbal remedy, and her symptoms went away. On the other hand, Marcie Richardson, the gynecologist I mentioned earlier, told me about a neighbor of hers who had heavy perimenopausal bleeding and thought it was from a fibroid. She wanted to avoid surgery and went to an acupuncturist. He examined her, then told her that her bleeding was coming not from fibroids but from endometriosis, and recommended that she see a surgeon. His diagnosis was correct. She had a hysterectomy and now feels much better. No competent practitioner will try to steer you wrong. Explore all of your options—the menu is vast.

TWELVE

For Prevention: First, Look to Your Lifestyle!

Menopausal symptoms, disrupting though they can be to your life, aren't dangerous. The diseases that you become more vulnerable to as you grow older *are*. Further, the methods you use to avoid these diseases often have their own dangers. And since prevention is a lifetime commitment rather than a short-term remedy, the implications of a preventive treatment are far different from those of a treatment for controlling symptoms.

In chapters 12 through 15, we're going to look at various ways you can try to prevent heart disease, osteoporosis, and other diseases of aging. I'm not going to give you "the" answers, because there aren't any definitive answers. Each of you reading this has her own set of needs, her own concerns, her own symptoms, her own history, her own lifestyle. Each of you will come up with your own approach.

As with our discussion in chapters 10 and 11 about the treatment of symptoms, I've divided the discussion of prevention into three categories and four chapters (12–15): (1) lifestyle changes, (2) alternative treatments, and (3) drugs and hormones. And as with the treatment of symptoms, what you choose to do for one problem may well have implications for others. The exercise you do to help your bones may also help reduce heart disease. The stress-reduction techniques you use to control mood swings will also help your heart.

Remember, none of this is either/or. You may decide to start an exercise program and take calcium. You make your own rules, and you reexamine them as you get more information and your needs change. And you can always choose to "manage" your menopause simply by living with it. Consider chapters 12 to 15 as a survey of all the possible approaches to prevention. Then, the last chapter—Chapter 16—will offer suggestions for incorporating all the information in the book into a personalized formula that you can use to help you determine what, if anything, you want to do.

TAKING STOCK

The least risky and most natural approaches to preventing disease are the same as those for symptoms—lifestyle changes. These changes can have great psychological, as well as physical, benefits. Menopause is, after all, a rite of passage. Your reproductive life is over; you've moved from one stage of your life into another, and you're a bit closer to mortality. This is a good time to take stock of your life—and, pragmatically, to begin to take better care of your body, so that it will continue to serve you well as you grow into old age. The great thing about the kinds of lifestyle changes we're talking about is that while they're helping to avert heart disease and osteoporosis, they're also helping your overall health and sense of well-being—so that something that starts off as an attack on high cholesterol levels can end up giving you an energy and zest for life that you've been missing for years.

If you're going to make lifestyle changes, however, you need to set reasonable goals for yourself and develop a reasonable system for meeting them. Changing a habit or habits isn't as easy as popping a pill every morning. If you smoke two packs of cigarettes a day, eat steak every night, and wash it down with a vodka martini, never exercise, and find the idea of meditating faintly embarrassing, you're not going to turn into a salad-chomping, teetotaling, nonsmoking, transcendentally meditating jock in the next two weeks. Some people need to change slowly. They should focus on just one facet and work on it for a month or two. Make an inventory of your habits, decide which habits you want to change, and then focus on the most important one. Start working on that one first: "For the next two months, I'll work on adding more fruits and vegetables to my diet." Others, like me, prefer to make big changes all at once. (I drive my family crazy when I suddenly make a major dietary change while the refrigerator is still stocked with last week's fad.) Either way, with a strong balance of self-discipline, self-awareness, and patience, you can make as much change as you want.

I recommend that you get a complete physical exam and blood-cholesterol check before you begin any new diet or exercise program. It's good to know what your general health is, and a checkup can help you decide where you want to focus your efforts and perhaps give you a sense of what limits you may need to impose on yourself. If you've been out of shape for years and have a sudden conversion experience, you'll need to know that you can't start running ten miles a day and lifting twenty-pound weights all at once.

DIET

"You are what you eat." We all know what good eating habits are—lots of green leafies and not much cheesecake. (No, cheesecake is not a good way to get calcium.) Most of us, however, are more likely to eat lots of cheesecake and go light on the green leafies.

With menopause, your metabolism begins to change, and some eating habits that haven't visibly affected you before may start to show up in your waistline and your digestive system. Sometimes, you may even find that your tastes are changing. So maybe it's a good time to look at your eating habits and change some of them. They all have an impact on both menopausal symptoms and the diseases of age that you're most likely to be worried about. Keep in mind that fad diets are not the way to do this. Diets that have very high protein and low carbohydrates, for example, may be good for short-term weight loss but are not particularly healthy over the long term.

I personally favor the DASH diet (page 361), which was devised with the support of the National Heart, Lung, and Blood Institute. The reason I like it so much is that it has actually been studied... drum roll, please... and found to work.[1] (Further, studies have been done on different subgroups including men, women, African Americans, and non–African Americans.[2]) Two randomized controlled studies showed the diet to reduce blood pressure across the board.[3] So it worked, not only in people with high blood pressure but in those with normal blood pressure as well. New studies have shown that even high normal blood pressure is a risk factor for heart attacks and strokes, and this diet is likely to prevent these diseases of aging.[4] It can be used for weight loss as well by just reducing the total number of calories. The core of the DASH diet is an eating plan that is low in saturated fat, cholesterol, and total fat and that emphasizes fruits, vegetables, and low-fat dairy foods. It also includes whole-grain products, fish, poultry, and nuts while reducing red meat, sweets, and sugar-containing beverages. For those with high blood pressure, reducing the sodium in this diet will reduce pressure even more. Since 80 percent of people in the United States age fifty or over have a blood pressure of at least 120/80, it is a diet we all should consider adopting.

Salt

When I was in surgical training, I was taught that salt was related to high blood pressure and all hospital food was bland and boring. Then I went to England for a year, where all patients had a salt shaker on their hospital tray. This just shows you the controversies that have raged over salt. Well, in fact, no randomized trial has examined the effect of salt restriction, independent of other components of diet. Many randomized studies show that lower-salt diets, with or without weight reduction, modestly reduce blood pressure and may reduce the need for medication. The more you reduce the amount of salt in your diet, the more you can reduce your blood pressure. And African Americans and people over forty-five have greater reductions in blood pressure with salt reduction than younger people and non–African Americans. Women may also be more sensitive to salt. I know that I have to put only a bit of soy sauce on my food and I will gain two or three pounds, just from the salt causing me to retain water!

Most of the salt in our diets these days comes from processed foods and restaurants. All you have to do is start checking the nutrition labels on your favorite packaged food to be shocked. The upper limit of the current recommendations of the Federal Government's National High Blood Pressure Education Program is 2,400 milligrams a day, or two level teaspoons. Better yet would be a diet with 1,500 milligrams a day of salt. If we could all wean ourselves off salt, we would be healthier, and, who knows, maybe restaurants would start making low-salt entrées.

Watch Your Fats and Cholesterol

A diet low in fat, especially saturated fat, and high in fiber is important for good health. To help prevent heart disease, you also want to maintain your cholesterol at a safe level.

What's a safe level? According to the American Heart Association, blood cholesterol of over 240 milligrams per deciliter (mg/dl) puts you at high risk of heart disease; 200 to 240 mg/dl is borderline. Thus less than 200 mg/dl is what you should aim for (see Chapter 6). Getting your cholesterol down isn't as easy as it may sound. It's not just a matter of avoiding foods with high cholesterol (although you should try to consume less than 300 milligrams a day). We've discovered that the cholesterol you eat probably isn't as dangerous as the cholesterol your own body makes.

Fat affects your cholesterol. Fats in foods come in three main varieties: polyunsaturated, monounsaturated, and saturated. Saturated fats are especially dangerous. Any fats that stay solid at room temperature are highly saturated. Some vegetable fats that don't have any cholesterol are high in saturated fats—such as chocolate and hydrogenated vegetable shortenings (corn oil). Although they don't have cholesterol, they create it—which is actually worse for you. So a diet low in saturated fats is probably more important than a diet low in cholesterol. Among foods high in saturated fat are meats, full-fat milk, eggs, cheese—foods high in animal fat. However, the problem isn't in the fact that something is an animal product; some animal products—skim (nonfat) milk and other nonfat or low-fat dairy products, lean meat, and egg whites—are fine. Even more important than the saturated fats, which we all have heard about, are the less-known trans-fatty acids. These are the "partially hydrogenated vegetable oils" you see on the nutritional labels of many snack foods and packaged baked goods. "Sat-fats" are also high in fast foods, especially when they are fried (and that's where much of the salt is hidden as well). The number of coronary heart disease deaths attributable to trans-fatty acids in the United States is thought to be substantial.[5] Other countries have made a conscious effort to reduce the amount of trans-fatty acids in their foods and often have had dramatic results: the Netherlands have seen a 23 percent decrease in coronary deaths.[6]

Polyunsaturated fats and monounsaturated fats are usually oils. Greeks and Italians are only half as susceptible to heart attacks as Americans, because the traditional Mediterranean diet is low in saturated fats and the fat most commonly used is monounsaturated olive oil. This kind of diet helps lower LDL ("bad") cholesterol and also helps protect against oxygen-free radicals, which help to oxidize the LDL when it's trapped in the artery wall. (Remember that rotting garbage next to the freeway in Chapter 6?)

When you use monounsaturated fats in place of saturated fats, you get a bonus: a lower risk of breast cancer. But don't go overboard. Monounsaturated fats don't lower cholesterol unless they're taking the place of a saturated fat in your diet. Too much fat of any kind is not good for you. Some people have interpreted the data on monounsaturated fats to mean that they should douse everything with olive oil. It doesn't work that way.

What you should do is eat a diet low in fat (I'd aim for no more than 30 percent of your total daily calories from fat, only 7 to 10 percent of it saturated), and when you need to use fat in cooking and salad dressings, use olive oil, canola oil, or peanut oil. And use it sparingly.

You should also avoid oils high in polyunsaturated fats such as corn, safflower, and soybean oils. The structure of the fat helps determine its function. They are omega-6 fatty acids, and there's some evidence that they weaken the immune system and increase the chance of getting cancer. (The fact that soybean oil falls into this category is ironic because, as you'll see shortly, soy itself is one of the best things you can possibly eat.) On the other hand, omega-3 fatty acids—such as those found in salmon, mackerel, tuna, bluefish, Atlantic sardines, herring, whole grains, flaxseed, beans, seaweed products, soy, shellfish, and fish oil— may prevent cancer as well as heart disease.[7] (Omega-3 fatty acids in fish are better absorbed, but those in soy and flaxseed have phyto-SERMs as well.)

In his book *Dr. Dean Ornish's Program for Reversing Heart Disease,* Ornish points out that a very low-fat (10 percent) vegetarian diet combined with exercise and stress reduction not only prevents hardening of the arteries but can even reverse it.[8] The Women's Health Initiative (the randomized controlled study of menopausal women's health) is specifically looking at the effects of a very low-fat diet on heart disease, osteoporosis, colon cancer, and breast cancer. This part of the study is not done yet but should give us some solid information on which to base our recommendations in the future.

Eat More Fiber

Fiber is found in whole grains, beans, fruits, and vegetables. Increasing the fiber in your diet helps you to decrease cholesterol and lower the risk of colon cancer. There are two kinds of fiber—insoluble and soluble. Insoluble fiber increases the bulk of stool your body produces. It helps to move things through at a faster clip, removing toxins in the process. Wheat bran is a major source of insoluble fiber. Notice that I said wheat bran—not refined wheat. The refining process strips away most of the fiber. Look for products that say "100 percent whole wheat."

Soluble fiber helps prevent the absorption of cholesterol by forming a gel in your intestine that traps some of the fat. Oat bran, rice bran, rolled oats, carrots, and guar gum (found in beans) are all soluble forms of fiber. They have been shown to decrease cholesterol and balance your blood sugar.

Aim for thirty to thirty-five grams of total fiber a day. Fiber is best found when a food is in its most natural state. Plenty of whole grains, fruits, and vegetables should do the trick. You get more fiber from eating a grapefruit than from drinking grapefruit juice. But I must caution you: if you start on your fiber kick all at once and load up the first day, expect to have a gaseous time of it. It's better to introduce fiber into your diet gradually so that your intestine has time to become accustomed to the change.

Animal Protein Versus Vegetable Protein

In the last edition of this book I warned about too much animal protein, saying that it increased excretion of calcium. It turns out I was incorrect. In fact protein, both animal and plant, appears to increase bone density. How could this be? The problem turned out to be with the choice of study subjects. The women on a high-protein diet who appeared to show more excretion of calcium in the urine all had very low levels of calcium in their diets to begin with. (It turns out that women with inadequate levels of calcium will have problems with a high-protein diet while those who are taking enough calcium will actually benefit from the high protein. And it doesn't matter which kind of protein it is.[9])

But before you run for the steak and bacon, remember all that fat! It still seems that the best way to get protein without the fat is a largely vegetarian diet (see the DASH diet). At this point in my life I find myself an "almost vegetarian" (I still eat an occasional hamburger). This shift to a plant-based protein diet has happened gradually, as I lost much of my taste for meat. It turns out that for once I may have developed a good habit on my own. (Also, much depends on the kind of vegetarian you are. My coauthor has been a vegetarian for years, but for a long time her protein consisted of cheese, cheese, and more cheese. This solved her moral dilemma and supplied protein, but it was as dangerous for her health as a solid diet of pork chops and steak.)

Soy: The Wonder Food

We spoke earlier (see Chapter 11) about plant selective estrogen receptor modulators, often wrongly termed plant estrogens. From all that you read these days, these appear to be close to a natural wonder drug—able to treat menopausal symptoms while helping to prevent heart disease, osteoporosis, and breast cancer. Remember those Japanese women who had lower rates of breast cancer, heart disease, and osteoporosis? They also had little trouble with hot flashes. One hypothesis is that this is because they eat a lot of soy, which acts as estrogen in some organs and blocks estrogen in others.

The discovery of the estrogenic effect of these plants is fascinating. It began in Western Australia in 1946, when sheep grazing on red clover became infertile.[10] Much to everyone's surprise, studies showed that the clover the sheep had been eating was high in plant estrogens. The estrogenic clover decreased sperm transport in rams and blocked ovulation in ewes.[11] Since then, animals as diverse as cattle, mice, and quail have been found to become infertile from dietary phyto-SERMs. In fact, one researcher, Claude Hughes, has gone so far as to suggest that plant compounds that can act like estrogens are defense substances produced by many plants to decrease the fertility and therefore the population of plant-eating animals.[12] Nature is pretty clever. (But don't be alarmed by these animal studies—soy doesn't cause infertility in humans, so your kids can eat it safely.)

Of course by now you are smart enough to notice that we have an observational study (women in Japan) and a biological rationale (all those animals) but have not proven cause and effect. This is absolutely true. These are studies looking at the key ingredients of soy as well as studies in petri dishes and lab animals, but since we have not done a large randomized controlled study over time, we really can't say what they mean in women.

Having said this, the soybean has a lot going for it. It's a high-quality protein supplying most of the essential amino acids needed by an adult or child. It has more protein and less fat than other beans. It's also a lactose-free, cholesterol-free source of omega-3 fatty acids and calcium (equal to one third the calcium content of milk). These characteristics alone would make it good to eat, and if it has other benefits as well, so much the better.

Soy and Your Heart

One of soy's proven benefits is in lowering cholesterol. As little as twenty-five grams of soy protein a day can lower cholesterol in people with high cholesterol. An article in the *New England Journal of Medicine* reported that an average intake of 47 grams of soy decreased total cholesterol by

9.3 percent, LDL by 12.9 percent, and triglycerides by 10.5 percent. HDL, "good cholesterol," went up a little (2.4 percent), though not a significant amount.[13] In a study of monkeys whose ovaries had been removed, the equivalent of a half cup of tofu a day was enough to produce a dilation of coronary blood vessels similar to that seen with estrogen.[14] Since soy does not cause blood thrombosis, it is probably good for our hearts. Of course, as was the case with estrogen, we need randomized controlled studies to be sure there is a cause and effect (see Chapter 6).[15]

Soy and Your Bones

What about osteoporosis? The isoflavones in soybeans may directly inhibit bone resorption. More important, they seem to help the body hold on to calcium.[16] In a study on rats whose ovaries had been removed, there was also evidence that soy helped increase the intestinal absorption of calcium, much as estrogen does. The rats had higher bone density as a result.[17] A soy-based drug called Ipriflavone is being used in Japan and Italy to treat osteoporosis (see Chapter 14).

Soy and Cancer

If soy helps the heart and bones, it must hurt the breast, right? Not clear. As more research has been done, we have realized how confusing this really is. By now, though, you know that nothing is ever entirely clear. The epidemiological data would suggest that dietary soy helps prevent breast cancer through several different mechanisms, but studies of isoflavones (genistein and daidzein), the "active ingredients," alone with cancer cells in a petri dish show that low levels actually stimulate estrogen-sensitive cells to grow, although high levels block both estrogen-sensitive and estrogen-resistant cancer cells.[18]

In animals fed high soy diets the data are also mixed, with some studies showing a decrease in induced tumors and others showing less effect.[19] In an attempt to answer the question of breast cancer survivors, studies have also looked at whether diets of soy will increase tumor progression in animals. This effect, too, is variable. In women the data are no less clear. Nicholas Petrakis studied pre- and postmenopausal women fed on a diet high in soy for five months. He found an increase in nipple aspirate fluid among premenopausal women and in postmenopausal women only among those on estrogen replacement. What this means is hard to decipher. While women with nipple aspirate fluid have a higher risk of breast cancer in general, this is an association and not cause and effect (as, for example, the sight of people with umbrellas usually suggests rain, but doesn't cause it). On the other hand, two studies have shown a decrease in mammographic density in women taking soy, a sign of decreased breast cancer risk. What is the answer? Well, it's certainly not clear. But most experts in the field feel comfortable letting women with breast cancer eat one or two servings of soy a day and are uncomfortable with isoflavone supplements or soy-fortified foods.

How Should You Eat Soy?

If you want to increase the amount of soy in your diet, how should you do it? Well, all experts agree that you are much better eating food composed of soy than taking isoflavone supplements or even foods supplemented with soy.

You can buy both fresh and frozen soybeans, especially in Asian grocery stores in the summer. Boil the pods for fifteen minutes in salted water and eat them by putting a whole pod in your mouth and drawing it through your teeth to free the beans. In Japanese restaurants this is called edamame. My local grocery store in L.A. actually carries frozen edamame! You can find canned soybeans in Asian markets and dried raw soybeans in health food stores and some supermarkets. Like some other beans, dried soybeans need to be soaked in water overnight and then cooked for three hours. They can be used in soups, casseroles, and salads. Soy sprouts are similar to mung bean sprouts.

Soynuts are made from soybeans. You can buy them in health food stores or make them yourself by soaking the beans for three hours and then roasting them in the oven for about fifteen minutes.

Soymilk is the liquid expressed from soybeans that have been soaked and pureed. You can get it in different flavors, as well as low-fat and nonfat.

Tofu, produced from curdled soymilk, is the most common form of soy. It's available in soft, medium, or firm, and it also comes in a low-fat form. You can use it in soups, stews, and casseroles. You can also puree it to use as a substitute for sour cream, to make mock mayonnaise, and to replace an egg in baking. You can slice and bake it, to use on sandwiches. One of my favorite forms of tofu is tempeh, a combination of fermented soybeans and grains. It has a distinctive taste and is a good substitute for meat in soups, chili, or stir-fry dishes. After marinating in soy sauce, it can be grilled like a burger. It comes in sandwich-sized squares and makes a good, easy lunch food.

Miso is fermented soybean paste, most familiar as a salty soup.

You can use soy flour in some baking. Soy flour is made from soybeans that have been hulled, cracked, and heat treated. It can be mixed with other flours, but it contains no gluten and inhibits rising, so it isn't good on its own for baking.

Unfortunately, soy sauce doesn't have an estrogenic effect, because the genistein is leached out in the processing. Other products that appear not to have much in the way of isoflavones are soybean oil, canned meal-replacement drinks, soy cheese, soy hot dogs, soy bacon, and tofu yogurt. Soy foods made from soy protein concentrate, such as veggie burgers, vary considerably in the amount of isoflavones they have, depending on the processing. Just because a product says "soy," then, doesn't mean that there are isoflavones in it. As with TVP (texturized vegetable protein), studies now taking place should tell us in a few years how valuable some of the processed soy products actually are.

Flaxseed

While soy's claim to fame is genistein, flaxseed has lignans—between seventy-five and eight hundred times more lignans than any other food. And there is growing evidence that this strange-sounding substance may have anticarcinogenic properties as well as the symptom-reducing properties of plant estrogens.[20] It also can lower LDL significantly and may prevent bone loss.[21] And flaxseed contains five times as much omega-3 essential fatty acids and alpha linolenic acid (see page 224) as any other commonly available plant food.[22] One tablespoon of flaxseed is roughly equivalent to one serving of soy. As with soy, you should pass up flax supplements and go for the food itself. As mentioned earlier, you can grind it up in a coffee grinder and sprinkle it on your cereal or soak it overnight and drink the liquid and seeds for breakfast. Preground seeds are available and are just as good but must be refrigerated. Flaxseed oil, which spoils quickly, should also be refrigerated. And note it is not good for frying. Finally, I should warn you that a few people are allergic to flaxseeds. If you try flaxseed and have an allergic reaction, obviously you should stop taking it.

How Much Flaxseed and Soy Should You Eat?

All plant foods—soy, flax, garlic, tomatoes, broccoli, and grains—are good for you. But their biggest benefit comes when they replace some of the foods that are not so good for you, like French fries, cheeseburgers, and cheesecake! One or two servings of soy and two tablespoons of flaxseed a day are safe and good for you. It doesn't pay to go overboard with these foods or any other. Too much of a good thing may not be so good.

On the other hand, many women in the United States find the idea of adding soy and flax to their diets quite daunting. I recommend that you start considering flaxseed and soy as ingredients rather than as endpoints in themselves. As Nina Shandler says, you have to think of tofu the way you think of flour. "It is not how tofu tastes straight out of the package that matters," she writes. "It's what I can do with the stuff."[23] Soy cookbooks are cropping up all over. Shandler's showed me how I could get all of my estrogen needs for the day satisfied by one serving of homemade flaxseed and soynut granola. I've become a convert.

If your family objects to this new cuisine, remind them that soy and flaxseed can help all of them. It helps to prevent prostate cancer and to lower cholesterol in men. Remember too that the immature breast tissue in girls is more sensitive to the carcinogens leading to breast cancer. Soy will help mature that tissue better than anything besides teenage pregnancy—with none of the drastic consequences of that condition.

Bringing your family around may not be easy, of course. My fourteen-year-old keeps making nasty faces at the tofu chocolate pudding I make her. (I'm not giving up, though—I've only gotten up to recipe number 52 in Shandler's cookbook.)

Get Enough Fluid

The axiom has been that you need at least eight glasses of water a day. But this is being reevaluated. Most adults who do not exercise probably do not need that much. What is the harm of drinking so much water? Nothing really except the fact that you will have to make more trips to the bathroom. The best gauge to the amount of water you need is thirst!

There's another benefit to water. One of my more delightful discoveries while doing this book is the fact that calcium can be found in some of the ubiquitous mineral waters so many of us drink these days. (Lest we forget, calcium is a mineral.) I even came across an interesting study funded by a mineral water company demonstrating that mineral water intake in young men can block bone loss.[24] Of course, men don't have a lot of bone loss, so I'm not sure how significant this is. Nevertheless, if you're going to drink mineral water anyway, check the labels. My local supermarket stocks Pellegrino, a naturally sparkling mineral water with 5 percent of your daily requirement of calcium in each eight-ounce glass. (A

German brand called Gerolsteiner Sprudel has 8 percent of the daily requirement.) Mineral water is surely not the main way to get your calcium, but if you're choosing between brands, you may want to drink the one with calcium in it. At least it makes me feel better about drinking mineral water.

Another addition to the guilt-reduction pool is a study showing that among women who drank two or more cups of regular, caffeinated tea (green or black) a day, the rate of cancer of the digestive tract and urinary tract was only 40 to 70 percent of the rate for women who drank tea infrequently.[25] Green tea and black tea are being studied to determine how they act to prevent cancer. This is, of course, observational data, and, so, who knows if it is the tea or the type of woman who drinks tea! Nonetheless, I feel better as I write this with a pot of tea at my elbow! Alcohol, in addition to its other dangers, can dry you out. Sugared drinks provide fluid but create other problems, so use them very sparingly. Low-fat and nonfat milk and soymilk are also excellent ways to get your daily fluid.

Get Enough Calcium

Calcium is very important for women, and it becomes even more important as you grow older. You need it for your heart, bones, and nerves. If you don't consume enough calcium, your body will steal it from your bones. Calcium absorption decreases naturally with age, and even more postmenopausally, so it's important to increase your intake to compensate. Getting enough calcium—along with exercising—will increase your bone density.[26]

Premenopausal women should get at least 1,000 milligrams of calcium a day (more if they're pregnant or nursing). Perimenopausal women should get 1,200 milligrams. Postmenopausal women should get 1,500 milligrams. According to government studies, however, the average woman consumes only 450 milligrams of calcium a day—a third of what she needs if she's perimenopausal, and only a bit more than a fourth of what she needs if she's postmenopausal. This alone could account for the 15 percent decrease in bone mass most women experience between ages fifty and sixty.

The best way to get calcium is in your food. Calcium is found in many foods, especially cheese, yogurt, and milk products. (Remember to use low-fat or nonfat dairy products whenever possible.) You can actually get 25 percent (350 to 400 milligrams) of your daily calcium needs from one cup of yogurt or milk, an ounce of hard cheese, or half a cup of ricotta cheese. Calcium is also found in many green leafy vegetables. One cup of cooked broccoli, kale, turnip greens, or mustard greens contains 200 milligrams of calcium. (Sadly, you won't get much calcium from some otherwise excellent green leafies: spinach, chard, beet greens, parsley, and rhubarb. They contain oxalate, which binds to calcium and makes it harder to absorb.)

Other sources of dietary calcium include shellfish, almonds (one cup equals 304 milligrams), Brazil nuts (eight nuts equal 50 milligrams), tofu made with calcium sulfate (check the label—one ounce equals 36 milligrams), and canned salmon or sardines with the bones (587 milligrams in 8 ounces).

Further, calcium has been added to some foods that don't naturally contain it. Minute Maid orange juice is one of these (one cup of Minute Maid contains 320 milligrams). Herbs such as valerian, nettles, peppermint, oatstraw, sage, raspberry leaf, and many others also contain calcium. I personally like the calcium chocolate chews available in the supermarket and drugstore.

Watch Your Weight

With middle age, your metabolism starts to slow down. You also tend to decrease your activity. Together, these two tendencies lead to the gradual increase in weight you see in most middle-aged people.

In this country, obesity—defined as being at least 20 percent over your healthy weight, or target weight—is a serious health problem. In the Nurses' Health Study, weight gain between ages thirty and fifty was the biggest risk factor for later breast cancer.[27] Certainly heart disease is higher in women who are overweight, as is diabetes. About the only advantage to being heavy is a decrease in hot flashes and osteoporosis. Thus it's important to stabilize your weight at a reasonable level for you.

Avoid Crash Diets

If you're 20 percent over your target weight, start trying to lose weight gradually and sensibly. You all know how to find your target weight: look at one of those horrible charts put out by the insurance companies, the ones where you always need to decide that yes, you are big-boned and deserve to be in the heaviest category. (It's amazing how many "big-boned" women I know!) Bit by bit, decrease the amount of food you eat.

This doesn't mean eating like a rabbit. Perimenopause is not the time for a crash diet. One of the causes of decreased peak bone mass is the continual dieting too many of us engage in for too much of our lives. Also, extreme dieting can lead to anorexia, a serious disorder that is certainly more dangerous than a few extra pounds. On average, you'll need four hundred fewer calories a day to maintain the same weight at age eighty than you do at age fifty. Make what you eat count nutritionally, cutting down on fat and increasing fiber, fruits, vegetables, and soy.

Avoid Late-Night Meals

It's also very important to consider when you eat. Many of you are probably like I used to be: you tend to eat a small breakfast or none at all, grab a quick lunch on the run, and nibble throughout the workday. When you get home, you're starving. So you sit down to a big meal at seven o'clock, finish at eight, and then go to bed an hour or two later. This is the worst way to eat, and there's a fascinating study about this.[28] Some researchers wondered why Japanese sumo wrestlers are so obese, when the Japanese diet is so healthy—low in fat and high in soy. So they interviewed a group of the wrestlers about their eating habits. It turns out that a sumo wrestler's diet is basically no different from that of the average Japanese man, except for two factors. Sumo wrestlers consume more calories and they make sure to eat a big meal just before going to bed. The latter appeared to be the most important factor in their weight gain. For a sumo wrestler, weight gain is useful, but if obesity isn't in your job description, you can help avoid it simply by shifting the timing of your meals.

A less colorful study showed why this happens.[29] Robert Superko at the University of California at Berkeley found that the triglyceride levels are highest four hours after a big meal. If you have that big meal during the day, you can burn up these triglycerides. If your triglycerides peak at two in the morning, however, they are stored as fat.

So you should either eat your larger meals earlier in the day, or just eat a number of small meals instead. This advice is difficult to fit into your lifestyle if you're working and your only time with your family is when you all sit together at the dinner table at seven o'clock at night. Still, you can decrease the amount you eat at the family meal while maintaining the ritual. I now eat a good breakfast and lunch. My biggest problem comes from not eating from 1 P.M. until 7 P.M., at which time I am famished. A healthy snack would help a lot!

Watch Both Fat and Calories

In the old days, the buzzword was *calories*. You were told to avoid any-thing that was high in calories, and that was pretty much all that mat-tered. Then we did a turnaround: it wasn't calories that mattered, it was high fat content. So the current style in dietary circles has been a diet low in protein and fat and high in complex carbohydrates. But as is so often the case, the baby got thrown out with the bathwater. Calories do make a difference—especially if you're overweight. The huge bowls of pasta we're eating aren't making us thinner. Pasta is a good food, but a lot of it has a lot of calories.

Further, since *low-fat* and *fat-free* are our current magic words, it's easy to see them jumping out at you in large letters on the front of the package and to ignore the rest of the label. Look very carefully at every label on the food you buy. Often the reason a low-fat product tastes so good is that it contains a lot of sugar. Sugar isn't fat, but it turns into fat in your body, so replacing fat with sugar isn't really improving anything. Also, beware our other magic word: *natural*. Many products boast that they have *all-natural* ingredients. Remember that sugar is a natural ingredient, and it's in a lot of those "healthy" foods.

A combination of choosing nutrient-rich foods and eating smaller por-tions more often may be a better choice than big platefuls of carbo-hydrates. Nutritionists disagree about that, as they do about some of the other finer points of diet. Everyone agrees, however, that we don't need a high-fat diet and that we all should eat at least five servings of fruits and vegetables a day.

What If You're Too Thin?

There are some women who are too thin. These are the ones who are at risk for osteoporosis and more hot flashes. For some, being underweight is a matter of metabolism alone. Others have dieted most of their lives to get to that weight, and for them the problems are worse. These women might actually consider gaining a few pounds to help them through the menopausal transition. I know this sounds like absolute heresy in our culture, which is obsessed with thinness and in which any weight gain is often accompanied by feelings of guilt and anxiety. We've been told our whole lives that gaining weight is the ultimate sin. But in reality, "middle-age spread" can have some good points. Susun Weed, in her book *Menopausal Years,* actually recommends that premenopausal women who aren't overweight begin to gain slowly—a pound a year—to prepare themselves for perimenopause.[30] She feels that ten "extra" pounds are the "best ally you can have on your menopausal journey." I find her argument persuasive. There may be a reason your body wants to gain weight for menopause: those extra pounds keep bones strong, reduce hot flashes, and cushion you against falls. Still, before you make a beeline for the cream puffs, remember that we're talking about a few pounds. And those extra pounds shouldn't be all fat—they should be a combination of fat, muscle, and bone.

The key here is that good old-fashioned virtue: moderation. It's important to avoid both obesity and fanatical weight loss. We spend much too much time on dieting and weight loss and not enough on good nutrition and a healthy lifestyle.

So how do you gain a little weight but not too much? If you're among the rare people who don't put on weight with middle age, add a bit more complex carbohydrate to your diet. You can have a bigger plateful of pasta than the rest of us or add an extra slice or two of bread.

Diet and Cancer Prevention

Eating foods high in antioxidants, beta-carotene, and retinoids will help you lower your risk of cancer. In addition to the leafy greens, go for the fruits and vegetables that are orange and yellow; they're highest in antioxidants. A low-fat diet high in soy protein, fresh fruits and vegetables, and antioxidants can help prevent breast cancer, colon cancer, and heart disease. This is important to all women, but it is especially important if you're on hormone therapy, which increases risk of breast cancer. A recent study in the *Journal of the National Cancer Institute* showed that women who eat a lot of fruits and vegetables (more than five servings a day) have less breast cancer than those who eat less than three servings a day.[31] (Interestingly, some studies have shown that supplements of beta-carotene, one of the antioxidants, don't have the same effect as the real thing.[32]) In other words, do what your mother told you—eat your vegetables, especially your broccoli and carrots.

Developing Good Eating Habits
Keep a Food Diary
It usually takes work to develop good eating habits—most of us are too used to a high-fat, low-fiber diet to switch smoothly into a healthier

mode. The best way to start on a diet like this is to keep a "food diary." Every day for a week, write down everything you eat. This means everything—not just what you eat at meals. The snacks and the little "extras" are usually what do you in. I suggest a week because one week is usually long enough to include all of the circumstances you're usually up against—including a weekend dinner in a restaurant or fast food at a ball game.

This dietary diary is for your eyes only, so you can be brutally honest. This kind of honesty can be very revealing: one well-known nutrition researcher told me that once he started keeping a food diary, he stopped eating his beloved chocolate eclairs. When you look at your own diary after a week and see everything you've been consuming, you're likely to be surprised—and maybe even appalled. When I started training for the marathon (more about that later), my coach had me keep a food diary. I find that the mere fact that I have to write things down (I actually keep it in my computer) makes me think twice about many foods.

Once you've written your food diary, use one of the many books or computer programs available to calculate exactly how many calories you're getting from fat, protein, and carbohydrates. (To calculate calories, for every gram of fat multiply by nine; for every gram of protein and carbohydrate, multiply by four.) Then calculate what percentage of your diet is fat, carbohydrate, and protein. You might want to keep this up for longer than a week. As a result of my food diary, I now know that when I travel my fat percentage soars, as does the sodium in my diet. I can keep the calories and protein stable, but the loss of control that comes from eating in restaurants does me in. If you eat out only occasionally, then it is fine to splurge... but when I am on the road, I eat out all the time and sabotage all my good habits.

The average American diet is 30 to 40 percent fat, when it should be 20 percent. For a diet with two thousand calories, this would be about 60 grams of fat. Once you see where you're starting from, it becomes easier to see how to get to this goal. Remember, don't get too low. You need those essential fatty acids in nuts, flax, and fish. In the Nurses' Health Study and the Iowa Women's Health Study they found that the more nuts a woman ate, the less likely she was to develop heart disease.[33] We provide several good sources of recipes and menus in Appendix 3. Although these can be helpful, they often don't take your individual circumstances into consideration, so you'll probably want to spend a little time tailoring them to your needs.

Other Techniques for Limiting Fat

A food diary is not the only way to develop better eating habits. If counting fat calories seems too obsessive to you, you can reduce fat to a certain degree simply by watching, and controlling, what you eat. Decrease the amount of meat or poultry you eat to one serving a week. (It's important to remember that a "portion" or "serving" is three ounces, or a piece the size of a pack of cards. Most Americans think a serving is two or three times that large.) When you do eat red meat or poultry, trim off the fat or skin. Eat fish and shellfish once or twice a week—most seafood is high in polyunsaturated omega-3 fatty acids, which help prevent heart disease. If you're a vegetarian, or an observant Jew who doesn't eat shellfish, you can increase your soy and nuts. Choose low-fat or no-fat dairy products. When you have to use oils or fats in cooking, use monounsaturated forms such as olive oil and peanut oil. Stay away from fast foods and processed meats.

As you decrease fat and animal protein, increase fresh fruits, vegetables, and plant protein—especially soy. A diet high in a variety of fresh fruits and vegetables will supply many of the vital vitamins and minerals women over forty need. (Sometimes you may want to take vitamin and mineral supplements; we'll discuss those in the next chapter.) Take a look at the DASH diet in Appendix 5 for a good guide.

ALCOHOL IN MODERATION

Sometimes improving your health is a matter of subtraction rather than addition. Alcohol is a ritualistic part of many of our lives, but many of us overuse it.

Moderate use of alcohol has mixed effects. One drink a day—a four-ounce glass of wine, a twelve-ounce can of beer, or one ounce of hard liquor—may help to decrease heart disease, Alzheimer's, and osteoporosis. Alcohol has bioflavinoids and phytoestrogens in it, so it presumably raises your estrogen levels. Not surprisingly, then, one drink a day will also increase your risk of breast and endometrial cancer—even four drinks a week increases the risk of breast cancer. And heavy drinking is always bad for your health, whether or not you're an alcoholic.

Unfortunately, alcohol is worse for women than for men. A woman's body doesn't metabolize alcohol as well as a man's, and so the damage to the liver per drink is higher for a woman. Problems from drinking include pancreatitis; cirrhosis of the liver; cancer of the esophagus, head, and neck; and cancer of the liver. New studies have shown that the combination of estrogen replacement therapy and alcohol can be worse than either alone. The women who took HRT had a 300 percent increase in their blood levels of estrogen after an alcoholic drink. So you may have to choose your poison.[34]

What constitutes "heavy drinking"? Less than you might think: you don't have to be falling-down drunk to be a heavy drinker. For a woman, more than two drinks a day is "heavy." If you find that you're drinking to that extent, you need to reevaluate the role alcohol is playing in your life. Are you using it to reduce stress? Then maybe you should try instead one of the techniques discussed later in this chapter. Are you using it to help you sleep? Alcohol can actually inhibit restful sleep. Try daily exercise or another method for improving sleep. One simple aid is to make sure you do something relaxing to wind down at the end of the day—watching light TV or reading a light novel, for example. If you need some kind of drink at night, make it chamomile tea, or the old standby warm milk. You could even make that warm soymilk. Is alcohol helping you tolerate a bad relationship? Then maybe counseling would be more effective.

I must admit this is an area I have difficulty with. I come from a large Irish Catholic family, and alcohol has always been part of my life. For me it's the easiest way to reduce stress, and I have to be continually on guard against slipping into the habit of drinking a glass or two of wine every night.

Unless you have a drinking problem, you don't need to give up alcohol completely. But it's really wise to keep it at no more than three drinks a week. This won't increase your risk of breast cancer, and it can still help lower your risk of heart disease. Save your drinking for specific times, and then savor it. Have a glass of wine with a special dinner. Celebrate with champagne when the occasion calls for it. Have a beer at the baseball game. And leave alcohol alone the rest of the time. If you don't drink, don't feel you have to start.

QUIT SMOKING

Why You Should Stop Smoking

There's no question that smoking is the single most dangerous thing you can do in terms of your overall health. Smoking increases infertility and the rate of miscarriage. It causes premature menopause (and wrinkles)—and that's the least of it.

Smoking is an enormous risk factor for heart disease. Among the women in the Nurses' Health Study, one of the most comprehensive studies ever done, it was the greatest risk factor.[35] If you quit smoking, your risk of heart disease will be reduced by 14 percent within two years, and after ten to fourteen years your risk is scarcely higher than that of people who never smoked.

Smoking also dramatically increases your risk of osteoporosis. In addition, it causes emphysema, cervical cancer, lung cancer, bladder cancer, cancer of the nose and mouth and throat, and cancer of the esophagus.

In some ways smoking is even worse for women than it is for men. A woman who smokes the same amount as a man is more likely than he is to get lung cancer. If you're on estrogen replacement therapy, you increase this risk even more.

How to Stop Smoking

Studies have shown that the most common reason women give for not quitting smoking is their fear of gaining weight. Smoking also serves many women as a major way to reduce stress. If you want to quit, you need to take this into consideration. It's important that you develop other methods of losing weight and reducing stress—such as exercise—before you try to quit smoking. In addition, give yourself permission to gain an extra eight or ten pounds, at least temporarily. If you deprive yourself of too much all at once, you're much more likely to go back to smoking.

Giving up smoking is never easy. You're giving up both a physical and an emotional addiction. It's a loss, and, as with any loss, you need time to grieve. You may be able to do it on your own, but you may also need some help. Look into comprehensive smoking-cessation programs to help you succeed. Seek out various methods. There are lots of them out there—nicotine gum and patches, support groups, hypnosis, acupuncture. And don't give up trying to quit if it doesn't work the first time. Try another approach. It often takes several tries before you can really quit.

I firmly believe you have to start by deciding in your heart of hearts that you want to quit. Then, you need to set a date. Next, you need to mobilize your friends and family to help you.

It can be done. I started to smoke heavily when I was twenty, and I kept it up for ten years. I decided to quit at age thirty because I felt I was then an adult. Besides, as a doctor I'd seen some of the horrors caused by smoking. I didn't succeed when I tried to quit on my own, however. So I made an appointment to see a hypnotist. On the way up to his office I smoked three cigarettes. They were my last. The most important thing the hypnotist said to me was that I would no longer think of myself as a smoker. It was hard, but the hypnosis, and my own determination, got me through it. I haven't had a cigarette in more than twenty years—and I no longer even crave cigarettes.

Of all the changes discussed in this chapter, quitting smoking will have the most profound effect on your health. If you're a smoker and you're concerned enough with preventing disease to read this book, you can quit. Your life is worth it.

EXERCISE

If there were a drug that had as many good effects as exercise has, we'd all be buying stock in it and getting rich. Yet most people don't take advantage of exercise. It's free, it's familiar, and it's not a chemical. So we don't trust this simple thing nature has made accessible to us.

Exercise and Your Heart

Exercise can affect almost all aspects of your life. Regular exercise will decrease your risk of heart disease by raising the level of good HDL and lowering bad LDL. Sedentary women are three times more likely to die of heart attacks than women who exercise regularly. If you're at risk for heart disease, you can reduce your chance of dying of a heart attack 50 percent by becoming physically fit. Studies have also shown that regular moderate exercise is as good as medication for lowering high blood pressure.

Exercise and Cancer

Exercise can also lower your risk of breast cancer. Premenopausal women who exercise 3.8 hours a week will decrease their risk of breast cancer by 70 percent if they have had full-term pregnancies and by 30 percent if they haven't.[36] Exercise may offer this protection in part because it lengthens your menstrual cycle, thus decreasing the overall amount of estrogen and progesterone your body is exposed to. Over time, this can add up to an enormous decrease, so it behooves every premenopausal woman to get onto a regular exercise program.

Studies have shown that there is a lowering of risk in postmenopausal women as well, although not quite as much (30 percent). It is never too late to start exercising.[37]

In addition, physically active women have less ovarian, uterine, and colon cancer than sedentary women.

Exercise and Your Bones

Women who have done a lot of muscle strengthening have stronger bones. This may have to do with increased estrogen production, especially since, as we saw in Chapter 11, women who exercise also have fewer symptoms of menopause. Until recently, it seemed that the only way to increase your own estrogen production after menopause was to gain weight. I always thought this was unfair. It *is* unfair—and what's more, it's untrue. My research has shown me that there are other possibilities. Like fat, muscle contains an enzyme called aromatase, which converts testosterone and androstenedione into estrone (a form of estrogen).

Researchers in St. Louis found that in less than twenty-two months women who exercised at least three times a week increased their bone density by 5.2 percent, while sedentary women actually lost 1.2 percent of their bone.[38] After twenty-two months, the exercisers in the study had increased their bone mass by 6.1 percent—which is comparable to the changes seen with a medication such as estrogen or Fosamax. A recently reported randomized controlled study from Canada found that subjects who exercised for sixty minutes three times a week for a year stabilized their bone mass, improved their cardiorespiratory endurance, and had a better overall sense of well-being than those in the control group.[39] However, as with estrogen supplements, as soon as the women stopped exercising for a week or more, their bone density began to decline. Bone will grow again when you start exercising again, so it's important to choose an exercise program you can stick with—as we discuss later in this chapter.

Combining exercise with enough vitamin D and calcium (see Chapter 13) can decrease your risk of fractures by 30 percent. In addition, by making you stronger and improving your balance, it will decrease your risk of the falls that lead to fractures.

To help your bones, you've got to do some exercise against gravity. Jogging, running, or walking are the best forms of exercise because they use large muscles and make you support your own weight. Bicycling and swimming are next best. Although it was once thought that swimming didn't benefit bones, it now appears that it does increase bone density in your back.

Steven Blair at the Institute for Aerobics Research in Dallas found that people who engaged in regular physical activity had lower death rates from all causes. Death rates declined from thirty-nine per ten thousand people per year among the least fit to eight per ten thousand people per year among the most fit.[40]

Getting Started with Exercise

Ah, yes, you sigh. I realize now that I should have been exercising all these years. But the damage is done; it's too late to start now. And you fall sadly but comfortably back into the depths of your overstuffed chair.

Well, you're wrong. Although it's true that exercise is most effective if you start young, it can help you at any age. Studies have found that ninety-year-old women in nursing homes can increase their fitness when they start exercise programs. And you don't have to become a jock! The biggest benefits come when you switch from doing nothing to doing something—that is, getting off the couch and walking a half an hour a day will reap huge benefits. There is less additional benefit to your health of going from a thirty-minute walk to running marathons (more about that later)!

Okay, you don't like to walk or you live in a place with an unsuitable climate much of the year. Before you assume that this means you're condemned to a daily visit to purgatory, stop and think about all the activities that involve exercise. Many women have an allergic reaction to the notion of exercise—they don't want to stand in front of the television set imitating the gyrations of some cheery health guru, and they see the health club with its fancy machines as a modern-day version of the Tower of London's torture chamber. But if you give it some creative thought, you may be able to identify some kind of exercise that you can enjoy—or at least tolerate. Exercise means getting your body moving and using your muscles. It can be tap dancing, ice skating, step aerobics, swimming, walking, bicycling, in-line skating, gardening, ballroom dancing, tennis, basketball, softball, soccer, ballet, hiking, cross-country skiing, jogging—any number of activities.

If you have arthritis and find all of these movements difficult (or even if you don't), you may want to look into water aerobics. Water is less stressful on the joints, and the resistance of water is great for strengthening muscles.

Even if there's no sport you really like, you can build exercise into your regular activities. My determinedly sedentary coauthor doesn't mind walking, so she works that into her daily life. There's a bus stop around the corner from her house that goes to her subway station—but she ignores it and walks ten minutes to the station and back. Often she gets off at the stop ahead of hers, adding another fifteen minutes to her walk. Adding this kind of exercise doesn't require any more time than the activity itself—no changing into sweats or going back and forth to the gym.

Of course, as I keep reminding my coauthor, not everyone hates to exercise. If you enjoy exercise, as I do, you're ahead of the game. Now you just have to make sure you do it regularly, and get in the basic kinds of exercise you'll need to stay in your best shape.

Creating an Exercise Routine

How do you start creating an exercise program suitable to your own goals? First, you have to identify those goals. The major goals include flexibility, increased muscle strength, and aerobic conditioning.

Stretching for Flexibility

Flexibility is best achieved by stretching. When you were a kid, you were flexible (I look at my fourteen-year-old sitting on the floor and marvel). But I don't have to tell you those days are gone. If you want to maintain flexibility, you need to work on it. Five minutes of stretching a day can increase your flexibility considerably and make you feel better. There are several books available that give you the outlines of stretching for a variety of activities. My couch-potato coauthor has grudgingly admitted that daily stretching exercises actually do make her feel better—more energized to focus on the reading and writing she prefers to spend her time on.

Stretching is often best done when your muscles are "warm." This means that you've been using them to exercise or at least move around a bit. You can combine stretching with the rest of your program by tacking it onto the end or doing stretches after you've warmed up a bit. Don't neglect stretching—the aches and pains that come after exercise are due as much to lack of stretching as to the exertion itself.

On the other hand, it's a good idea to add more stretches to your life. I thought I was stretching until I started yoga . . . now, *that's* stretching. I was amazed how hard it was and how much better I felt afterward. And I do it only once a week.

Building Muscle

Muscles have a tendency to weaken with age, adding to overall frailty and the tendency to fall, so you'll probably want to do some muscle-building exercises. These can also help increase bone density; bone attached to a muscle being exercised will increase in density. For example, squats increase the bone mass in your hips. Although all exercise will strengthen some muscles, it's best if you strengthen all of them. Jogging, for instance, increases the muscles in your legs but doesn't do much for your arm muscles.

The best way to strengthen your muscles is with weight-resistance training. You can do this with machines, like those in a gym or health club, or by using free weights (small dumbbells of different weights) at home. There are books and videos that can help you get started, or you can hire a trainer for a lesson or two. Once you're in a routine, it becomes easy. You should start with muscle strengthening three times a week, every other day. (Take off Sunday.) Daily weight training doesn't give your muscles enough time to recuperate between efforts.

Aerobics

Cardiovascular training is also important. You can think of it as exercising your heart. This means aerobic exercise, which will get your heart rate into the target range. Aerobic exercise can take the form of walking at a brisk pace, bicycling (either outdoors or on a stationary bike), swimming, or any other activity that will get your heart beating faster.

Your target heart rate (beats per minute) is calculated by subtracting your age from 220, and then multiplying the resulting figure by 0.6 to 0.8. So, for example, if you're 50, subtract that from 220 and you get 170 beats per minute. Multiply that by 0.6 and you get 102; multiply by 0.8 and you get 136.

You can check your heart rate by feeling for the pulse in your neck, counting the beats for ten seconds, and multiplying by six. Your heart rate should be between 102 and 136. This formula is fairly accurate for premenopausal women, though according to Morris Notelovitz, it underestimates the target range for women in their sixties by 6.9 percent and for women in their seventies by up to 16 percent.[41]

A breath test is an easier way to determine whether you're exercising aerobically. You should be able to sing the words "God bless America, land that I love" before taking a breath. (If, like my coauthor, you loathe "God Bless America," pick a song line that takes the same amount of time. She's settled on "Come to me, my melancholy baby.") If you can go on to the next line without taking that breath, you're exercising too little; if you need to catch your breath between words, you're working too hard. You shouldn't be panting, but you should have some feeling of exertion.

How Much Exercise Should I Do?

To keep your heart in shape, you need to exercise twenty minutes a day, three or four times a week. If you're interested in weight control as well, increase that to forty-five minutes every day. To build bone mass, you need twenty to thirty minutes a day of antigravity exercise—such as walking, jogging, or bicycling—two or three times a week. Add upper-body weight training (fifteen minutes of lifting two to three times a week). For stress reduction, thirty to forty minutes of brisk walking every other day will work wonders.

Yoga is a wonderful way to incorporate many of these elements and stress reduction, too. Many women find it is a perfect way to maintain their fitness.

More Thoughts on Exercise

If you've been sitting on your duff for the past twenty years, let me remind you that you should have a physical examination before starting an exercise program. This should include tests for cholesterol level and blood pressure, which you can then use as a baseline. After six months of exercise, you can recheck them to see if your new habits have had an effect.

There are lots of aids available for exercising. There are videos for aerobics, for muscle toning, for flexibility, and for all three combined (see Appendix 2). If you prefer to exercise in the privacy of your home, videos may be the perfect choice. There are also audiotapes: I use music tapes on which a beat is maintained at a set pace to keep me going when I walk briskly or jog. You can get everything from rock to big band music to country and western, and from three to ten miles per hour.

If you prefer to work out with others, you can join a health club. Or you can get a group together to walk early in the morning, during lunch breaks, or after work in the evening. Often working out with a group, or even just one friend, can motivate you on those days when you're tempted to stay home and watch TV. (If you prefer, you can stay at home and watch TV—on your treadmill or exercise bike. You can even build in bribes to yourself: my coauthor does her weight lifting exercises while watching *Hollywood Squares*—no weights, no Whoopi Goldberg!)

But how do you put all these things together into a cohesive program? A one-hour program might include a five-minute warm-up (walking slowly or stretching) followed by fifteen minutes of weight training on machines or free weights, then thirty minutes of aerobics (brisk walking, running, bicycling, dancing, climbing stairs), followed by a ten-minute cool-down (stretching). A thirty-minute routine could alternate muscle strengthening one day with aerobics the next. But again, make sure you pick something you know you can stick to. It may be easier for you to break up your exercise. Walk to and from work, for example, and do your weight training every other evening.

The more research I did for this book, the more I became convinced that regular exercise was the most important lifestyle change I could make. Although I've been involved with athletics throughout my life, I've also had intermittent periods of being fairly sedentary. This book started me back on a regular program. In my usual fashion I went gung ho and started doing everything right away. Before I knew it I had an injury and had to start all over again. I find I do better when I have a goal and some guidance. In an attempt to avoid further injury, I joined the L.A. Leggers, a local running club. I was appalled to find out that they were training to run the L.A. marathon. Before I could run away in horror, I got hooked. The two features that seduced me were the fact that they alternated five minutes of running with one minute of walking and the fact that I had to run only thirty minutes twice a week on my own and then do a long run early Saturday morning with the group. This sounded doable. Lo and behold, seven months later I ran the L.A. marathon (slowly) and astonished myself and my family. I have since done another marathon in Dublin and find that I enjoy the structure of training and the goal. I now do weight training and yoga once a week and run every other day. I feel much better, sleep better, and definitely feel a sense of moral superiority. This works for me. Not only does it make me feel healthier, but it gives me a sense of control over my body when being in perimenopause makes me feel out of control in so many other ways. You don't have to run, but maybe you'll want to join the Master's swim team or a local softball team.

We don't get a chance to measure our progress as much as we age, and competition, even if it is only against yourself, can be a real morale boost.

I realize that my approach isn't right for everyone. Some of you might be closer to my end of the spectrum; some might be closer to my co-author's. She wants to do as little as she can possibly do and still get some benefit from it. As we worked on this book, she finally broke down and got some three-pound weights and a video; she has started to do weight training for fifteen minutes a day, alternating upper- and lower-body exercise days, which she's added to her walking and stretching. She's been sticking with it, and she's even beginning to enjoy it, much to her chagrin.

And that's the key. If my coauthor tried my heavy routine, she'd quit in a week. If I used her mild routine, I'd be bored to death. You have to find what will work for you. Remember, you're not just trying to find an exercise pattern for the next six weeks to lose an extra five pounds—your goal is to get fit and stay fit for the rest of your life. It's better to do a little less and stick with it than to do a killer regime for a couple of weeks and then drop it in despair.

There are also a number of small things you can do—with or without a regular routine—that can incorporate exercise. Use the stairs instead of the elevator or escalator. While I was still at UCLA, I got into the habit of walking the five flights of stairs to the clinic. At first I'd arrive huffing and puffing and dripping with sweat, but soon I could do it while remaining cool and collected. Walk to the store instead of driving (harder to do in L.A.). At home, don't save yourself steps by waiting for things to stack up before taking them upstairs—make all of those extra trips; they'll work your muscles. Look for ways to be active. Even standing up four hours a day can increase your bone density. Every little bit counts.

I like to think of exercise as a medical treatment without side effects, but that's not always the case. You have to be careful not to overdo it, especially if you're just starting. And you need to be conscious of your body's messages to you. Jogging and squats can be hard on the joints. If you're feeling frequent pain in your joints, check with your doctor and modify your routine. One of my friends walked around for months with pain in her foot, which her doctor said was nothing. She finally found a podiatrist who discovered a tiny stress fracture in her ankle: she'd gone from no exercise to strenuous walking without giving her body time to build up to it. I suddenly switched from walking to jogging in the hills around my house. Running downhill turned out to be too hard for my legs, but as soon as I changed to the relatively flat beach, I was okay. This doesn't mean that the slightest muscle ache should be your excuse to give up forever, but it does mean you should be sensible. Moderation counts, even here.

REDUCING STRESS

One of the worst threats to health is chronic stress. It increases blood pressure, respiratory rate, heart rate, and oxygen consumption. Stress isn't a bad thing in itself: it's the body's way of alerting you to danger, so you can do whatever is required to escape. But when it becomes chronic, it interferes with the body's resistance to illness and its ability to repair itself. When you're stressed, your body has a "fight or flight" reaction, pouring out epinephrine and norepinephrine, causing your heart to race and mobilizing your body for action. This reaction, which is great if you have to run away from an attacker, isn't the best way to handle sitting in traffic on the freeway. The results of chronic stress are heart disease, high blood pressure, and cancer.

I hate it when well-meaning friends tell people to cut out the stress in their lives, as if it were something you could remove surgically. Stressful situations are part of everyone's life, and, as we discussed in Chapter 3, the years when you're approaching or beginning menopause are often the time when new stresses are added to your life: the loss of aging parents, the departure of kids for college or jobs, and more responsibility at work. What you can do, though, is change the way you deal with stress.

Health Benefits of Stress Reduction

Reducing stress—or dealing with it better—sounds like motherhood and apple pie. Of course it's a good idea. Of course you feel better. But did you know that in randomized controlled studies it has been found to lower blood pressure? There is even some evidence, which I'll discuss in Chapter 13, that it might affect the progress of life-threatening diseases like cancer and heart attacks. And as we saw in Chapter 11, it can reduce hot flashes.

Reducing Stress by Taking Time for Yourself

I met Susun Weed, author of *Menopausal Years: The Wise Woman Way,* when we both spoke on a panel on hormones in Philadelphia, and I was impressed with her view of menopause.[42] She sees this stage of a woman's life as no less than a metamorphosis, a complete change from one stage of life to another. She says that the first step of menopause is a need for isolation. She uses a wonderful metaphor: a caterpillar who's been munching leaves with all of the other caterpillars until one day it looks up and says, "I don't want to munch another leaf. In fact, I don't even want to hear leaves being munched anymore!" So it moves away and finds a place to weave its cocoon.

We need our own version of that cocoon, Weed says, and she uses another image for the time menopausal women need—a "crone's year away." For a particular woman, that "year" may be only a month, a day, or even a few minutes, but we all need some time to ourselves, especially around perimenopause. The enormous physical changes we go through may be our body's way of telling us to wake up and readjust. Maybe irritability and mood swings are the body's attempt to drive away everyone so that we can have the time we need alone.

While I was writing the first edition of this book and wiping off the perspiration from my hot flashes, I suddenly realized that I needed a break from my medical practice. I'd been caring for patients for almost twenty years; I needed to take a break to focus on caring for myself. As a result, I retired from seeing patients. I have many activities I'm still involved in, from research, teaching, lecturing, and writing to going back to school to get my M.B.A. Maybe I'll go back to patient care at some point, maybe not. I hadn't really thought that this change had anything to do with approaching menopause until I heard Susun Weed on that panel. But doing this for myself has made an enormous difference in my level of stress.

Your own "crone's year" may not involve anything as drastic as quitting your job. But it could include some major change—moving to a new home, taking a long-dreamed-of trip. On the other hand, it could be something as simple as finding a way to create time for yourself and to bring peace and relaxation into your life. Byllye Avery, the founder of the National Black Women's Health Project, suggested (in a speech I heard in Provincetown) that all women give themselves an hour a day when they don't have to answer to anyone but themselves. You can meditate, exercise, pray, or listen to music—but do it alone. Above all, don't use your hour as a chance to catch up on chores or other work. Have a family meeting and announce that this will be your hour, and no one is to interrupt you. I know I just told you to find time for exercise, and now I'm telling you to find yet another hour from a day that's already too busy.

But adding exercise and "alone" time will recharge your batteries, so you'll do the other things in your life more efficiently and more whole-heartedly. Just as menopause is a wake-up call for nutrition and exercise, it should be a wake-up call for incorporating techniques for stress reduction into your life.

Mind-Body Techniques for Reducing Stress

It's not hard to convince people that the mind can have a powerful effect on the body. Any woman knows that all she has to do is worry that she might be pregnant, and her period will be late. We all know of people who stay alive against all odds until a special event has occurred and then, as soon as they're ready, die.

Effects of mind-body have been inadvertently demonstrated by scientists in an interesting way. Remember the cholesterol studies we discussed in Chapter 6, in which even the control group, who took a placebo, experienced a change in HDL levels? This change was less than that among the groups that took hormones, but it occurred. The only explanation is that some of the subjects believed they were getting a remedy. This was hardly an isolated event: many studies find a significant change in subjects who receive placebos. Norman Cousins called the public's attention to this in his 1979 book *Anatomy of an Illness*, in which he advocated a conscious use of the placebo effect to heal illnesses—and reported that he himself had done so.[43]

The most common self-administered mind-body methods of stress reduction are meditation, mental imagery, autosuggestion, progressive relaxation, breath therapy (discussed here), and mindfulness (discussed later in this chapter). These are all variations on a single theme: getting in touch with your inner core.

The most important of these techniques is meditation. Herbert Benson, a doctor who has studied many alternative forms of healing, calls his own version of meditation the "relaxation response."[44] This was the basis of his work as director of behavioral medicine at Deaconess Medical Center in Boston. With his colleagues, he ran several groups for people with a variety of diseases. One of the doctors who worked for a time in the group for cancer was the oncologist Leo Stolbach, who reported positively on the results. "What the relaxation response can do," Stolbach said, "is to slow down or even stop the continuous chatter the mind is constantly putting us through. It gives the mind a rest from those thoughts and then a chance to deal with the issues they raise." He described a number of physiological responses to the relaxation response: a decrease in pulse, blood pressure, respiration rate, oxygen consumption, and overall metabolism—all of which helped reduce stress.[45]

Meditation is easy to describe, although it's harder to do. There are many different ways to meditate, coming out of many different traditions. All of them are said to induce the relaxation response.[46] One of the most popular begins with finding a quiet, comfortable place where you can spend fifteen to twenty minutes. The next steps include repetition of a word, sound, phrase, or prayer, and a passive return to the repetition whenever thoughts intrude. The famous *om* is one such word—it comes from Eastern traditions—but you can use any word that has meaning to you, like peace, or a phrase from your favorite prayer.

There's good evidence that meditation measurably reduces stressful reactions in the body. One study compared meditation and exercise to see which had the stronger effect on beta endorphins (chemicals that act like narcotics in the brain) and corticophin-releasing factor (a hormone from the brain that tells the adrenal gland to release cortisol). They found equal effects in elite runners and experienced meditators, showing that you don't have to sweat to get a "runner's high."[47]

In my favorite study, researchers quantified the effect of adding meditation to a "happiness enhancement program." Those who meditated scored highest on the "happiness" measure.[48] I can't think of a greater role for any lifestyle change, any alternative, or any drug than "happiness enhancement." Excuse me while I go meditate.

Mental imagery—also known as visualization—can be used with meditation or on its own. We've already discussed the use of mental imagery for symptoms such as hot flashes. It can also work for generally calming yourself, and to bolster your system against future disease. This ancient technique, rediscovered in recent years by "new age" devotees, has as its basis the belief that if you create strong mental pictures of what you want, while affirming to yourself that you can and will get it, you can make virtually anything happen. It involves imagining that the changes you want to happen in your body (or in your life) are actually happening. For example, you might imagine that your bones are sturdy, rocklike structures impervious to decay. Or you might visualize one of your concerns metaphorically—LDL as an army advancing through your arteries toward your heart, and HDL as a defending army, defeating the LDL, for example. There are many, many ways you can envision a problem and its solution. This technique has actually been found to increase immune function and to achieve some remarkable cures. (You can also use it to help achieve other goals, from getting a job to finding a parking space. Maybe you've always wanted to go to Paris: take part of your "alone" hour and visualize yourself walking along the Seine. This may sound like hocus-pocus, but if you tell your mind something will happen, you open yourself to the possibilities that may have been there all along without your seeing them.)

Autosuggestion (also called affirmation) is similar to visualization, but it is a verbal rather than a visual approach. You use phrases rather than images to describe the changes you want. When the changes are health related, you focus on the area of the body involved as you form words (in your mind, or out loud, depending on which you're more comfortable with and where you are). The phrase can be very simple—"I am calm and serene," or "My heart is strong and healthy." Whenever your mind wanders, bring your attention gently back to the phrase.

For autosuggestion to be effective, two things are very important. One is to use the present tense rather than the future: "I am healthy," not "I will be healthy." If that feels too discordant—as it sometimes does when you're feeling very uncomfortable and can't persuade your mind that you feel great—you can phrase it in terms of a choice: "I choose to be healthy." Formulating your wish in the future pushes it away from the present. As the song says, tomorrow is always a day away.

The second essential thing is to use positive, not negative, phrasing: "My bones are strong" rather than "I won't get osteoporosis." You don't want to insinuate into your mind the very idea that you're trying to program it against.

If you want to try working with mind-body techniques on your own, there are a number of audiotapes and videotapes on relaxation and imagery that might help you. If none of these tapes is exactly right for you, you can try creating your own. In *The Road Back to Health,* the psychologist Neil Fiore suggests a model for creating your own visualization tape.[49] Progressive relaxation involves tensing each muscle for a count of ten and then releasing for a count of ten before moving on to the next muscle.

Breath therapy induces the relaxation response by concentrating on slow, deep diaphragmatic breathing.

Laughter and Stress Reduction

When Norman Cousins set about to cure himself of a degenerative illness, he came up with a creative form of therapy. This rather formidable intellectual decided to laugh his way back to health. "I discovered that ten minutes of genuine belly laughter had an anesthetic effect and would give me at least two hours of pain-free sleep," he wrote.[50] He researched and found the medical basis for this: laughter can stimulate endorphins.

Several of my patients have used laughter as an important part of their healing process. One woman had breast cancer twice, and laughter was an integral part of her treatment. "I told people I wanted to laugh. Friends sent me funny books, cut out cartoons, called me and said funny things," she reported. Eventually she died of her cancer, but her multilevel approach to fighting her disease had given her the strength she needed to live her life fully to the end—and to help launch the breast cancer political movement. Laughter can help heal, as it did with Cousins; and it can help improve the quality of your life, as it did with my patient. I have no doubt that, together with other approaches, it can help prevent disease as well.

Integrating Stress Reduction into Your Everyday Activities

Some techniques for reducing stress can be used during your normal life, apart from your special "hour apart." You can use deep breathing at any time, for instance, to work on a specific symptom as it's occurring (this is what makes it so good for hot flashes), or simply to program your mind to relax. Similarly, you can say "affirmations" at any time, and for any length of time. One technique—mindfulness—is actually designed to work as part of everyday activities, rather than in a particular, set-aside time. Mindfulness is really a form of meditation. You become mindful of whatever is happening at the moment and focus on it—whether it's washing the car, sharpening a pencil, or reading a bedtime story to your children. Whenever thoughts intrude, you bring your mind back to its focus.

Making meditation, the relaxation response, or some other stress-reduction technique a habit can be one of the most important steps to improving the quality of your life and to preventing disease. On the other hand, not every technique is good for everybody. Lawrence LeShan, in *How to Meditate*, emphasizes that meditation is something you have to work at, and that it needs to feel right for you.[51] Meditation, he says, should "make you feel better when you do it than when you don't do it." If it doesn't, you should stop doing it.

I would go a bit further. There are times in your life when you have enough you need to work at, and the thought of one more pressure, one more obligation, is too much to deal with. If that's how you feel, even meditation or visualization, for instance, may be the worse possible use of your "crone time." Sometimes the most healing things can be the most apparently trivial ones. Your "alone" hour might be best used listening to music, reading a romance novel, or watching a sitcom and laughing. Or maybe you just need to sit and stare out the window, letting thoughts flit through your mind without paying much attention to them. The worst thing you can do is get all stressed out about the need to fight stress. Find what works for you—and if it stops working, find something else. "Cronehood" is a very creative state.

SOCIAL SUPPORTS

There is growing evidence that supportive interpersonal relationships are strongly related to better health. We're social beings; we need contact with others to survive. It's unrealistic, particularly during a time of transition such as menopause, to expect your spouse, partner, lover, or best friend to be all things to you. You may want to find a support group where you can discuss the changes going on in your body and mind. A night out with your friends, a religious club, a reading group, or an exercise class may also help serve your need for like-minded companions. In one randomized study of women with metastatic breast cancer, the women who were assigned to a support group lived on average eighteen months longer than those who weren't.[52]

CREATIVITY

Another important aspect of lifestyle is creative activity. The end of biological fertility can be a good, symbolic time to stress other forms of creativity. You may want to take up painting, music, or writing. Or you might want to run for political office, or do volunteer work for a cause you believe in. Involve yourself in something you're passionate about. Your soul, like your body, needs exercise.

Although I'm suggesting a lot of changes that, in most cases, take a lot of self-discipline, I think it's equally important to be a bit self-indulgent. Life needs to be enjoyed. You need generally healthy habits, but you also need room for the occasional exception. I generally eat a low-fat diet based on fish and vegetables—but I've decided that chocolate is a vegetable. I try to exercise six days a week—and sleep late on one. Having fun is vital to your emotional health. The goal isn't to prolong life at all costs—it's to live a joyful, vigorous, healthy life for as many years as you're given.

THIRTEEN

ALTERNATIVES: FROM ACUPUNCTURE TO HERBS

Ideally, we'd all exercise regularly, eat a perfect diet, develop terrific stress-management techniques, never touch tobacco or booze, and sail through life in vigorous health, meeting a peaceful and painless death at the age of a hundred. But life isn't always ideal. Some people would find the elements of creating a completely physically healthy lifestyle so difficult they wouldn't want to live to a hundred. And for others, even the most rigorously healthy regimen doesn't always provide enough of a sense that they're doing all they can to prevent osteoporosis and heart disease.

In this chapter we're going to look at some of the supplements, herbs, and alternative treatments used for prevention of disease. I'll talk about vitamin therapy, Western herbal traditions, and traditional Chinese medicine (which includes herbs, acupuncture, and other treatments), among other methods. All of these involve more risk than making lifestyle changes but less risk than taking drugs.

As we mentioned in Chapter 11, the medical establishment is becoming increasingly interested in these alternative approaches. At the 1996 meeting of the American Association for Cancer Research, there were several reports of studies on ginseng and dong quai, as well as on soy and green tea. All were being studied in a vigorously scientific way in animal models to see if they have a beneficial effect on cancer.

My plan in this chapter will be to describe the different alternative approaches to health that I believe can be helpful in restoring balance at this challenging time of life. Part of this involves looking at how each approach views menopause to demonstrate alternative ways to frame the experience. I'll also review what I think are the most tried and true herbs and remedies and give you references in case you want to explore anything more thoroughly.

A FIRST STEP: FINDING A GOOD PRACTITIONER

My original intention in this chapter was to describe herbs and other treatments that could be used as alternatives to Western preventive drug therapy. As I became immersed in the research, however, I realized that picking bottles of herbs off the health food shelf and trying them without supervision or prescription could be as ridiculous as sampling drugs off the pharmacy shelf. This is important even when you're considering such treatments for short-term control of symptoms, as discussed in Chapter 11. When you're thinking about them for long-term use in preventing disease, it's still more important, for the same reason that it's important with Western medicines. The longer you take a substance, the more vulnerable you're likely to be to its side effects.

The initial research is something you can do on your own by checking out the literature on these healing techniques or talking with friends who have used them. But before you decide to start using an "alternative" healing method, you should consult with a qualified practitioner. It's not as simple as saying, "This herb is good for this symptom, so I'll take it." Just as you need a Western medical doctor to get a prescription for estrogen, you should see the appropriate practitioner to obtain the correct prescription for a given alternative therapy. If anything, alternative practitioners tend to individualize their therapies more than Western providers; and for most of these treatments, you'll need to be evaluated personally if you're going to benefit.

In Western medicine, we treat everything as if one size fits all. (For example, most doctors who put you on estrogen will automatically give you 0.625 milligram of Premarin regardless of why you're taking hormones, or what your height and weight are.) But many of these other traditions treat the person rather than the symptoms, as they try to restore balance. This requires that you see a diagnostician who can individualize a regimen for you. In addition, although many of these approaches can be complementary to Western (allopathic) medicine, they often don't work together. Chinese herbs may have one aim whereas Ayurvedic herbs may be trying to achieve something entirely different, for instance. Practitioners of each approach can help you decide which herbs will work together and which will counteract each other—as well as which will work with or counteract whichever Western medications you're using.

I also strongly recommend you keep all of your health care providers and practitioners informed about every drug or remedy you may be taking. You should be careful not to mix and match without help.

MINERAL AND VITAMIN SUPPLEMENTS

Not all alternatives are unfamiliar, exotic, or "new age." In fact, some you probably use already—such as mineral and vitamin supplements.

There's no question that the best way to get the vitamins and minerals you need is in food. That way they come packaged with all of the other factors that can help them work. For example, while beta-carotene may be the most "active" carotene, taking it alone in a pill does not replicate the benefits of consuming foods rich in all eight hundred carotenes and one thousand–plus carotenoids. This has been recently demonstrated in studies that found that adding a supplement of beta-carotene to the diet of smokers and asbestos workers did not prevent lung cancer, as had been hoped, but may have actually made it worse.[1] On the other hand, eating a diet high in fruits and vegetables does help prevent cancer. Maybe we haven't isolated the right active ingredients, or maybe the active ingredients need to be taken along with certain other substances (cofactors). Thus I think we need to be careful about equating supplements with what we can get from our diet.

Having said that, I must still acknowledge none of us is perfect. There may be certain vitamins or minerals that you chronically miss in your diet. Take another look at your food diary (see page 236) and make some calculations for a few typical days, to see what you're really getting in your diet. This will give you a better idea of whether you need a supplement and if so, how much. The women who are most likely to be missing some vitamins or minerals are those who smoke, are dieting, are under stress, have heavy menstrual bleeding, are vegetarians, or have digestive problems. One study of both men and women found that girls and women were getting less than 80 percent of the "recommended daily allowance" (RDA) of calcium, magnesium, iron, zinc, copper, and manganese.[2] In another study—a two-year study of women—about 70 percent of the subjects consumed less than 70 percent of the RDA for calcium and iron, and about 40 percent of these women didn't get enough vitamin B_6 or magnesium.[3] This may be even more serious than it appears, since the recommended daily allowances were set to prevent deficiencies, not to promote health. The metabolic changes of menopause can require different amounts of some vitamins and minerals than you needed when you were younger. For example, you'll need more calcium than the RDA to help prevent osteoporosis, colon cancer, and high blood pressure.

Minerals

Calcium Supplements

As we said in Chapter 12, calcium is important for our hearts and bones, and possibly to help prevent colon cancer. A meta-analysis of calcium and bone mass in adult women suggested that women could add 0.8 percent bone mass per year with calcium supplements. The author speculated that "up to half of the women who take calcium supplements might prevent the usual 2% loss in bone that occurs with aging, and . . . high calcium intake could benefit women in their early postmenopausal years."[4] Calcium (along with vitamin D) has been found to reduce the incidence of colon cancer in a study of men.[5] Though there haven't been studies of its effect on colon cancer in women, it's likely that such an effect exists. Calcium and vitamin D also lower blood pressure in women.[6]

Calcium supplements come in a variety of formulations. Calcium citrate (Citracal) is the easiest to absorb on an empty stomach. But calcium carbonate (Tums, Os-Cal, and their generic equivalents) is the most commonly used. It's absorbed well when chewed and taken with meals. It's also the least expensive and has the highest concentration of calcium. (And it's very well advertised—with a catchy tune borrowed from *Dragnet* and an ad campaign that seems strongly focused on women.) My new favorite is Viactiv, which is calcium carbonate in a chocolate chew. It is just tasty enough to make sure that I have one at lunch and dinner. Calcium gluconate and lactate are less concentrated, so you have to take more tablets to get the same amount of calcium. You want to avoid dolomite, bonemeal, and oyster shell, since they're generally contaminated with lead and other minerals.

Calcium, calcium carbonate, calcium citrate, calcium lactate, and calcium gluconate are all forms of calcium. But it isn't just overall calcium that matters—it's the amount of elemental calcium a supplement contains. Read the label carefully. For example, the label for one generic calcium says: "Each tablet contains 500 milligrams of calcium carbonate or 200 milligrams of elemental calcium, which is 20 percent of the USRDA for calcium." Since the RDA underestimates your real need, this means that you'd need to take seven or eight tablets to get your daily requirement if you have none in your diet. Since you probably eat some foods with calcium, taking two or three tablets in the morning and two or three before bed is probably about right (800 to 1,200 milligrams).

Up to 2,000 milligrams of calcium daily is probably safe for most women, but more than that can increase the risk of kidney stones, as well as potentially increase your intake of harmful trace metals (manganese, lead, cadmium, aluminum copper, and arsenic) commonly found in antacids and supplements.

Calcium supplements are best taken as divided doses, as only about 750 milligrams can be absorbed at once. According to Susun Weed, 500 milligrams taken morning and night provides more calcium than 1,000 milligrams taken at one time.[7] But if you take calcium only once a day, do it at night, when your body needs more calcium. You could argue that taking Tums at night is triply good, since it gives you calcium, prevents heartburn, and helps you sleep. (My more frugal coauthor prefers her drugstore's own brand, which is fine—but you need to read the label and make sure it's got all the same ingredients as Tums, not one of the other, aluminum-based antacids. Make sure it says "calcium carbonate" on the label.)

To absorb calcium, you also need vitamin D, magnesium, and boron (see page 261).

Magnesium

One study suggests that magnesium may be even more important than calcium for building bones.[8] Magnesium depletion causes bones to stop growing, decreases osteoblastic and osteoclastic activity, and results in low bone density and increased fragility. Not only is magnesium important for the absorption of calcium, but low magnesium can cause vitamin D resistance. One study found that women who combined calcium and magnesium were actually able to build bone, as opposed to simply stopping its loss.[9]

Luckily, most foods high in calcium are also high in magnesium. (You should aim to have calcium and magnesium in a ratio of 2 to 1.) If you're taking 1,500 milligrams of calcium, you should take 750 milligrams of magnesium (not the laxative magnesium citrate) along with it. If you're not getting enough of one in your food, you won't be getting enough of the other, either. Foods high in magnesium include nuts, legumes, cereal grains, dark green vegetables, and seafood.

Other Minerals

Calcium and magnesium aren't the only minerals important in the menopausal and postmenopausal years. If you have heavy bleeding, you may be losing a lot of iron, so you'll need to increase your iron intake, which may mean taking supplements. On the other hand, after menopause, when you're no longer bleeding, you need less iron and can decrease your consumption. Overly high levels of iron have been associated with heart and liver disease. One way you can keep iron levels in check postmenopausally is to donate blood. You help other people and yourself at the same time (unless, of course, you're anemic, but they'll check your blood count before you're allowed to give blood). Iron can be found in red meat, fortified cereals, fish, green leafy vegetables, poultry, and beans. Most nutritionists recommend 15 milligrams a day for women under forty and 9 milligrams a day for those over forty.

Zinc is a trace element that's needed for adequate immune function. You need about 30 milligrams of zinc a day. Larger doses can interfere with copper metabolism, and doses over 2 grams (2,000 milligrams) are toxic. Sources of zinc include pumpkin seeds, oysters, and spirulina. Herbs containing zinc include sage, wild yam, and nettles, to mention just a few.

Copper helps build bones, lower cholesterol, and strengthen muscles. The best sources of copper are seafood, organically grown grains, beans, nuts, leafy greens, seaweeds, and bittersweet chocolate. (I always knew that chocolate was good for me!) A supplement of 2 milligrams daily is enough. Herbs containing copper include skullcap and sage.

Boron also helps keep bones healthy. It's found in green leafy vegetables, grapes, raisins, apples, nuts, wine, and cider. If you don't eat enough of those, you can take a 3-milligram supplement. Boron is found in all organic garden weeds, such as chickweed, nettles, and dandelion.

Chromium helps reduce cholesterol and therefore is another useful trace mineral. You can get it in brewer's yeast, wheat germ, whole grains, brown rice, beans, cheese, beer, and meat. A supplement of 100 micrograms a day is reasonable. (A microgram is one-millionth of a gram, or one-thousandth of a milligram.) Chromium is found in such herbs as oatstraw, nettles, red clover, wild yam, and black cohosh.

Selenium in the diet has been linked to a lower risk of breast cancer and heart attacks. Although there are no definitive data, a few provocative studies have found that regions with low levels of selenium in the soil have higher rates of cancer and heart disease.[10] Selenium is found in seafood, liver, kidneys, grains, chicken, mushrooms, and garlic. A supplement of 50 micrograms is reasonable, although (as with beta-carotene supplements) it may not have the same effect as it does in foods.

Manganese is good for bones, hearing, and prevention of diabetes. Recent studies of women with osteoporosis showed that they had manganese levels 29 to 75 percent lower than other women.[11] This mineral is found in seeds and leaves grown in healthy soil, and in seaweeds. Herbal sources include raspberry leaf, chickweed, ginseng, wild yam, nettles, and dandelion. A supplement of 5 micrograms daily is sufficient.

Phosphorus is important in the formation of bones and teeth. But it can be harmful, too. Some animal studies have shown that a low calcium-to-phosphorus ratio leads to bone resorption.[12] Women who consume little in the way of dairy products and green vegetables can have a calcium-to-phosphorus ratio as low as 1 to 4. Most junk foods and sodas are very high in phosphorus and should be avoided. The recommended daily allowance of phosphorus is 800 milligrams, but supplements aren't usually necessary, because virtually all of us consume adequate amounts in our diet.

To summarize, if you're over forty, you should be sure you're getting (daily) 1,500 milligrams of calcium, 750 milligrams of magnesium, 30 milligrams of zinc, 2 milligrams of copper, 3 milligrams of boron, 100 micrograms of chromium, 50 milligrams of selenium, and 5 milligrams of manganese—while keeping your iron intake down to 9 milligrams, unless you're losing a lot of blood. Should you get a blood test to see if you're getting enough? Not really. Most of these minerals are bound in the body, so that blood levels may not reflect the true amount you have or need. A minimal supplement that provides the amounts we have listed won't be toxic even if you're getting enough in your food. Megadoses of minerals (and vitamins) are a different matter and should only be taken under a practitioner's supervision. More isn't necessarily better and can even be harmful.

Vitamins

As with minerals, the advantage of obtaining vitamins from food is that they come automatically combined with the appropriate minerals and cofactors that make them easiest to absorb and most functional. Rather than take up a lot of space about which vitamins are in which foods, I'll just give an overview here. The detailed information is available in many other places. And there are few surprises. Except for vitamin D, you can get most of the vitamins you need by eating lots of fruits, vegetables, and whole grains. (I told you there were few surprises!)

Vitamin D

Preliminary studies have found that aside from helping absorb calcium, vitamin D may help protect against colon cancer and breast cancer. This vitamin is found in your skin, and it's activated by the sun. Fifteen minutes in the sun daily without a sunblock will supply it. Unfortunately, the same ultraviolet rays that give you the vitamin D also cause skin cancer. This means that you need a sunblock, but you'll get less vitamin D when you're wearing a sunblock and may need to be out in the sun longer. Morris Notelovitz and Diana Tonnessen did a study showing that women living in Florida had twice as much vitamin D in their blood during the spring as did women living in Finland. They also cite another study, which found that half of a group of postmenopausal women living in Boston were deficient in vitamin D during the winter months. However, those who took a supplement of 220 IU (International Units) of vitamin D a day blocked seasonal fluctuations in parathyroid levels.[13] In Chapter 5, we talked about how parathyroid hormone regulates the amount of calcium in the blood. If your calcium levels are low because an insufficiency of vitamin D is keeping your body from absorbing it, your parathyroid will go into action and leech calcium from the bone in an attempt to remedy the situation.[14]

If possible, therefore, walk or exercise outdoors (not at high noon, though, and not without an adequate sunblock). Try to make sure to get outdoors even in cold weather—you can still get vitamin D from winter sunshine, and you're less likely to get skin cancer. Vitamin D is hard to find in food, but some foods do have it—fatty fish (salmon, tuna, and mackerel), liver, and eggs. In addition, milk is supplemented with vitamin D, as are many cereals. Most multivitamins supply the 400 units of vitamin D you need each day. And those of you living in an area with cold, gloomy winters (I've gotten very smug about weather since I moved from Boston to L.A.!) should take a vitamin D supplement during that season if you don't spend much time outdoors. You can overdose, however, so you should avoid taking more than 1,000 units a day.

Antioxidants

Antioxidants are probably the most important vitamins for women who are aging. These include vitamins A, C, and E, and beta-carotene. As we noted in Chapter 6, it's the oxidation of LDL that is the first step in the hardening of the arteries. The oxygen-free radicals created in this oxidation process are now thought to be related to wrinkles, liver spots, rheumatoid arthritis, and cancer. Vitamin E is the best at neutralizing these free radicals before they can do too much damage. It reduces tissue damage after a heart attack, decreases damage caused by inflammation, and increases resistance to cancer cells. An adequate dose of vitamin E is 400 IU. Vitamin A and carotenoids (found in green and yellow vegetables) are also important sources of antioxidants. Beta-carotene decreased the incidence of heart attack and stroke by 50 percent in a group of male doctors (I know, I know) who took it every other day for six years. There has been some speculation that beta-carotene can prevent lung cancer in smokers, but as I mentioned, recent studies of supplements have been disappointing.

Vitamin A is also important for vision, and it can improve night vision, which often decreases as we age. You remember all those old jokes about how rabbits don't wear glasses because they eat all those carrots? Well, carrots are a great source of vitamin A. For a supplement, women need about 5,000 IU of vitamin A and 3 to 5 milligrams of beta-carotene daily. (Don't overdo it—15,000 milligrams a day may be toxic over time and can cause birth defects.)

Vitamin C also works with vitamins E and A to prevent oxidation of LDL, and it helps the immune system as well. As a million commercials have told you, there's a lot of vitamin C in orange juice—and, as you might have guessed, there's also a lot in oranges. It can also be found in broccoli, hot peppers, green peppers, tomatoes, cabbage, green leafy vegetables, strawberries, and grapefruit. If you take a vitamin C supplement, divide it into three daily doses. You don't need a whole lot—between 500 and 1,500 milligrams a day.

B Vitamins

Vitamin B isn't a single vitamin but a whole collection—thiamine, riboflavin, niacin, pantothenic acid, pyridoxine (B_6), folic acid, cyanocobalamin (B_{12}), biotin, para-aminobenzoic acid, inositol, and choline. Vitamin B_6 is said to relieve PMS in premenopausal women, but there are no randomized controlled studies. A few clinical studies have shown that vitamin B deficiency may be the cause of some postmenopausal anxiety and irritability. B vitamins should usually be taken together as a B complex in order to achieve the best balance. If you're over forty, be sure you're getting at least 100 milligrams of niacin.

Recent research on high homocysteine as a risk factor for heart disease again points to the importance of enough vitamin B. Make sure your multivitamin contains at least 3 milligrams of vitamin B_6, 6 milligrams of vitamin B_{12}, and 400 micrograms of folate.

Multivitamins: Can One Pill Do It All?

A multivitamin supplement will often supply what you need and is a good idea for most menopausal women.[15] But how do you choose the right one from the multitude that are on the shelves? Sherry Sultenfuss offers advice in her book *A Woman's Guide to Vitamins and Minerals.*[16] First read the label. As with calcium supplements, you can get confused. It's important to see if an ingredient is listed plainly or in parentheses. If a label says "zinc picolinate 50 milligrams," this means that 50 milligrams is the combined weight of the zinc and the picolinate. If it says "zinc (picolinate) 50 milligrams," this means that there are 50 milligrams of zinc. Since you want to know how much actual zinc there is, you'd do better with the latter. Taking a balanced supplement with vitamins and minerals is important. Inappropriate combinations can be a problem, as we saw with phosphorus.

Natural versus synthetic probably doesn't matter as much as you would think. Most natural vitamins contain other ingredients—such as rose hips, which include not only vitamin C but also flavinoids, fructose, malic acid, sucrose, tannins, zinc, and vitamins A, B, D, and E. You may be surprised to hear that a vitamin can (legally) be labeled "natural" if as little as 10 percent of its ingredients are natural.

Be sure to look at the expiration date on a bottle of vitamins before you buy it. Many vitamins and minerals can lose their potency quickly.

Finally, Sherry Sultenfuss says that it is better to take your supplement three times a day than all at once: the water-soluble vitamins have a greater chance of being absorbed. (Of course, you can't do that if you have one capsule a day, but taking timed-release formulations may help in this situation.)

So do your research. A vitamin ad may claim to have "everything a woman needs," but that doesn't mean it's true. Once you find a combination that truly provides you with the appropriate supplements, stick to it, while you keep trying to improve the variety and healthfulness of your diet. You can't lose.

HERBS

I discuss the use of herbs for symptoms at length in Chapter 11. In this chapter I'll focus on those herbs that are generally used for prevention. These herbs, as opposed to some of those we considered earlier, are not known to be estrogenic and therefore are considered safer for women with breast cancer. They are generally considered nourishing rather than medicinal herbs. I have not been able to locate any traditional scientific literature supporting their use. Therefore, you should consider these recommendations as unproved but probably not risky.

Horsetail (Equisetum arvense)

Horsetail picked in the spring is said to be especially good for preventing or reversing osteoporosis because it is rich in minerals, especially magnesium. It's also said to prevent clogged arteries by virtue of its silica, chromium, flavinoids, saponins, and astringent agents. It can be combined with stinging nettles for an even stronger effect. It also provides potassium and iron, which help increase energy and decrease fatigue.

Horsetail can be used in soup or dried for teas. The dosage is one cup (250 milliliters) daily of tea made from dried spring-gathered herb. (Ready-made teabags are less reliable in the amount and potency of the herb you will get. Nonetheless, they are probably safe.) Don't use horsetail if you experience sensations of nervous sensitivity or urinary irritability after drinking it.

Oatstraw (Avena sativa)

Oatstraw does indeed come from oats, just like oatmeal. It is rich in calcium and has a reputation for building tough, hardy bones. It also reduces cholesterol and therefore the risk of heart disease. The dosage is one cup or more of dried-leaf, stalk, and grain infusion daily. I bought some oatstraw tea, and I've found it very tasty.

Seaweeds

Seaweeds contain high levels of almost every mineral you need for good bones. They are also said to lower blood pressure and cholesterol. They have abundant antioxidants, which can help prevent heart disease as well as cancer. You can buy seaweeds in an Asian grocery store or a health food store. You can use them as a condiment daily and also as a vegetable. Try them with pasta, grains, eggs, salad, and popcorn. Because they're high in iodine, however, you should be careful if you're hyperthyroid.

Stinging Nettle *(Urtica dioica)*

Stinging nettle herb is a good source of calcium, magnesium, potassium, silicon, boron, and zinc, as well as vitamin D. It's therefore likely to be of some help in preventing osteoporosis. It can be eaten as greens all spring, when nettles are fresh; the dried plant can be drunk as a tea the rest of the year. The dosage is one cup or more of dried-leaf infusion daily.

CHINESE MEDICINE AND ACUPUNCTURE

Chinese medicine covers a variety of related systems of healing. It has been practiced for more than two thousand years in China and since the 1700s in the United States. It's based on a paradigm completely different from that of Western medicine.

One of the key principles involves yin and yang. These are generic concepts, representing any two opposite aspects within a single object that are interdependent and in constant flux. In the human body, health is a relative balance of yin and yang that's never static. Although they've been misinterpreted in the West as representing male and female, in nature yin and yang correspond to the natural principles of fire and water. The ultimate goal of Chinese medicine is to balance yin and yang. Marie Cargill describes this in *Acupuncture: A Viable Medical Alternative:*

> Yin and yang are dynamic states that continually create and regulate one another through many subtle transformations.... [They] define and constrain one another by striking a balance between excess and deficient energy levels. They are fluid states of beginning, acting, changing, resting—in short, the entire repertoire of balances that constitutes being.[17]

Another principle is *ch'i* (or *qi*), the "life force energy." *Ch'i* is thought to be responsible for the movement and transformation of the bodily fluids.

Finally, there is *jing*—the vital physical essence of the body. According to Honora Lee Wolfe, in *Menopause: A Second Spring,* menstrual blood is the outward physical manifestation of *jing* in women, as semen is in men.[18] In Chinese medicine, menopause, although it is a sign of aging, actually slows down the aging process by preventing unnecessary loss of blood and *jing*. Therefore it's a necessary, vital, stabilizing mechanism in a woman's body, slowing down the loss of *jing* and thus allowing the woman another twenty to thirty years of relative good health.

This view of menopause leads to a different approach. You're dealing not with a disease needing treatment, but with a stabilizing force that may need balancing. This balance relates to the individual's constitution and is affected by stress, overwork, emotional upset, and any illness. For this reason, there's no single treatment appropriate for all menopausal women. Each prescription is individualized.

Treatments in Chinese medicine include acupuncture, Chinese herbs (some of which are described in Chapter 11), massage (acupressure, shiatsu), and *chi kung*. One of the martial arts, *chi kung* is also a type of mind-body medicine that combines elements of meditation, relaxation training, visualization, movement, postures, and breathing exercises. It serves both for physical fitness and for self-healing.

Chinese Herbs

There are several ongoing studies funded by the National Institutes of Health on the use of Chinese medicine in the United States. Some studies have already found that Chinese herbs can decrease symptoms resulting from chemotherapy and radiation treatment for cancer. Chinese herbs have also been found to reduce heart disease and cancer.

We've already discussed how Chinese medicine can be used to treat the symptoms of menopause. It's also used to help prevent future problems. Some of the Chinese herbs are the same as the ones used by herbalists in the United States, while others are unique to China. Because the literature about them is mostly in Chinese, I've been unable to evaluate it fully. I suggest you consult a traditional Chinese doctor if you're interested in pursuing this course further. (There are, by the way, a large number of American practitioners of Chinese medicine, many of whom have studied in China. It isn't nationality or race that's important; it's the study of the discipline.)

Also, as we mentioned in Chapter 10, you need to be careful about the source of any herbal treatment or formula. There have been some reports of adverse reactions, usually involving herbs that contained other prescription medications or contaminants. These complications have included kidney failure, liver failure, coma, and death. Most of these drugs used in the United States come from Hong Kong, where there is no regulation. For example, in 1994 there was a report of two deaths following the use of an herbal formula containing aconitine, which is used for relief of minor muscle pain. When the herbal preparations were analyzed, it was found that the amount of aconitine was greatly in excess of the maximum recommended in the pharmacopeia of the People's Republic of China.[19] Analysis of another Chinese herbal medication that had led to complications found that the herbs had been adulterated with a nonsteroidal anti-inflammatory drug (mefanamic acid) and Valium.[20] I don't want to imply that all Chinese herbal formulas are dangerous. In fact, a study done in Hong Kong of 1,701 patients admitted over eight years to two general medical wards at Prince of Wales Hospital found that only three patients had been admitted for complications from Chinese herbal medicines.[21] I could find many more reports on serious complications of aspirin. Still, I do want to remind you that even though something is an herb, it may not be entirely safe. The best approach is to go to a reliable practitioner who will know the best and most reliable sources of these remedies, and the proper dosages. Also, keep your provider informed about all the medications and treatments you're taking.

Panax ginseng, as I mentioned in Chapter 11, is the Chinese herb that has been studied the most. It has been found to increase HDL and reduce total cholesterol and triglycerides in rats and humans. It was also able to decrease the stickiness of platelets (the component of blood that leads to blood clots), much as aspirin does.[22] It has also been found to inhibit the growth of cancer cells.

Salvia miltiorrhiza (a cousin of garden sage) has been found to dilate blood vessels, especially in the coronary arteries. It was studied in comparison to nitroglycerin and found to be better at improving cardiac function.[23]

Tochu bark extract was found—in a randomized controlled study of rats whose ovaries had been removed—to increase the absorption of calcium and increase bone density and muscle weight, and so might help prevent osteoporosis as well.[24]

Acupuncture

Acupuncture has been used for the prevention of heart disease, osteoporosis, stroke, cancers, and many other diseases of aging. I was not able to find any Western scientific literature supporting its efficacy for these purposes, however.

AYURVEDA

The Ayurvedic system of preventive medicine and health care in India dates back more than five thousand years. It has recently gained popularity in the United States because of the work of Deepak Chopra. He describes the purpose of Ayurveda in his book *Perfect Health:*

> The guiding principle of Ayurveda is that the mind exerts the deepest influence on the body, and freedom from sickness depends upon contracting your own awareness, bringing it into balance, and then extending that balance to the body. This state of balanced awareness, more than any kind of physical immunity, creates a higher state of health.[25]

Ayurveda accepts that the body is always changing but holds that some of this change can be controlled by a mind-body approach. Rather than seeing the body as simply a group of cells, tissues, and organs, this discipline views it as a "silent flow of intelligence, a constant bubbling up of impulses that create, control, and become your physical body. The secret of life at this level is that anything in your body can be changed with a flick of an intention."[26]

Ayurveda—like traditional Chinese medicine—has a concept of vital energy, which it calls *prana. Prana* can be absorbed through the breath; thus breathing and breathing exercises hold an important place in this tradition.

The goal of Ayurveda is to promote and enhance health. Diseases can also be treated within this tradition, but the approach generally is to work on a person's overall integration, balance, and harmony. Ayurvedic doctors try to increase your resistance rather than to treat your symptoms.

The core of Ayurvedic treatment is meditation. In the strict tradition of the Maharishi Ayur-Ved, the development of consciousness through transcendental meditation is the basis of this science of mind–body. Other Ayurvedic practitioners also use meditation but feel that there are various ways it can be carried out. Both approaches, however, use a combination of meditation, diet, herbs, exercise, breathing exercises, aromatherapy, yoga, massage, and chronotherapy (paying attention to natural metabolic rhythms).

There is a body of scientific study on Ayurvedic medicine in India, and some initial studies are now being done in the United States. However, since this is a very individualistic approach, in which the treatment being proposed is specific to the individual rather than the disease, Western-style studies are difficult to perform. There is no readily identifiable end-point to measure. Ayurveda does appear to be helpful in treating chronic diseases and preventing disease. It's less effective for acute or advanced diseases. Its emphasis on prevention and enhancement of health makes it an ideal approach to menopause. It can provide an individualized lifestyle approach that can help many women achieve the balance they need for the second half of their lives.

Ayurvedic practitioners in the United States aren't as well organized as practitioners of traditional Chinese medicine. In India, the training lasts five and a half years, and the degree is called bachelor of Ayurvedic medicine and surgery. A few Western (allopathic) schools offer specialization in Ayurveda. In the United States, there are no strict criteria for training, but there are several training centers, which are listed in Appendix 1. The best way to select practitioners is by asking about their training and experience, getting recommendations from friends, and interviewing them.

Ayurvedic herbs have been found to decrease cholesterol-induced atherosclerosis in rabbits.[27] Other drugs and herbs that have been studied and found effective include *Terminalia belerica,* Maharishi Ayur-Veda herbal mixtures, and modified Anna Pavala Sindhooram.[28]

In addition to its herbs and medicines, the transcendental meditation used in Ayurveda has been found useful for patients with coronary disease in a randomized controlled study.[29] Another study compared transcendental meditation with muscle relaxation as a means of reducing stress in a group of older African–American men and women with high blood pressure. These researchers found that the group using transcendental meditation did much better at controlling their high blood pressure.[30]

NATUROPATHY

Naturopathy combines natural treatments from a variety of traditions, including those we've been discussing. In the 1980s the American Association of Naturopathic Physicians articulated the basic philosophy, taken from Hippocrates: "The body heals itself, and the task of the physician is to support this inherent healing potential."

There are six basic principles in naturopathy. First, respect the healing power of nature: the practitioner's job is to remove the blocks to healing and bolster the body's own ability to heal itself. Second, treat the whole person: health is a result of interactions of physical, mental, emotional, genetic, spiritual, environmental, social, and other factors. Third, do no harm. Fourth, use the least invasive treatment that will help the patient. Fifth, identify and treat the cause of the illness—by which naturopaths mean not bacteria or carcinogens but rather the patient's lifestyle, dietary habits, and emotional state. Sixth, prevention is the best cure. In all of this, the doctor is a teacher. The practitioner's role is to educate the patient and to encourage responsibility for oneself. Many of these principles have been absorbed by Western (allopathic) medicine, as "holistic" medicine becomes more and more popular. They make a lot of sense.

Naturopathic practitioners may use any of a number of methods, including clinical nutrition; physical medicine such as therapeutic manipulation, massage, and bodywork; homeopathy; botanical medicine; Chinese medicine; Ayurveda; and psychological counseling. There are no modalities that are the exclusive province of the naturopath; these practitioners hold that what distinguishes them is their adherence to the six principles.

There have been many studies of naturopathic treatments, though their connection with naturopathy isn't always noted. We've seen numerous studies of the results of diet and nutritional additives and their effect on the risk of cancer, heart disease, and other chronic diseases.

There is growing interest in natural approaches to prevention and treatment, not only because of their effectiveness but also because they're inexpensive. William Collinge, author of *The American Holistic Health Association Complete Guide to Alternative Medicine,* reports that in Germany, naturopathic services have been found so cost-effective that the government now requires conventional doctors and pharmacists to receive education in naturopathic methods and botanical medicine.[31]

According to naturopathic medicine, there are several main "gateways" in a woman's life. These include puberty, establishing a stable relationship, pregnancy and childbirth, and menopause. At any of these transitions, personality and health have an opportunity to undergo great change, for better or worse. Menopause can be a time of relief from troublesome periods, but it can also be a source of new problems if you're overextended. If you take care of your health during this transition, you can improve your constitution and enjoy the next phase.

Naturopathic medicine has much to offer the menopausal woman. It takes the best of many disciplines and treats the whole woman. And, like most of the other alternative philosophies, it views menopause as a time of transition, not a disease—a refreshing change from the attitude of Western medicine.

Naturopathic doctors are licensed in thirteen states in the United States and Canada. You can contact the American Association of Naturopathic Physicians to find out the situation in your state, and to help you find a naturopathic physician. Other resources are listed in Appendix 1.

MIND-BODY TECHNIQUES

In Chapter 12, I talked about several mind-body approaches you can use on your own—although for most of them, you're likely to do better if you have a few sessions, alone or in a class, with a practitioner. There are two mind-body techniques, however, for which a practitioner is essential: hypnosis and biofeedback.

Hypnosis puts you into a highly focused state that allows you to use imagery, relaxation, or autogenic phrases in a more powerful way. It's good for changing bad habits, such as smoking and overeating. We've had years of sitcom jokes about people being hypnotized and ending up quacking like ducks in the middle of business meetings; and a crime drama occasionally has a plot in which an innocent pawn is hypnotized into committing a murder. But hypnosis is unlikely to turn you into either a fool or a murderer—it can simply help you let your mind know you're serious about making a health-related change. I told you in Chapter 12 how I quit smoking through a hypnosis program. You do need a qualified practitioner, however. Amateurs playing around with stuff they don't know about can have a frightening effect on your mind.

As noted in Chapter 10, biofeedback is a method for learning to regulate certain bodily functions by using physical measurements. It can help control a number of symptoms, including headaches, chronic pain, asthma, and muscular problems.

MASSAGE THERAPY AND BODYWORK

Massage is one of the oldest forms of therapy, and it is a component of almost all healing traditions. There are more than eighty different types of massage or bodywork, but they all have some principles in common. The first principle is that improving the circulation of the blood and lymph is good for health. A second principle is that release of tension and toxins promotes greater relaxation and well-being. A third principle is that mind and body are related: as the body is relaxed, the mind can also relax. This also leads to reduction of stress, and a fourth principle is that most modern chronic illnesses are related to stress. Many of the approaches to bodywork also use the concept that massage increases the flow of energy or opens up new channels for energy.

Although there is no direct correlation with or prevention of disease, massage plays an important role in treating various joint and muscular aches and pains, which is useful in helping you keep up an exercise program, since sore muscles can be discouraging. It can also help in stress reduction.

The best way to find a massage therapist is through the American Massage Therapy Association. Other types of bodywork are mentioned in Appendix 1.

There are many other alternative approaches, but in a book this length, I couldn't begin to cover them all—nor can I do full justice to those I've described. If you're considering treatment for menopausal symptoms or trying to prevent heart disease or osteoporosis, I would strongly recommend that you look into some of these before you try Western drugs. There are fewer dangers, and for the most part equally good effects.

FOURTEEN

DRUGS: OTHER MEANS OF PREVENTION

We can talk all day about the benefits of a healthy lifestyle and the advantages of herbs, but there will always be women who need or want to go to the third and most risky level. One approach at this level is drugs. Side effects are inevitable with drugs, but this doesn't mean that drugs are never appropriate for prevention of potential illnesses. There are drugs that will lower your cholesterol when changing your diet doesn't work. New drugs are being developed to cure and even prevent osteoporosis.

We discussed surgery—which is also a third-level approach—in Chapter 11. In this chapter, I'll discuss the use of specific drugs for treating and preventing osteoporosis and heart disease. I will include the new category of Selective Estrogen Receptor Modulators, which tend to be more specific in their effects than HRT. Because HRT/ERT drugs are the ones that were most commonly used to prevent these diseases in women in the past and are the most controversial at present, I'll devote Chapter 15 to the topic of HRT in all of its guises.

DRUGS FOR OSTEOPOROSIS

Bisphosphonates

Bisphosphonates are drugs that act by binding to the osteoclasts (the cells that resorb bone), preventing them from functioning; this decreases bone loss in menopausal women. The fact that these drugs decrease bone loss, however, doesn't mean that they actually build bone. Also, although we know that they decrease fractures in the short term, we don't know what they do in the long term. Because they interfere with the balance between resorption and buildup, they may eventually affect the architecture of the skeleton.

Three bisphosphonates are already on the market: Didronel (etidronate) and Actonel (risedronate) from Procter and Gamble and Fosamax (alendronate) from Merck. The bisphosphonates—like estrogen—can give the illusion of creating bone growth, because bone growth already in progress doesn't stop: it completes its particular growing project. In Chapter 5, we drew an analogy with building a house. In terms of that image, it's like looking at one room that has been partially redone. The work on that room continues till it's finished, and it looks as if the house is getting nicely rebuilt. In fact, though, no more rooms are being added; it's just that a room that was already started is getting completed. This leads to an increase of bone of about 5 to 10 percent—the figure you see in most reports. But the growth continues for only a couple of years, after which bone activity levels off; and then it all stops—both growth and resorption.

That's why we're leery of long-term use of bisphosphonates. Your bones continue remodeling throughout your whole life. If you gain weight in the hips, they need to shore up the bone density in your pelvis and legs to be able to carry the extra weight. If you have arthritis and start walking differently (leaning to one side, say) to avoid pain in the hip, your bones need to shore up that hip and leg. What if you break a bone? You need to be able to repair it. So you don't want to block all bone turnover.

This concern led doctors to give the original bisphosphonates, such as Didronel, intermittently. You'd take them for three months and then stop for three months. There have been some reports of osteomalacia (soft bones) in women who took this etidronate for four years. Newer bisphosphonates such as Fosamax are less tightly bound by bone, and so it's thought—though not confirmed—that they can be given continuously.

A study done in the Netherlands examined some aspects of bone turnover in women who took an early form of bisphosphonate for five to nine years and then stopped.[1] The researchers found that the suppression of bone turnover was reversible once the drug was stopped, but that the beneficial effect on bone density and rate of fractures persisted for at least two years. As of yet we don't know what the correct duration of use should be, but this study suggests that it does not have to be indefinite.

The benefits of bisphosphonates are real. The Fracture Intervention Trial (FIT) first looked at women with low bone density and previous vertebral fractures. Fosamax (alendronate) reduced the risk of hip and wrist fractures by about 50 percent and all clinical fractures (symptomatic) by 28 percent.[2] However only 10 to 15 percent of postmenopausal women have vertebral fractures, so they added a second study looking at four years of treatment in postmenopausal women with a low bone density but no vertebral fractures. This study demonstrated that four years of alendronate decreased the risk of all clinical fractures, hip fractures, and vertebral deformities in women with osteoporosis as defined by bone density (T score less than −2.5) but not in women with osteopenia (T score > −2.5).[3] This finding emphasized the fact that bone density is only one component of fracture risk. The fragility of the bone is as important. Women who've already had a fracture have proven that their bones are fragile. Women who have very low bone density are also at risk, but those with slightly low bone density may not be as fragile. As a result of these data, most experts are no longer recommending bisphosphonates for women with osteopenia. This is based not only on the lack of benefit but also on the unknowns about how long you need to take alendronate and how long it is safe. Much of the antifracture effect of alendronate may be from blocking bone loss, which occurs early and does not increase over time. Alendronate accumulates in the bone and recirculates when bone containing it is resorbed. This may be a good thing if recycling of the drug means that you don't have to take it after a certain period of time. But it could be harmful if there are long-term side effects we don't know about that would be continually exacerbated by its endless presence in the body. We just don't know enough about these drugs to use them in a group of women for whom the benefit is not proven.

Are there any women with osteopenia who might benefit? A study of another bisphosphonate, risedronate, gives us some insight into this question. The study sought to determine whether a bisphosphonate could reduce the risk of fracture in elderly women identified on the basis of risk factors other than bone density. The findings were basically exactly what the FIT study showed. Hip fractures were reduced in elderly women with confirmed osteoporosis but not among those selected by other risk factors.[4]

All this does not mean that these are not good drugs, but rather that they should be saved for the women who have osteoporosis or have had a fracture, rather than being given as prevention.

Another point for limiting their use is the side effects. Ever since Fosamax was approved by the FDA, there have been reports of one particular side effect: Fosamax can cause severe ulcers of the esophagus if it's not taken in exactly the right way.[5] You have to take it with six to eight ounces of plain water immediately after you wake up; studies suggest that the problem can occur if you don't swallow the pill completely—you should take it as soon as you're upright. Then, you shouldn't lie down for at least half an hour afterward. You shouldn't eat or drink anything for thirty minutes after you've taken Fosamax. This includes vitamins, calcium supplements, mineral water, coffee, tea, or juice. Although this doesn't sound too hard if it's helping you cure a disease, it's a bit much for prevention.

There are other, though rare, side effects as well—abdominal pain, nausea, heartburn, vomiting, difficulty swallowing, bloating, constipation, diarrhea, and gas. In addition, some patients have reported muscle pain, headache, and an altered sense of taste.

The initial dosage of Fosamax was taken daily, but there is now a weekly version, which is certainly more convenient. And research is ongoing on a once-a-year shot.

As we pointed out in Chapter 5, this field is rapidly changing as new studies are being done.

Although I think it's great that we have alternatives to estrogen that are specific for treating osteoporosis, I'd still be careful about using them purely for prevention at this stage. For now, Fosamax is probably best used by women who are five years out of menopause and have very low bone density or have already had a fracture.

Calcitonin

Calcitonin, a hormone made by your thyroid gland, inhibits bone breakdown. There's a version made from salmon that you can take to help block bone loss. It's been tested only in women who already have osteoporosis, and it's most effective in women with the highest bone turnover. In two-year studies, it's been found to increase bone density by 5 percent when taken with calcium; in comparison, women who were given calcium and a placebo had a 2 percent decrease in bone density.[6] It's not really clear whether the effect of calcitonin will persist beyond two or three years. There are data, however, indicating that women who took calcitonin had two thirds fewer vertebral fractures in those first few years.[7] As of yet we don't know whether calcitonin can build bone or just prevent its loss. Interestingly, a study directly comparing alendronate and calcitonin showed that the calcitonin had significantly less effect on bone density and bone resorption markers.[8] Whether this means it doesn't work as well is not clear. Remember, bone density is only one part of osteoporosis, and calcitonin may be having its effect on the fragility part of the equation.

One of the more dramatic effects of calcitonin is the decrease of pain caused by vertebral fractures from osteoporosis.[9] This alone may make it a good choice in certain situations.

Calcitonin is not absorbed very well orally, but there's a new nasal spray version, Miacalcin, that's been approved by the FDA. It appears to be especially good for women over sixty-five with vertebral fractures. The only reported side effect is nasal irritation.

Parathormone

As I write this, parathyroid hormone (PTH) has been clinically evaluated and is awaiting FDA approval. Like calcitonin, it is based on a naturally occurring hormone. Interestingly, the high levels seen in hyperparathyroidism (when the parathyroid glands are overactive) cause a decrease in bone, but low intermittant doses have been shown to produce an *increase* in bone. A randomized controlled study of two doses of PTH compared to placebo was done in women who already had a vertebral fracture. Daily injections increased the bone density of the spine by 9 to 13 percent when compared to placebo. New vertebral fractures were reduced by 65 to 69 percent, nonvertebral fragility fractures by 53 to 54 percent, and all nonvertebral fractures by 35 to 40 percent.[10] These exciting findings were tempered a bit by an increase in bone cancer in rats. So far there have been no cases of bone cancer in women or in monkeys. It is hoped that this drug will be a great boon to women with osteoporosis who need to build bone.

Ipriflavone

Ipriflavone, which is based on soy, is a variant on the bioflavinoids we mentioned in Chapter 13. It's been approved in Italy and Japan for the treatment of osteoporosis and has been found to increase bone density in the wrist and stabilize the lumbar spine after one year of treatment.[11] A large randomized controlled study, however, showed that it did not prevent bone loss or vertebral fractures. Nor did it affect the markers of bone absorption. And it caused lymphoctyopenia (a decrease in one kind of white blood cells) in a significant number of women.[12]

SELECTIVE ESTROGEN RECEPTOR MODULATORS: TAMOXIFEN AND RALOXIFENE

Tamoxifen was first introduced as a fertility drug. It then found a role in breast cancer treatment as an estrogen blocker. Much to everyone's surprise, when it began to be used over a period of years, it turned out to be more complex. (If you think this is a recurrent theme of this chapter, you're right). It acts like estrogen in some organs and blocks it in others. So instead of causing osteoporosis as we had suspected, it actually helps to maintain bone. The downside is that it causes hot flashes, blood clots, and uterine cancer. Although the benefits are worth the risks in women with breast cancer where it will reduce the chances of recurrence, this is not true for healthy women.[13]

In an attempt to improve on tamoxifen, a new SERM, raloxifene (or Evista) was developed. When it was first introduced, I was dubious that it would do everything that was claimed, but the data have supported its utility. It has been shown in a large randomized controlled study to reduce bone loss and prevent spine fractures in women with osteoporosis.[14] So far it has not been shown to reduce other clinical fractures. Interestingly, it has more of an effect on fractures rates that you would expect from its reduction in bone loss. This is yet another example of how bone density and fractures are not exactly the same. It did not increase heart attacks the way estrogen does or increase uterine cancer as tamoxifen does. This means that it can be taken without adding progestin. The good news is that in women with osteoporosis it decreases breast cancer significantly. The STAR study is comparing tamoxifen to raloxifene in women who are at high risk for breast cancer with the hope that it will be an even better form of chemoprevention. The RUTH study is looking at its effects on heart disease. Unfortunately raloxifene increases hot flashes and blood clots. Nothing is perfect. Its best use is in women who are past the symptoms of menopause.

As we start to understand how these drugs work, I am sure many more will be developed in hopes of getting just the right mix. And the increase in options and research will serve women well in the future. It's important to realize when we talk about drugs meant to prevent something that won't happen for twenty to thirty years that before that time has elapsed, we'll probably have much better treatments. At the rate pharmaceutical research is going, we should be able to rebuild your whole skeleton as well as identify the women destined by their genes to get into trouble, so we can head it off at the pass. So I worry about settling for the limited drugs we have now as prevention in women who aren't definitely at serious risk.

Tibolone

This drug has been available in Europe, where it is known as Livial, for well over a decade. It is used both to prevent menopausal symptoms and to reduce bone loss. It is not a hormone per se but more like the SERMs discussed above. In fact, it has been described as a "prodrug" because after ingestion it is quickly metabolized in the gastrointestinal tract to two estrogen break-down products, which then circulate in an inactive form until a particular tissue activates them.[15] It, therefore, has different actions in different tissues, acting variously as a weak estrogen, progestin, and androgen. It seems to be safe in the breast, at least according to the evidence of such markers as mammographic density and its ability to stop breast cancer cells from growing in a petri dish.[16] It does not stimulate the uterus and so does not increase uterine cancer.[17] This means that, like raloxifene, it can be taken without a progestin. Though it has been shown to increase bone density when compared to a placebo, there are no studies yet proving that it can reduce fractures.[18] Further studies of this drug are ongoing, and it is anticipated that it will be available in the United States sometime in the near future.

DRUGS FOR HEART DISEASE

Cholesterol-Lowering Drugs

When diet, exercise, and other lifestyle changes aren't enough to keep your cholesterol down there are cholesterol-lowering medications you can take. These range from drugs that block cholesterol absorption to drugs that block the body's system for manufacturing cholesterol. When one drug alone doesn't work, you can take combinations.

Cholestyramine (Questran) and Colestipol

The treatment of high cholesterol usually begins with the drug that has the fewest side effects. Cholestyramine and Colestipol bind bile in your intestine, making it harder for your body to absorb fat. The liver stores of cholesterol go down, and the liver takes some from the blood to make up for it. This lowers your LDL. It may also increase the good HDL while, unfortunately, also increasing the more harmful triglycerides. Initial doses have been found to decrease LDL cholesterol 10 to 15 percent; the highest doses reduce LDL by 15 to 30 percent.[19] In addition, these drugs have been around long enough that we know they can reduce heart attacks.

Since these drugs aren't absorbed, their side effects are limited. Most of the side effects, not surprisingly, relate to the digestive system; they include constipation, bloating, stomach fullness, nausea, and gas. They can also interfere with the absorption of some medications and so should be taken one hour before, or three or four hours after, other drugs such as antibiotics, beta blockers, digoxin, phenobarbital, thiazide diuretics, thyroid hormone, and coumadin. Long-term use can also interfere with the absorption of the fat-soluble vitamins A, C, and E.

The usual starting dose of cholestyramine is 4 grams once or twice a day with a maximal dose of 24 grams per day. It's available in a standard powder formula, a low-fat formula, and a flavored bar. Colestipol is a standard powder, usually given as 5 milligrams twice daily; the maximal dose is 30 grams.

This type of drug works best on women with moderately elevated LDL cholesterol and normal triglyceride levels.

Niacin

The other drug that has been proven to be both safe and effective in treating heart disease is niacin. (Although this is commonly thought of as a vitamin, at these dosages it is truly a drug.) It isn't clear how it works, but it has been shown to reduce LDL by 15 to 30 percent; it is available as 100-milligram and 500-milligram tablets as well as sustained-release formulas. The usual starting dose is 100 to 250 milligrams per day, with a gradual increase in the daily dose up to 1.5 grams per day. The maximum dose is 6 grams per day. It can't be used by women with ulcer disease, liver disease, or gout, and it should be used cautiously by women with diabetes. The main problem with niacin is its side effects, chief of which are flushing and itching—just what every peri-menopausal woman needs. You can prevent the flushing by taking aspirin or nonsteroidal anti-inflammatory agents before you take the drug, by taking the drug with meals, or by using the more expensive sustained-release formula. The flushing generally stops after several weeks. You can treat dry skin and itching with moisturizers, and you can avoid gastrointestinal side effects by taking niacin with meals. The best thing about niacin is its low cost. It's the cheapest cholesterol-lowering drug available. It is the first-line drug for those with elevated LDL and low HDL or high triglycerides.

Hydroxymethylglutaryl Coenzyme A Reductase Inhibitors

These drugs are the newcomers on the block. They work by preventing the manufacture of the body's own cholesterol, which, as you'll remember from Chapter 6, is the source of most of the cholesterol in your blood. As a result, the liver pulls back some cholesterol that's already in the blood to shore up its stock, just as it does with cholestyramine. These drugs include Lovastatin (Mevacor), pravastatin, simvastatin (Zocor), and flura-statin. In women, lovastatin can decrease LDL cholesterol by 24 to 40 percent as well as increase HDL slightly (7 to 9 percent) and decrease triglycerides somewhat more (9 to 18 percent).[20] The usual starting dose of lovastatin is 20 milligrams with dinner. If necessary, you can increase it to a maximum dose of 80 milligrams per day. With pravastatin, you start at 10 to 20 milligrams and go up to 40 milligrams. With simvastatin, you start at 5 to 10 milligrams and go up to a daily dose of 40 milligrams. For flurastatin, you start at 20 milligrams and go up to 40 milligrams. These drugs are generally well tolerated. The side effects include some digestive problems, muscle aches, tiredness, headache, insomnia, and rash, although none of these effects are common.

This whole field got a tremendous boost recently when a large double-blind randomized prospective study in men and women with established coronary artery disease found that these drugs not only lowered cholesterol but also decreased the rate of heart attacks.[21] This is important because the reason to lower cholesterol is to prevent heart attacks. Statins may also have an effect on C reactive protein which could be a second mode of action.

Gemfibrozil (Lopid)

This recently developed drug is especially good at decreasing high triglyceride levels and even increases HDL. In women with high triglycerides, it can reduce LDL by 10 to 15 percent. Researchers don't completely understand how it does this. The recommended dose is 600 milligrams twice daily one half hour before meals. It has few side effects. It does, however, increase the ability of the bile to form stones, and you should therefore not use it if you have gallbladder disease. It's the best drug for women and/or diabetics with high triglycerides.

There's been some concern that the cholesterol-lowering drugs have the potential to increase cancer. While this is still hypothetical, it emphasizes the fact that we should use them only when nothing else works.

Aspirin

Aspirin doesn't lower cholesterol, but it seems to prevent heart attacks and strokes by decreasing the blood's ability to clot.[22] You should take a daily half-aspirin for this purpose only under a doctor's supervision. Aspirin may be common, but it's still a drug, and it can have serious side effects when taken over the long term.

As with osteoporosis, I have confidence that we'll eventually have better and better ways to treat coronary heart disease and to predict which women are at risk. Only if you have heart disease or have very high cholesterol levels that don't respond to exercise or diet changes do you need to be on drugs.

Blood Pressure–Lowering Drugs

Luckily we have three types of drugs that have been shown in randomized controlled clinical trials to reduce the chances of a heart attack in women with high blood pressure.[23] The first step is usually a low-dose diuretic. These pills will block fluid retention and thus lower blood pressure. Beta-blockers and Angiotensin-converting enzymes (ACE) inhibitors are also used to treat high blood pressure that is unresponsive to lifestyle changes and have been shown to reduce the risk of heart attacks.[24] Interestingly, calcium channel blockers, which have been shown to reduce blood pressure, do not reduce the risk for heart attack and heart failure. As with osteoporosis, it is better to use drugs that not only improve the risk factor such as high blood pressure or low bone density but also prevent the disease!

FIFTEEN

HORMONES: THE MENU OF OPTIONS

While other drugs are worth thinking about, the drugs most commonly taken to alleviate the symptoms of menopause are still hormones. They're also the drugs that have been the most commonly taken by women to prevent heart disease and osteoporosis in the past.

You might wonder why I refer to hormones as drugs when they're made naturally by our bodies. The answer is that, first, it's not "natural" for us to have them in high levels after menopause; and, second, many of the hormones used in hormone therapy are not the ones our bodies make naturally, either before or after menopause. As I said earlier, calling hormones "replacement" therapy implies that we're just restoring something that's missing. The problem is that it's not what would be present, even if you were thirty-five; and when you're fifty-five, it's extra. And "extra" isn't always good.

Some of you may also be surprised to see "natural hormones" in this chapter, rather than in Chapter 11 or 12, where "alternative" approaches are discussed. But natural hormones (not to be confused with the phyto-SERMs in some vegetables) are still hormones, and, as such, they're drugs.

HOW WE THINK HORMONES WORK

Hormones are powerful and complex, and we don't yet know nearly enough about how they work. For example (as noted in Chapter 7), we've known for a while that for a hormone to work, it needs a receptor to get into the cell. This receptor is like a lock and the hormone is the key that fits it and opens the door. Researchers originally assumed that every drug that fit a given receptor would cause the same effect—open the same door. But further research has revealed that some drugs seem to fit a receptor (or lock) without opening the door. Instead, they block another hormone from getting in. These are antagonists or hormone blockers. Tamoxifen, which is used to treat breast cancer, is a good example, as is RU 486, which blocks progesterone in the uterus. So researchers refined their theory and came up with a nice simple model: drugs act either to cause an effect or to block it.

However, the more studies we did, the more complicated the model got. For example, our original assumption was that tamoxifen would not only block estrogen in the breast but would also increase osteoporosis and heart disease by blocking estrogen everywhere. But it turned out that it didn't work that way. Much to our amazement, tamoxifen, though it does indeed block estrogen in the breast, acts like estrogen in the uterus, bones, and liver. Tamoxifen causes uterine cancer and it prevents bone loss and high cholesterol, much the way estrogen does (though it doesn't work quite as well as estrogen in reducing bone loss).[1] This isn't simply an either/or phenomenon, then, but something much more complicated.

So we've developed a new model to explain how hormones work. We now say that some drugs like tamoxifen are selective estrogen receptor modulators (SERMs).[2] It's likely that most of the plants that have hormonal effects are SERMs as well. We're starting to figure out how SERMs work. It turns out that the locks aren't the same in every organ. Progesterone, for example, has two possible receptors. The receptor in the uterus is completely different from the one in the breast. So progesterone may block estrogen in the uterus and stimulate it in the breast.

In addition, some cells may have a double lock. And in that case it may matter which one you turn first. One drug may fit one lock or part of the receptor, causing one effect, while another may fit another area and have a completely different effect. Some drugs will fit both spots and have a third effect. In fact, different drugs acting through the same receptor can induce different receptor conformations—that is, actually change the shape of the lock—and this results in different reactions.[3] And finally the other natural compounds that are recruited by the drug to help can have either activator or repressor effects.[4]

To make matters more confusing, we have two different estrogen receptors to contend with (see page 139). And remember Tibolone (see last chapter), a drug used in Europe that gets converted into different hormones (estrogen, progestins, and androgens) depending on the organ.

Are you totally confused? Good! You're starting to get my point—that none of this is simple and that we're only beginning to understand how all of these hormones work. We can't assume that natural progesterone and progestin, a synthetic cousin, act the same; and we can't assume that horse estrogen and synthetic estrogen act the same. Nor do we yet assume that any of these are safe for postmenopausal women.

Scientists are hoping to use some of this new information to design the perfect hormone: one that will protect the uterus and breast from cancer, stop hot flashes, and prevent osteoporosis and heart disease. It would be lovely—could it do housework, too?—but I'm skeptical. It would still be a drug. And I have yet to see a drug that doesn't have some side effects. We'll see.

Meanwhile, I'm going to take you on a tour of the currently available hormones. If you decide to take hormones to address symptoms you have, one size rarely fits all. Your decision should take into account your body and its metabolism, your lifestyle, and the reason you're taking these drugs.

The commonly used hormones are forms of estrogen, progesterone, and sometimes testosterone. These are often mixed and matched in a variety of ways and delivery systems. As I've pointed out, most of the studies on prevention have been done on Premarin, taken by mouth, without added progestin or testosterone. You have to be careful about extrapolating these data to all hormones or to all methods of taking them.

NATURAL OR BIOIDENTICAL VERSUS SYNTHETIC HORMONES

The word *natural* is fashionable. Somehow we think that anything is better and safer if it's natural. There are two ways to interpret this word with regard to hormones.

First, *natural* can mean that a hormone is most like the hormones we have in our bodies, either postmenopausally or premenopausally. With this interpretation, Premarin, which is made from the urine of pregnant mares and is in fact horse estrogen, isn't natural—unless you're a horse. Does this really matter? It's possible that the ingredient producing some of the observed effects of Premarin has nothing to do with horses. But on the other hand, these effects may have nothing to do with estrogen. The effects may come from some other, as yet unidentified, factor indigenous to horses. Maybe it's the soy the farmers are feeding them!

Another definition of *natural* is that a hormone is made from natural ingredients rather than in a laboratory. In this case, Premarin does qualify as natural, since horse urine isn't synthetic. But most other commercial hormones are made from progesterone, which is synthesized in a lab from diosgenin obtained from the wild yam or from soybeans. This includes progesterone that is "natural"—in that it's the same as the progesterone our bodies make—and "unnatural" in the form of Provera.

Is a drug "natural" because it's made from a wild yam, or is it "unnatural" because it's then synthesized in a laboratory? The whole thing becomes ridiculous. It makes me laugh to see that the makers of estradiol are now advertising it as "plant-based estrogen." Needless to say, each pharmaceutical company is going to use the definition that allows it to call its own product "natural." Calling drugs "natural hormones" may make them sound less like drugs, but don't let anyone kid you—these are all drugs.

In order to get around the "natural" problem, some alternative doctors talk about bioidentical hormones. By this they mean hormones that are more like the ones our own bodies make. Several pharmacies in the United States still compound their own drugs, as opposed to using only drugs made by large pharmaceutical companies. These pharmacies are able to make micronized progesterone, estradiol, or estriol to fill a doctor's prescription. They do much of their business by mail order. In fact, in some compounding pharmacies you can get Triest (estrone, estradiol, and estriol), which is a combination of the three types of estrogen meant to mimic the ratio found normally in *premenopausal* women. Thus the prescribers have fallen into the old assumption that women need to be converted back to their premenopausal condition. They are not "bioidentical" to what a postmenopausal woman makes, which is primarily estrone. Other doctors will titrate your dose of hormones by your salivary or blood levels. Claims for this approach are unsubstantiated, with no studies in the medical literature. In fact, we don't even know what normal should be for a postmenopausal woman. Nevertheless, many books and practitioners claim that if the hormones are bioidentical, they will be safe. I need data. Having said this, however, I must admit that short-term use of hormones, whether they are bioidentical or not, seems to be relatively safe. If you feel better using a compounded formula, then by all means do it, to get you over the hump of symptoms. But just as with synthetic hormones, consider tapering off after three to five years.

The real benefit from the "natural" movement is that it has spearheaded a move away from the "one size fits all approach" that has been the norm in the past. If you are taking HRT and it is not helping your symptoms, there are many different formulations, routes of administration, and doses available.

DELIVERY SYSTEMS

How a drug is delivered to your bloodstream can vary. You can take a drug by mouth, under your tongue, through your skin, or through your vagina—even through your nose.

If you take it as a pill, it has to be digested before it reaches your bloodstream. Some drugs are better digested than others. Premarin probably works in part because it has to pass through your liver before it reaches the bloodstream. On the other hand, progesterone isn't very well digested, which means that you need very high doses to achieve adequate blood levels.

Any delivery other than the mouth is called *parenteral*. The skin is an excellent parenteral channel for absorbing a drug, and the drug then bypasses the digestive tract. Patches, creams, and gels applied to the skin go directly into the bloodstream. It's even easier to absorb drugs through mucus membranes (the wet linings of the different entrances to our bodies), so rectal suppositories and vaginal creams and suppositories are good ways to get hormones directly into the bloodstream (as are nasal sprays, such as the calcitonin spray we mentioned in Chapter 14). Finally, you can get a shot or have a drug implanted under your skin for delayed release.

Because there are so many different drugs and ways to deliver them, the choices for hormone therapy are like options on a restaurant menu. You can have one from column A and one from column B. Too often, a gynecologist will prescribe one drug or one combination as if that were the only choice. I'll try to sort out the most common types of drugs so that you at least feel you've seen the menu—and can insist that your "waiter" give you what you order.

ESTROGEN

As we mentioned in Chapter 1, three main forms of estrogen occur naturally in our bodies, all made from cholesterol in the ovary and the adrenal gland or converted from testosterone and androstenedione in individual organs. Estradiol predominates in premenopausal women. Estrone is the dominant estrogen postmenopausally. Estriol is a third, less potent, form, which is highest during pregnancy. Estradiol can be converted to estrone, and estrone can be converted back to estradiol. Estriol participates less in this interchange. All of them fit the estrogen receptor equally, but, as you might expect, they don't have the same effects. Estradiol is the most potent. Estrone and (as just noted) estriol are weaker. Because of this, high levels of estrone or estriol can bind with the receptor and have the potential to act as antiestrogens—to keep the more potent estradiol from binding.[5]

Oral Estrogen

Premarin

The most common method of taking estrogen is in a pill. Premarin, as I mentioned, is the most frequently used in the United States. Its "conjugated equine estrogens" are absorbed through the intestinal wall, where they begin to turn into estrone and estradiol. Then the compound continues on to the liver, as does everything you swallow. It reaches the liver at a very high concentration—much higher than the level of estrogen that the normal premenopausal ovary sends to the liver.

Not surprisingly, this super-high level of estrogen affects the liver. The estrogen stimulates some of the proteins that are made in the liver. This may be responsible for some of its good effects on cholesterol.

After the estrogen is metabolized, it's released into the bloodstream at a much lower level—more like the level found in a premenopausal woman (although there's still more estrone and less estradiol than a premenopausal woman would have).

As I said earlier, most of the studies on estrogen therapy in the United States have been done on Premarin, and mostly with women who have had hysterectomies. It's very good for hot flashes (although it may not eliminate them completely), and for many women it reduces insomnia. It also relieves vaginal dryness, although some women need to use a vaginal treatment as well. It decreases bone loss and fractures. It probably increases breast cancer risk and definitely increases endometrial cancer risk and heart disease.

PROBLEMS WITH PREMARIN

The effects of Premarin on the liver don't appear to be limited to digestion. Even when it's given vaginally, which means that it avoids the digestive system, Premarin has more of an effect on the liver than non–horse estrogens do. There may be something else in the horse urine besides estrogen that causes some of this additional effect.

Another problem is that the level of estrogen produced in the blood of women on Premarin is probably much higher than normal. This is because Premarin consists of three major components. The first is estrone sulfate, which makes up 50 to 60 percent of the preparation. This is a hormone found in both horses and humans. Then there are two horse estrogens that aren't made by humans—equilin sulfate, which is 20 to 30 percent of the preparation, and 17 alpha dihydroequilin sulfate, which is 15 percent. The levels of the equilin estrogens in these pills are many times higher than our bodies' normal levels of estradiol or estrone.[6] What effect does that have? The pharmaceutical companies haven't told us that. And no one else has studied it. We simply don't know.

A third problem with Premarin is that you might not be comfortable with a medication based on the urine of pregnant mares. To begin with, it isn't a particularly appealing notion. As my coauthor exclaimed when she first learned of the derivation of Premarin, "You mean I'm swallowing horse piss every morning?" But there's also the more serious issue of the way the horses are treated. We've become increasingly aware in recent years of the moral issues raised by the abuse of animals in laboratories, at racetracks, and even in homes. For the reader who tries to buy "cruelty-free" products, the treatment of the animals used for her hormone pills might be of interest.

To get the urine needed to make Premarin, about fifty thousand mares are impregnated each year. For seven months of her eleven-month pregnancy, each mare is kept in a tiny stall, barely large enough to hold her. She wears a harness with a device to collect her urine. In order to make the urine more concentrated, she is given only minimal water to drink.

The foals that are the offspring of these pregnancies are sold as pets, or kept to be used in their turn to produce more urine for Premarin, or—most commonly—slaughtered for their meat.

Most of the 480 Pregnant Mare Urine (PMU) farms are in Manitoba, Canada; a few are in other parts of Canada and in North Dakota. When a team from the World Society for the Protection of Animals (WSPA)—including Joe Silva from the Massachusetts Society for the Prevention of Cruelty to Animals (MSPCA)—was invited to inspect thirty-two of the Manitoba farms, it found that the animals were given little to no exercise, had no space to lie down or move around, and were often neglected when they were ill.

When the company that produces Premarin, Wyeth-Ayerst, was confronted with the results of the WSPA inspection, it promised to make a few changes, but WSPA considered these inadequate and unconvincing.

Needless to say, the animal rights movement has taken on the treatment of these horses as a cause. It has called attention to the unpalatable ingredients in this popular pill by parodying a currently popular ad for milk: the anti-Premarin ad shows a cheery actress whose grin is capped with a yellow mustache.

On the other hand, a colleague of mine checked out this matter, and she reports that the mares are actually kept as well as any horses bred for uses other than racing or pleasure. Horses, my colleague points out, don't normally lie down. The mares do get out to exercise and are actually treated well, since each one is an important investment for the farmer.[7]

Although this controversy is unlikely to be settled soon, it is important to know about it as you consider your options. There is now a generic, non-horse formulation of conjugated estrogen called Cenestin.

HOW MUCH PREMARIN SHOULD YOU TAKE?

Premarin comes in several different doses. The most common dose (typically, daily) is 0.625 milligram. A higher dose—1.25 milligrams—is sometimes prescribed, particularly for young women who have especially severe symptoms after hysterectomy. Since the risk of breast cancer is related to the strength of the dose as well as to how long estrogen is taken, this higher dose is probably the cause of some breast cancer. (It was also the dose used in the studies we mentioned earlier on men with heart disease.)

Almost all of the data we have are based on the 0.625-milligram dose. This is really quite amazing. It's almost certain that women's metabolism, their size, and the amount of their own hormones will make a difference in their absorption of the drug, and yet there's rarely any attempt to modify the dose to fit a particular woman's needs. (I guess that is just our fate as women: our clothes come in only a few set sizes as well.) I recommend that you take the lowest dose that will take care of the problem you want to treat. If it's symptoms or osteoporosis, this might be 0.3 milligram. (If your symptoms aren't decreasing enough, you can always increase the dose.) If that's not enough but 0.625 seems too high (for example, if you're experiencing breast tenderness), you can try 0.625 milligram of Premarin during the week but not on weekends. (This will often relieve you of breast tenderness.)

Most women who currently take Premarin have been told that they are on the lowest dose. This was undoubtedly true when they started, but now lower doses—0.3 or even .15 milligram—are also available. This is not unlike the situation with oral contraceptives thirty years ago, when I first took them. We took industrial-strength levels of hormones compared to what is used today. Over time we realized that smaller doses would do the job. Bruce Ettinger at Kaiser Permanente in Oakland, California, demonstrated that most women over fifty-five can safely switch their HRT regimen from the standard dose of HRT to low-dose estrogen and progestins every six months. This new regimen controls symptoms, prevents bone loss, and does not cause bleeding.[8]

Many women start on Premarin after hysterectomies for relief of symptoms and just go on taking it for the rest of their lives. They may well want to reevaluate this with all of the new data and either reduce their dose or taper off entirely. Others take it for a short time after the surgery, or until the normal age of menopause, to tide them over and then slowly taper off, mimicking a more natural menopause. Finally, others get started to combat symptoms and just never stop.

SIDE EFFECTS OF PREMARIN

The side effects of Premarin get very little press, but they do exist. The most common are breast swelling and tenderness, PMS, rash, increased growth of facial and body hair, intolerance of contact lenses, migraine, dizziness, headaches, depression, changes in libido, and reduced tolerance of carbohydrates. (This last effect is a warning sign that you're on your way to diabetes. Diabetics have problems with sugar, and carbohydrates turn into sugar in the body.) Premarin doubles the risk of gallbladder surgery. It also raises triglyceride levels. This could be a real problem if you have a disease characterized by high-triglyceride levels to start with, since that is a serious risk for heart disease. Interestingly, the package insert for Premarin also describes as a possible side effect blotchy skin, especially on the face, which may be permanent. (So much for enhancing your beauty.)

Women who are on the standard dose of Premarin alone won't get regular periods, but 25 percent will have some bleeding. There is a risk of endometrial hyperplasia, so any bleeding or spotting should be checked out immediately, and you may need an endometrial biopsy to rule out any problems (see page 57). Some gynecologists suggest a yearly endometrial biopsy for all women with a uterus who are on Premarin alone. One study found that, compared with a woman who is not on estrogen, a woman who still has her uterus and takes estrogen alone has eight times the chance of bleeding, a five times greater chance of having a D and C, a 6.6 times greater chance of having a hysterectomy, and a seven times greater likelihood of uterine cancer.[9] Nowadays, most women with a uterus will be given a progesterone or progestin to prevent these problems.

TAPERING OFF PREMARIN

If you want to consider getting off Premarin at any time, you should consider tapering off. (There's no medical problem with stopping cold turkey, but about half of women experience severe withdrawal symptoms.) Researcher Deborah Grady suggests stopping cold turkey and finding out whether you are going to have symptoms.[10] If you feel fine, you are done. If you do have hot flashes and sweats, you can go back on and taper off. Although not scientifically studied, there are two ways to taper off. You can do it by time or dosage. The dosage approach, which I favor, means alternating one pill with half a pill (or a pill of a lower dosage) for four to six weeks. Then go to half a pill (or reduced dosage) every day for four to six weeks. Then go to half a pill every other day for four to six weeks. Finally, stop. (The pills aren't scored, so you need to break them either with a sharp knife or an inexpensive pill-cutting tool, which most pharmacies carry.) The time approach is to take the pills Monday to Friday and skip the weekends. If this works, you can drop Wednesday and so on until you are off. If at any time you experience severe symptoms, you're tapering off too fast and need to slow down. A few women find that they just can't tolerate the symptoms. In that situation they are probably better off using the lowest dose that will maintain their comfort. Let your health care provider know if you decide to taper off.

Other Kinds of Oral Estrogen

One other form of oral estrogen is micronized estradiol (Estrace). This is "bioidentical" in the sense that it's the same chemical formula as your own body's estradiol—the estrogen that's highest in premenopausal but not postmenopausal women. *Micronized* means that it's been suspended in very fine droplets to aid its absorption in the digestive tract. Other plant-based estrogens used in the United States include esterified estrogens (Estratab) and estropipate, or piperazine estrogen sulfate (Ogen). Any one of them will work. You may want to experiment with one of these other formulations. Everyone's body is different and responds differently to medications, so it's fortunate that there are options.

There is very little research comparing the different estrogen formulations head-to-head, especially long term. The manufacturers of Premarin want to say that the others are not the same, while the manufacturers of the others want to say that they are all the same. The published data, not surprisingly, reflect the point of view of the company sponsoring the research. In response to the recent report of the Women's Health Initiative, all the same companies will be trying to point out how different they are from Prempro, implying that makes them safe. I would be wary of any claims unsubstantiated by data.

In Europe, the most commonly used oral estrogen is estradiol valerate (Progynon). Another form of oral estrogen used in Europe provides a combination of estrone, estradiol, and estriol. Estriol alone is also used in Europe for hormone therapy, and it's gained some popularity among alternative health care practitioners in the United States, since it's less potent than estradiol and estrone and may have some antiestrogenic effects. Some research done on rats and mice in the 1970s found that estriol protected them against breast cancer.[11] In addition, there are some epidemiological data suggesting that women in countries with higher rates of breast cancer have lower levels of estriol in their urine.[12] I would not take estriol in the hopes of preventing breast cancer, however. Since estriol is the least potent of the estrogens, it has much less effect on the uterine lining, yet it can still reduce menopausal symptoms. Unfortunately, though, high doses (12 milligrams daily) of estriol are necessary to prevent osteoporosis. It therefore is a better choice for controlling symptoms than for prevention.

There are also synthetic oral estrogens. Their chemical structure is very different from that of human estrogen, but they have some estrogen effects. These include ethinyl estradiol (Estinyl), diethylstilbestrol (DES), and quinestrol (Estrovis). These are rarely used today.

The Estrogen Patch

USING THE PATCH

Recently in the United States the estrogen patch has been prescribed more commonly than in the past—in Europe, they've been using it for years. Estrogen delivered through the skin is absorbed better, since it doesn't have to go through the liver and intestine.

The most common patches (Climara, Vivelle) are a matrix—a thin adhesive film with estradiol inside it under a translucent liner. It looks like a piece of clear plastic with a sticky side. It now comes in three dosage forms: .025 microgram, 0.05 microgram, and 0.1 microgram a day. It's about the size of a half dollar. Once you remove it from the foil package, you need to apply it immediately. It lasts for seven days. You can bathe, shower, and swim while wearing it. As with oral estrogens, there has been increasing research on lower doses of the patch. A patch with a dosage of .025 microgram is as good as one with .05 in relieving hot flashes.

The blood levels of estrogen available vary but are usually similar to those of a premenopausal woman in the first half of her cycle. After the patch is applied, the estrogen levels gradually go up and then reach a steady state in about two hours. These levels last for a couple of days, then start to decline.

The patch may be perfect for women who have had hysterectomies. The patch still stimulates cells in the endometrium, so you need to take some progestin to avoid uterine cancer or other problems. Right now, the best route is to use the patch for most of your cycle, and then take a progestin pill toward the end. This is, of course, less convenient than taking a single pill that gives you both estrogen and progestin (such a pill is being used in the United States; see page 307). There is a patch called Estrogest that combines estrogen and norethindrone, a synthetic progesterone, which is available in Europe. It has the same effect as oral estrogen on bone, hot flashes, and vaginal dryness.

The patch doesn't affect the liver, so it might be better for women who smoke, or have high blood pressure, or those with a tendency toward blood clotting (thrombosis). It won't promote gallbladder disease or cause nausea, as Premarin sometimes does. Thus for women who have gastrointestinal problems, gallstones, or high triglycerides, the patch has some real advantages.

Like Premarin, the patch can cause breast tenderness, headaches, migraine, dizziness, depression, an increase or decrease in weight, reduced tolerance of carbohydrates (which can be a precursor to diabetes), fluid retention, and change in libido.

TAPERING OFF THE PATCH

The patch is great for tapering off hormones. You can cut a quarter off the actual patch and use that dosage for a month, then cut it in half, then cut off three quarters, etc. As with pills, if you experience withdrawal symptoms, you should go more slowly. Tell your health care provider you're tapering off.

Other Parenteral Methods of Estrogen Delivery

In countries other than the United States, an estrogen gel in an alcohol base is sometimes used; this is rubbed into the skin. You apply it over a large area of your abdomen and thighs and let it dry for two or three minutes before you put on clothes. It's odorless and isn't sticky. It's absorbed into your skin and gradually released into your body.

The gel is similar to the patch in that it uses estradiol (Oestrogel) and works by slow absorption. It's a bit trickier to use, though, because it's a little harder to be sure of the dose. The gel is absorbed fairly well, and like the patch, it doesn't go through the liver. It has slightly less effect on HDL and LDL, but it's basically just as good for protecting against osteoporosis. It doesn't irritate the skin as the patch can, because it doesn't contain any adhesives. Unfortunately, it's not yet available in the United States.

In the United Kingdom, Australia, and South Africa, women can use a crystalline implant of estradiol, both for prevention and for treatment. It works somewhat like the contraceptive Norplant. It's inserted under the skin in a minor surgical operation. Blood levels rise to a peak once a month, plateau for two to four months, and then decline. There are similar implants that add testosterone to the estrogen. The problem with implants is that they initially produce very high levels of estrogen, which can fall fairly rapidly, causing symptoms like hot flashes when they're first inserted. Since the pellets are under the skin, the dosage can't be changed until the next implant. But there are a number of advantages: an implant eliminates the inconvenience of taking a pill; over time, it produces more constant blood levels of hormone; and it produces stable changes in the lipids and bone.

Parenteral estrogen is easily absorbed. Since it doesn't go through the liver as a first step, the amount that eventually reaches your liver is similar to what would get there if your ovaries were making it. So it's more physiologic—more the way the body normally works. Parenteral estrogen doesn't cause an increase in your triglycerides, and it doesn't have as much effect as oral estrogen on lipids, LDL, or HDL, although there is some effect after six months to a year. It also results in a more stable level of hormones.

In general, the alternatives to oral estrogen, including the patch, deliver estrogen in a constant manner, produce higher physiologic estrone and estradiol levels than oral estrogens, and avoid the liver-protein effect. And the lower-dose vaginal methods (discussed on page 207) are certainly a good alternative if your only concern is vaginal atrophy (dryness). Unfortunately, they're more expensive.

So the effect of estrogen really depends a lot on the type, the dose, and how you take it. They're not all equivalent—the patch isn't equal to the Premarin, which isn't equal to vaginal estrogen. Does this mean that the risks are less with other formulations? There are no data at this time. In the absence of data, it is wiser to assume that they are all dangerous than that they are safe.

Vaginal Estrogens

There are several different applications of vaginal estrogen, including creams, vaginal rings, and vaginal tablets. These often work better for vaginal dryness than the parenteral drugs. The creams are very well absorbed and increase the blood levels of estrogen. Women who need to avoid estrogen should be careful with them. If you are going to use them, you want to use a much smaller amount than is recommended on the package insert. Applying a dab of cream in the opening of the vagina every day for two to three weeks and then once a week thereafter should do the trick. Even more convenient are the new vaginal inserts. Estring is a vaginal insert that releases a very small amount of estrogen over a long period of time. It does not increase systemic levels of estrogen and so is thought to be safe in women with breast cancer (no long-term studies, however). Vagifem is a vaginal tablet that also acts locally.

When You Shouldn't Take Estrogen

If you have undiagnosed vaginal bleeding, or if you might be pregnant, you absolutely shouldn't take estrogen. It's also a bad idea if you have a history of breast cancer, endometrial cancer, or ovarian cancer; a history of deep-vein thrombophlebitis or pulmonary embolus; a blood-clotting disorder; an active liver or gallbladder disease; heart disease; or high triglycerides.

PROGESTERONE AND PROGESTINS

Progesterone is very different from estrogen, because your body produces almost all of its own progesterone only when you're premenopausal: it's produced by the corpus luteum after ovulation. The adrenal gland also produces a very small amount, but that's usually used as a building block for other hormones, such as testosterone. If you're not ovulating, then, you have virtually no progesterone.

As we discussed in Chapter 2, progesterone and progestins have only recently become part of hormone replacement therapy. Initially, the only hormone "replaced" was estrogen. Then, when postmenopausal women on estrogen began to develop uterine cancer, progesterone and pro-gestins came into the picture. Their addition to estrogen for a few days at the end of the cycle causes the uterine lining to be shed, preventing buildup and minimizing the risk of uterine cancer.

But progestins do other things as well. When added to estrogen, they can cause or intensify many symptoms of PMS: headaches, depression, irritability, bloating, fluid retention, abdominal cramping, and breast tenderness. In addition, progestins have their own effects on the liver and the blood vessels. In the liver, they lower triglycerides and block the helpful estrogen-derived increase in HDL. In the blood vessels, they block the helpful vasodilation of the coronary arteries induced by estrogen. Progestins may even counteract any potential benefit estrogen may have on libido. And now we know that the combination of estrogen and progestin increase breast cancer more than estrogen alone. Therefore, we just can't assume that "HRT" is the same as "ERT."

Kinds of Progesterone and Progestins

As with estrogen, there are different forms of progesterone and progestins, and different methods of delivery, each of which influences its effects.

"Natural" progesterone isn't very well absorbed when taken by mouth (because it's broken down in the liver). Until recently, therefore, the only way it could be given was by vaginal suppository or by a skin cream. Vaginal suppositories allow progesterone to be absorbed without passing through the liver. It is a good delivery route but sometimes messy.

The skin creams have become somewhat controversial lately. There are a number of them on the market, claiming to contain progesterone and to decrease hot flashes and increase bone density. Many of these actually have very little progesterone. The assumption is that because they're made from wild yam, they'll have the same effect as progesterone, which is also made from wild yam.

A better development for advocates of progesterone is micronized progesterone, created by breaking progesterone up into very small pieces. Since it's taken orally, it's broken down by the liver. Thus in order to get blood levels of progesterone that were considered adequate, the original prescriptions called for high doses (200 milligrams), taken twice a day. But in the PEPI study (see Chapter 6), researchers decided to investigate whether 200 milligrams once a day of oral micronized progesterone added to estrogen would be adequate. They found that it was still effective at protecting the uterus and did not greatly interfere with the effect of estrogen on the lipids.[13] Other studies have shown that micronized progesterone (Prometrium) is very good for preventing osteoporosis and may even build bone rather than just stop resorption.[14] It can also treat hot flashes without the use of estrogen.

Natural (Bioidentical) Progesterone Cream

This approach to menopause has been popularized in books by John Lee, M.D., and Christiane Northrup, M.D. Unfortunately the science is not as definitive as they would have you believe.

The creams are formulated from a vehicle—a "base" of a fatty or oily substance. It also has an active agent—in this case, micronized natural progesterone. Micronized natural progesterone is extracted from *Diascorea*, a variety of wild yam. Thus it is considered a supplement rather than a drug and therefore does not require FDA approval. The creams are produced by compounding pharmacies, which make their own prescriptions rather than dispensing products manufactured by drug companies. As a result, the creams aren't standardized, and there is no guarantee of the amount of progesterone in a cream. Nor is there much information about a cream's effectiveness, because the pharmacies aren't required to conduct clinical trials to test the product.

As with all creams (even those approved by the FDA), the amount of drug delivered throughout the body is unpredictable, because the drug has to be absorbed through the skin into the blood. The amount that gets into circulation for distribution to other parts of the body depends on skin thickness and temperature and therefore varies markedly from individual to individual, making it hard to predict the effect it will have.

DOES IT PREVENT BREAST CANCER?

Some laboratory studies indicate that progesterone stimulates the growth of breast tissue. Others suggest that it curtails tissue growth by triggering apoptosis (programmed cell death). One theory is that intermittent doses may stimulate growth, and constant doses may suppress it.[15] While researchers try to determine how progesterone works on breast cells, epidemiologists are looking at the relationship of progesterone use and breast cancer. Most observational studies have indicated that the addition of a progestin to hormone replacement therapy increases the risk of breast cancer.[16] The Women's Health Initiative confirmed this when it was halted early because of the increase in breast cancer risk to the women on estrogen plus progestin (see page 142).

While progestins are not natural progesterone, they are synthetic cousins that have many of the same effects. In concert, the studies hardly constitute a ringing endorsement for progesterone as a breast cancer preventive. In fact, they don't rule out the possibility that it may even *increase* breast-cancer risk. Researchers have discovered that breast cell proliferation is higher in the second half of the menstrual cycle, when progesterone levels are higher.[17] This has led them to assume that progesterone stimulates breast tissue. To investigate this further, a study was done on women who were about to undergo breast-reduction surgery.[18] (This meant that the breast tissue removed in the operation could be examined afterward.) Each woman applied progesterone to one breast every day for two weeks. After the reduction surgery, the pathologists examined the breast tissue that had been removed and found that the progesterone had decreased cell division. This has been interpreted as demonstrating that progesterone prevents breast cancer. Again, though—as in the case of estriol—the data are provocative but not yet definitive. The PEPI study, which compared estrogen alone, estrogen and natural progesterone, estrogen and Provera cyclically and estrogen and Provera continuously, showed that progestins (both Provera and progesterone) blocked the beneficial effects of the estrogen on cholesterol. Provera was worse than progesterone, but progesterone was worse than estrogen alone. Another interesting finding was the fact that all of the estrogen and progestin combinations, including natural progesterone, showed an increased mammographic density in almost a third of women.[19] Mammographic density has been shown in many studies to indicate an increase in breast cancer risk. In addition, the women taking both estrogen and a progestin (Provera or progesterone) had more breast pain, a sign of breast stimulation.[20] These both correlate with the recent study of Premarin and Provera showing that adding Provera to the estrogen increased the risk of breast cancer eightfold. In addition, in petri dishes progesterone causes breast cancer cells to proliferate or grow.

But things get more complicated. It may be different if you give progesterone with estrogen or alone. In cell culture, progesterone primes the cells and gets them ready to grow, and estrogen then causes the growth. It is possible that progesterone alone may get the cells ready but not actually cause them to grow if there are no stimulants around (estrogen is not the only one).[21] Thus, it is theoretically possible that progesterone without estrogen in a postmenopausal woman will neither increase nor decrease breast cancer. When I asked one of the foremost researchers in the field of progesterone in the breast (Kate Horwitz at the University of Colorado), she said it was possible—but only hypothetically. The dose of progesterone and the method of giving it, as well as the schedule, she said, can have very different effects, and it is not clear which, if any, are safe.

For example, one study done in France looked at the use of a cream of 19-nortestosterone (a synthetic progestin) in premenopausal women and found a decrease in breast-cancer risk, while none of the other progestins had that effect.[22] So are the over-the-counter creams safe? Not clear. Although there are published reports on the levels of progesterone in the creams, they are not required to be standardized, so one batch could have one level and the next something different. The absorption of the creams depends in part on which part of the body they are applied to. Luckily there is a commercially available natural progesterone pill called Prometrium, which is probably a safer way to take it.

At this point in time, I think we can say that the effect of progesterone on the breast is unknown. When given with estrogen, it causes breast cancer, but when given alone it may be neutral—i.e., it will not cause or prevent breast cancer. I think the real question is whether it is ever really "alone." Since we still produce estrogen postmenopausally, there is always some around, especially in the breast. In addition, the notion of taking progesterone to balance high levels of estrogen should cause it to increase breast-cancer risk, not decrease it. Although you can use the limited data to support either opinion, the real answer is that we don't know.

DOES IT HELP HOT FLASHES?

The one randomized controlled study conducted to determine whether progesterone cream controlled hot flashes indicated that it was effective. In this trial, 102 healthy postmenopausal women were randomly assigned to one of two groups. One group applied a quarter teaspoon of progesterone cream to their skin daily; the other group did the same using a placebo cream (the cream base without the progesterone). At the beginning of the study thirty women in the first group and twenty-six in the second said they were bothered by hot flashes. A year later twenty-five (83 percent) of the first group, but only five (19 percent) of the second reported that their hot flashes were less intense or gone.[23]

DOES IT BUILD BONE?

One of progesterone cream's strongest proponents, Dr. John Lee, claims that progesterone cream actually reverses osteoporosis. However, he has published only one study in a medical journal. Although he reports that the women who used progesterone cream had increased bone density, he doesn't indicate whether they were also taking estrogen—which has been proven to increase bone density. In other words, it's likely that the positive effect was due to estrogen, not progesterone cream. A few randomized studies have been conducted and none has found that progesterone cream increases bone density.[24]

SHOULD YOU USE PROGESTERONE CREAM?

We certainly can't give it a blanket endorsement. There is no evidence that it increases or preserves bone density, so it would be a poor choice for women whose major concern is preventing osteoporosis, especially when there are other agents like alendronate, calcitonin, estrogen, and raloxifene that are proven bone builders.

There is also little solid evidence that it prevents breast cancer and some suggestion that it may contribute to breast-cancer risk. Whether it increases or decreases risk, the effect isn't likely to be huge. Nevertheless, it would be smart to hold off until there is a lot more research in this area.

Based on the single study cited, progesterone cream does work in controlling hot flashes. Although women who use it may incur a slight increase in breast-cancer risk, short-term use probably won't make much of a difference. If you've tried all the other nonhormonal approaches and nothing seems to work, it may be worth a try. But if breast-cancer risk is high on your list of anxieties, it may not.

Progestins

Progestins in pill form are still also commonly used. Progestins are all related to androgens, the male hormones. Some of them have more of an androgenic effect than others. The two main types are C19 and C21 progestins. (The numbers relate to the chemical formula.)

C19 progestins tend to be more androgenic, so you're more likely to get acne, greasy hair, and greasy skin. They also tend to lower triglycerides, an effect that can be beneficial, since estrogens cause triglycerides to rise. Examples of C19 progestins include norethindrone and norethindrone acetate. Norethindrone is very potent, so you need smaller doses. It's used more frequently in Europe than in the United States.

C21 progestins are less androgenic. Provera (medroxyprogesterone acetate), the progestin most commonly used in the United States, is one of these. Provera is given in pill form, either continuously (see below) at a low dose or cyclically in the first half of the cycle. It has less effect on triglycerides than norethindrone or norethindrone acetate, and it blocks some, though not all, of the beneficial effects estrogen has on cholesterol. As discussed in Chapter 6, the PEPI study found that estrogen alone had the best effect on lipid levels, and estrogen with micronized progesterone was second. Provera was definitely third, although it didn't cancel out all of the beneficial effects of the estrogen.[25] Norethindrone is a reasonable alternative for women for whom Provera produces intolerable symptoms.

Ironically, the greatest advantage of the progestins is also the source of women's greatest complaints about them. As I discussed in Chapter 8, estrogen alone can cause endometrial cancer because it thickens the uterine lining over and over again. Progestins allow the body to slough off the lining; this helps ward off uterine cancer, but it means that you have to deal with menstrual bleeding. Twenty-five percent of women taking estrogen alone will have some bleeding, but 85 percent of women who take Premarin plus Provera will get periods again. These periods are usually light, predictable bleeding lasting four to five days every cycle. Even if you opt for the continuous approach described below, you could still get periods for six months to a year, though they should ultimately stop once your uterus becomes atrophic (see the next section).[26] This is the main reason most women don't stay on hormones. No one wants to be buying tampons or pads any longer than she has to. Sometimes, at my most cynical, I think it's all a plot by the manufacturers of menstrual products, who don't want to lose sales when all of us baby boomers stop bleeding.

Progestosert

There's now an intrauterine device called Progestosert that gives out a very low, steady dose of progestin. Like the lower doses of the vaginal creams, it's not enough to be absorbed into the body as a whole. This is based on the very sensible idea that where you really want the progesterone is in the uterus, so that it can protect the endometrium. There isn't any known need for it in the rest of the body, so why not deliver it just where it's needed and avoid the side effects? This approach would eliminate the need for oral progestin. As currently designed, the device stops vaginal bleeding and works for five years, after which it would need to be replaced. As of yet we don't know what the long-term effects would be.

ESTROGEN PLUS PROGESTERONE OR PROGESTIN

Cyclical Versus Continuous Therapy

Estrogen and progesterone can be combined in various ways (see Table 15.1). In cyclical therapy, you take estrogen daily, add progestin for the first twelve days of the month, and then stop the progestin. You'll get a period as soon as the progestin is stopped.

Because women were complaining about bleeding, doctors began experimenting with a new strategy, *continuous therapy.* In this kind of therapy, women take estrogen and progestin continuously, but use a lower dose of progestin. The hope is that the continuous level of progestin will be too low to cause bleeding but high enough to block the stimulating effects of the estrogen. This approach causes much less bleeding than the cyclical approach, but, as we've discussed, it doesn't wholly eliminate bleeding. There's still a 60 to 70 percent chance that you'll have some breakthrough bleeding, or at least spotting. This wouldn't be too bad except for the fact that uterine cancer also shows up as breakthrough bleeding. This means that if you bleed for longer than six months or have heavy bleeding, you'll need an endometrial biopsy to be sure you don't have uterine cancer. On average, most women on continuous combined therapy have two or three endometrial biopsies. Even though the bleeding usually stops within six months to a year, some women continue to have periods. They then have to decide whether to stop hormone therapy completely or switch to just estrogen alone and take their chances. It's no

TABLE 15.1

Ways of Taking Hormone Therapy

DAY	CYCLICAL		CONTINUOUS	
---	Estrogen	Progestin	Estrogen	Progestin
1	X	X	X	X
2	X	X	X	X
3	X	X	X	X
4	X	X	X	X
5	X	X	X	X
6	X	X	X	X
7	X	X	X	X
8	X	X	X	X
9	X	X	X	X
10	X	X	X	X
11	X	X	X	X
12	X	X	X	X
13	X		X	X
14	X		X	X
15	X		X	X
16	X		X	X
17	X		X	X
18	X		X	X
19	X		X	X
20	X		X	X
21	X		X	X
22	X		X	X
23	X		X	X
24	X		X	X
25	X		X	X
26	X		X	X
27	X		X	X
28	X		X	X
29*	X		X	X
30*	X		X	X
31*	X		X	X

*Depending on how many days there are in the month

wonder that gynecologists would rather take the bothersome, bleeding uterus out and be done with it—and that you end up with a hysterectomy you don't need.

It's important to note that the bleeding occurs only if you're also on estrogen. If you're taking progesterone or Provera alone, you usually won't bleed.

If you elect to take estrogen alone, you of course still need to have your endometrium monitored. (What you don't want to do is skip the Provera and not have your uterus monitored.) In the PEPI study discussed in Chapter 6, the women who took estrogen alone had a 30 percent chance over three years of developing endometrial hyperplasia, which was detected on routine endometrial biopsy. This means there is a 70 percent chance that it won't happen in the first three years. (We have no studies to determine what happens after that.) You may decide to see if you can tolerate estrogen alone and take progestins only if you develop hyperplasia—precancer. (If you've had a hysterectomy, you're already protected from endometrial cancer, since there are uterine cells only in the uterus itself, unlike the case with the breast and the ovary.) This approach is not currently recommended by most physicians, because of the chance of endometrial cancer; but only you can weigh the risks in your own case.

Prempro

Prempro delivers continuous estrogen and progestin in one pill much the way the oral contraceptive does. (In the cyclical form, it's called Premphase.) Prempro contains the same dosages of hormones that most women in the United States are taking separately. It is the formulation that was tested in the Women's Health Initiative and the HERS study.

TESTOSTERONE

Understanding Testosterone

As we've noted, the normal postmenopausal ovary and the adrenal gland produces testosterone as well as androstenedione and low levels of estrogen. It should come as no surprise that women whose ovaries have been surgically removed experience a rapid decline in testosterone levels. In addition, postmenopausal women who take estrogen seem to have lower testosterone levels.

The question is what effect these lower levels of testosterone have. How significant is this? There's some evidence that osteoporosis may be related to testosterone as well as estrogen. It's not clear what effect testosterone has on cholesterol.[27] In addition, there's conflicting evidence about the effects of testosterone on the libido (see Chapter 11).

Testosterone is rapidly metabolized to estrogen in the body by fat, muscle, and possibly the breast. Serum levels of testosterone are correlated with an increase in breast cancer risk. Methyltestosterone (a variant of testosterone) isn't as easily converted. And it's important to note that testosterone appears to have effects only on women whose blood levels of testosterone are low to begin with. Nonetheless, there's a growing trend to add testosterone to the hormone mix in women who are complaining of inadequate libido.

The FDA has approved two combination pills of estrogen and testosterone. Estratest is a combination of estradiol and methyltestosterone and comes in two doses: regular and half strength. The other is Premarin plus methyltestosterone (the testosterone here is four times as strong in the Premarin version). In addition, you can get "natural" testosterone (like the kind in our bodies) or methyltestosterone in either a pill or cream, but it has to be made at one of the compounding pharmacies licensed to make drugs to specifications for individual physicians.

Side Effects of Testosterone

As with progesterone, doctors too easily assume that this potent hormone will have no effects other than the desired ones. Some women on testosterone have complained of rages of anger, however. Other side effects include acne, facial hair, weight gain, and liver disease. In addition, there is evidence that testosterone counteracts the lipid changes that estrogen can create. And it can compound the carcinogenic effect of estrogen on the breast and uterus. The Nurses' Health Study saw an increase in breast cancer in women taking androgens.[28]

In her popular book *The Hormone of Desire*, Susan Rako, a psychiatrist in Boston, suggests that there's a sensitive "window" of dosage that works best for women.[29] In her own experience, she has found that if the dose is too high, women may feel worse—agitated and depressed. On the other hand, on a much lower dose (one quarter to one half the dose of Estratest HS), they regain their sense of well-being and libido.

An ad for Estratest in the medical journals pictured a dejected-looking woman, while the copy described the new product as helping "where estrogen alone may not be enough" and "because she wants to feel like herself again." The implication is that this woman's libido is gone, and with it her sense of well-being. On the other side of the page, which reproduces the copy from the package insert, it says that the pill "should only be used for a short period of time because we don't know what the long-term effects are." But the implication of the ad itself belies this small-print message (which is there only because the law requires it). If you're taking this combination of estrogen and testosterone to increase your libido and sense of well-being, you're not just taking it for three months, unless you're planning one last desperate fling before settling into a life of loneliness and gloom. Presumably that's not what the Estratest manufacturers have in mind.

If you decide to take testosterone to increase your libido, you need to know that very little research has been done on it and that you may be risking serious side effects in the future.

DHEA has been touted in the popular press as the answer to aging. At this point there are no data to support this claim nor any safety information.

SALIVARY HORMONE TESTS

As I have mentioned, blood tests for hormones are notoriously variable. Because of this, some labs will test hormone levels in the saliva. Although this may be a good way to measure them, there is no published data to suggest what the right values are for a postmenopausal woman. There is no optimal estrogen level—only the one that feels right for you. The dose of hormones you take should be balanced against your symptoms and not some arbitrary laboratory number determined in blood or saliva.

Although symptom relief is best measured clinically, there are beginning to be some data regarding the serum level of estrogen necessary to prevent subsequent diseases. It's lower than we thought. Bruce Ettinger, M.D., from Kaiser Permanente in Oakland, California, reported a study of elderly women not on HRT, showing that those with estrogen levels between 5 and 25 picograms had half the fracture rate of those with levels less than 5 picograms. Maybe someday we will be able to give just the right amount to those who need it and none to those who don't.

WHAT YOU REALLY WANT TO KNOW: WHAT'S BEST?

Is one form of estrogen better than the others? I doubt it. Is continuous combined hormone therapy better than cyclical therapy? If anything, it may be worse for heart disease, but it will produce less bleeding. Is it safe to take testosterone? Many answers will be forthcoming from the further analysis of the Women's Health Initiative and other ongoing studies. Meanwhile, any woman continuing to take hormones has to realize that she's part of a large experiment.

SIXTEEN

DECISIONS: WHAT SHOULD I DO?

DECISION MAKING

So what now? You've got hot flashes and you can't decide whether to stock up on herbs, buy a bike, or take a pill. Or maybe you should do all three? Your doctor told you to go on hormones years ago to prevent osteoporosis, and now you aren't sure whether to stop. You agree that menopause is just a normal phase in your life, but that doesn't mean it's comfortable. How are you going to "manage" it? It would be nice if you could just say, "Of course I'll take hormones" or "Of course I'll stay on the hormones I've been taking for years." But then you wouldn't be reading this book. As you've realized by now, it's not a simple decision. The ambivalence that women have toward hormones, as I said at the beginning of this book, is well warranted. Hormones can do a lot of good, and they can do a lot of harm.

I hope I've been able to help you clarify the various factors involved in the hormone dilemma. I know, however, that you have one of three questions at this point: Should I start? Should I stop? And what *should* I do for prevention? Post WHI there is only one reason to consider starting on menopausal hormone therapy, and that is for the treatment of severe symptoms that are interfering with the quality of your life. These symptoms vary from woman to woman and any use of hormones carries a risk, so everyone needs to decide whether her own experience warrants treatment. Since the symptoms of perimenopause and early menopause are for the most part transient, women who take hormones for this reason alone will probably want to take them for four to five years at most and then taper off.

The second question of when to stop depends on how long you have been on hormones and why. For women who take estrogen after surgical menopause there may be some benefit in taking hormones initially. Still there are some data that estrogen alone will increase heart disease and blood clots in women who are at risk, and we anticipate the estrogen-alone arm of the WHI will answer whether this is also true for healthy women. We also know there's a cost for all women—a potential increased risk of breast cancer and possibly even of ovarian and lung cancer.

You've seen in this book that there are lots of options for the prevention of the diseases of aging such as osteoporosis and heart disease. In this chapter, I'll clearly outline the risks and benefits in a variety of situations and suggest ways to help you decide on the best approach for yourself.

Before you read any further, let me emphasize what may be the most crucial fact about this decision: *it's not a one-time deal.* You should always reevaluate your choice as your situation, the data, and your thinking change. This has certainly become clear, as you read this new edition, since you'll see that some of the "facts" have changed. You could have very reasonably decided to take HRT for prevention five years ago and have just as reasonably decided to stop this year after hearing of the increase in heart disease, stroke, and breast cancer in the HERS and WHI studies.[1] And there are plenty of other studies going on that will give us even more information. The rest of the Women's Health Initiative will be out in 2006 and will include not only the estrogen-alone study, but also one on low-fat diet, another on calcium and vitamin D supplementation, and an observational study. These, in addition to further analysis of the estrogen and progestin arm, will be a gold mine of information that could change our approach going forward. So it becomes very important that you keep reevaluating your decision, whatever it is. Set a certain time aside to do this, every September, maybe, or on your birthday. You don't want to be second-guessing yourself with every newspaper article, but you do want to recheck your decision periodically. Your health may change, and new information about hormones and other options will probably continue to come out. What makes sense for you today may not make sense five years from today—or even six months from today.

COMPARATIVE RISKS AND BENEFITS

There are many ways we could present the known data to help you get a clear sense of the risks and benefits for the general population of women—keeping in mind that your own situation may or may not fall into that category. I am including several ways to look at the data in the hopes that one will work for you. I must warn you, however, this is the numbers section. If you enjoy looking at data, read on. If you don't, just know that in all situations and at all ages, the risks outweigh or are equal to the benefits of HRT. Now you could skip ahead to the next section on values.

One approach that can help you visualize the magnitude of the potential risk or benefit is to consider what's happening with a hypothetical group of 100 women at age fifty.[2] The number of fifty-year-old white women who would be expected to get hip fractures from osteoporosis over the rest of their lifetime is fifteen out of one hundred (see Figure 16.1). Osteoporosis is one third as common in African-American women. Six out of one hundred African-American women get hip fractures (see Figure 16.2).[3] According to the WHI, estrogen and progestin will decrease hip fractures by five per ten thousand per year. Taking the average life expectancy to be seventy-eight this would be a reduction of 140/10,000 or 1.4/100 fewer fractures bringing the risk to thirteen or fourteen out of one hundred.

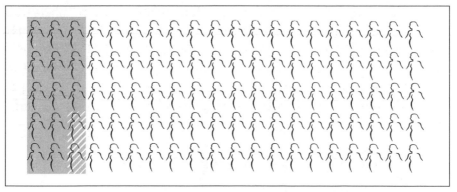

Figure 16.1 Hip fractures: White women.

Although we used to think that estrogen had its full effect on bones only while a woman was on it and quickly disappeared once she stopped, new data from the PEPI study have shown that this may not be true. In examining women who had stopped their HRT and comparing them to women who never took it, they found that bone was not lost at an unusually fast rate after discontinuation, and that use of HRT over three years did not lead to additional bone density gain.[4] So to get these benefits you may not need to take estrogen starting at age fifty and continue on well into your seventies to eighties—about twenty to thirty years. Short-term use for symptom

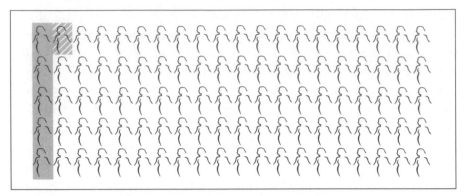

Figure 16.2 Hip fractures: African-American women.

Shaded area: Women with hip fractures

Striped shaded area: Decrease in hip fractures on estrogen

relief may also give you some help for your bones. As we mentioned in Chapter 5, it is better to treat osteoporosis than to try to prevent it at this time, so long-term use of HRT for bones just doesn't make sense.

Of those same 100 fifty-year-old white women, the number who would be expected to get heart disease is 46 (see Figure 16.3). The WHI would suggest an increase in heart disease of 7 per 10,000 per year. Again using an average life expectancy of seventy-eight, this would mean 196 additional cancers per 10,000 or about two more heart attacks per hundred women. This disease is the biggest killer of women, and when

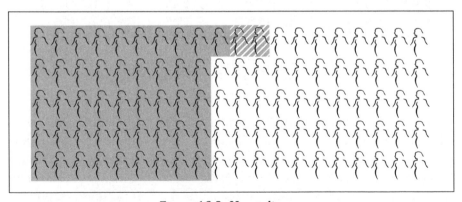

Figure 16.3 Heart disease.

Shaded area: Women with heart disease

Striped shaded area: Women whose heart disease would be prevented on estrogen we thought that ERT/HRT would reduce this, it made it all worthwhile. Now that we have evidence of the reverse, the arguments for using HRT for prevention have all but disappeared.

This is especially so because ten out of these same one hundred fifty-year-old women would normally get breast cancer. (This isn't the familiar one-in-eight chance over your lifetime you're used to hearing, but the number of women out of 100 fifty-year-olds.) WHI would suggest that there would be eight more breast cancers/10,000 women per year (see Figure 16.4). Over a lifetime that would be two more per hundred women. Since the effect appears to be cumulative, this is probably an underestimate. Using the observational data you might expect seven more cancers per hundred in the women on both estrogen plus progestin and two more for the women on estrogen alone. Approximately thirty percent of fifty-year-old women with breast cancer will die of it.

Finally, the number of fifty-year-old women who would naturally get endometrial cancer is three out of one hundred (see Figure 16.5). If these hundred women took estrogen alone for more than five years, twenty-two of them would get endometrial cancer—nineteen extra cases. If the hundred women took both estrogen and progestin, only three of them would get endometrial cancer. In fact the WHI did not show any increase in endometrial cancer.

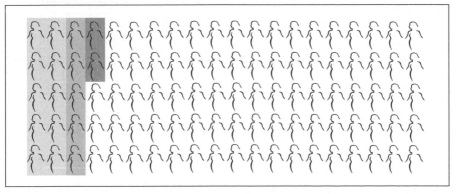

Figure 16.4 Breast cancer.

Light area: Women with breast cancer
Dark area: Additional cases of breast cancer in women on estrogen, based on observational study
Darkest area: Additional cases of breast cancer in women on estrogen plus progestin, based on observational studies

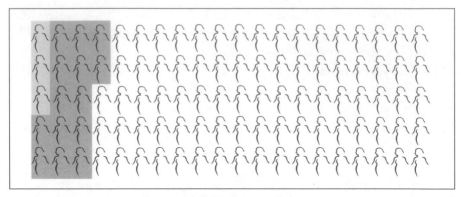

Figure 16.5 Endometrial cancer.

Light area: Women with endometrial cancer
Dark area: Women with endometrial cancer on estrogen

The other risks include about two more strokes, and two more pulmonary emboli per one hundred women who take hormones between the ages of fifty to seventy-eight. The other benefit is a reduction of colon cancer with two fewer cases per hundred women over their lifetime.

Because it is hard for us to put all this together, the investigators of the Women's Health Initiative developed a global index that combined all the risks and complications, giving more weight to the more serious ones. This global index demonstrated an absolute excess of risk of events of nineteen per ten thousand women per year. (Don't try to get to this number by just adding the risks and benefits mentioned above. It is based on a complex formulation used in the study.) But this information by itself is incomplete. You also need to look at the ages at which the diseases affected by hormone therapy typically occur. The average age at which osteoporotic hip fracture is diagnosed is seventy-nine. The average age at which breast cancer is diagnosed is sixty-nine.

The U.S. Preventive Services Task Force has done a great job showing the different risks of HRT at different ages (see Table 16.1).[5] They do this not just for the results of the Women's Health Initiative, but also for a large review they did of all the available studies combined together. Not surprisingly, the findings from the WHI were not that different from the previous work except for the heart disease risk. The table points out that the risks of HRT are bigger the older you are but so are the benefits, especially for fracture prevention. Still in most healthy women who have

TABLE 16.1

Hormone Therapy Use in 10,000 Women: Benefits and Harms per Year from United States Preventive Services Task Force and the Women's Health Initiative

BENEFITS	AGE 55—64		AGE 65—74		AGE 75—84	
	USPSTF	*WHI*	*USPSTF*	*WHI*	*USPSTF*	*WHI*
Hip fractures	3	4	9	13	33	47
Vertebral fractures	32	27	57	49	91	78
Colon cancer	2	3	4	7	7	12.5

HARMS	AGE 55—64		AGE 65—74		AGE 75—84	
	USPSTF	*WHI*	*USPSTF*	*WHI*	*USPSTF*	*WHI*
Coronary heart disease	0	6	0	9	0	11.5
Strokes	1	4	3	9	6	19
Breast cancer	7–11	8	10–15	11	11–17	12
Thromboembolic events (bloods clots in lungs and legs)	1.5	1.4	1.5	1.4	1.5	1.4

Note: The U.S. Preventive Services Task Force (USPSTF) is a meta-analysis of mostly observational studies, and the WHI is the first randomized controlled study of healthy women.

undergone a natural menopause, the long-term use of estrogen and pro-gestin will cause more harm than good.[6]

What if you're not exactly healthy? What if you're at high risk for osteoporosis or colon cancer: is it worth taking postmenopausal hor-mones then? Deborah Grady reviewed these questions at a National Institutes of Health conference in October 2002. She looked at the risks and benefits of the average woman in the Women's Health Initiative for several outcomes and simply added them together to get a net risk of benefit or harm (Table 16.2).[7] She also included the number of women

TABLE 16.2

Risks and Benefits of HRT in All Women over Five Years

	Events/1000/ Five Years	Number of Women Needed to Treat for Five Years to Have One Event
Harm		
Coronary heart disease	3.5	285
Stroke	4	250
Pulmonary emboli (clots)	4	250
Breast cancer	4	250
Benefit		
Hip fracture	−2.5	400
Colon cancer	−3	333
Net events	10	100

Note: Minus numbers indicate harm.

who would have to be treated with HRT for five years for there to be one event of benefit or harm. Ten events per thousand women over five years may not sound like much, but if six million women take HRT for five years it is sixty thousand!

Then she calculated the net benefit or harm if you had osteoporosis on bone density, had osteoporosis and had had a fracture, or had a family history of colon cancer. She found that at best the situation was neutral when you were at very high risk for fracture. In no situation was there a benefit of taking hormones for prevention (Table 16.3).[8]

This is interesting, but what about the risk for a fifty-year-old woman taking menopausal hormones for five years for symptom relief (Table 16.4)?[9] Even in this situation there is a net harm of six events per thousand women over the five years. She repeated the calculations for a woman who had a family history of breast cancer, who was a smoker, or who even had her own history of heart disease. For this table she had to

TABLE 16.3

Net Events of HRT over Five Years in Women at Risk

	Events/1000/ Five Years	Number of Women Needed to Treat for Five Years to Have One Event
Average risk	10	100
Diagnosed with osteoporosis	7.5	133
Osteoporosis plus a fracture	0	
Family history of colon cancer	7.0	142

extrapolate the risks for these women from several databases and used the HERS data to calculate the cardiac benefit since this study specifically studied women with heart disease. Somewhat more speculative, this table still gives us some insights. In each of the situations there was more risk than benefit for disease prevention. Obviously each woman has to decide whether symptom relief is worth this relatively small but real risk.

TABLE 16.4

Net Events of HRT in Young Women (50–55) with or without Risk Factors

	Events/1000/ Five Years	Number of Women Needed to Treat for Five Years to Have One Event
Average risk woman (50–55)	6	166
Family history of breast cancer	7.5	133
Smoker	10	100
History of Heart Disease (HERS)	7.0	142

You can well argue that the WHI was limited to one formulation of estrogen and progestin and that these numbers may not be valid for others such as bioidentical hormones. I think at this point we have to assume that they are all equally dangerous until we have randomized controlled data to suggest that they are safe or beneficial. We got into trouble assuming that HRT was safe before we had data, and we should learn from that error.

VALUES

All these numbers and comparisons are great, but your decision always boils down to how you feel—how you feel physically and how you feel about the different approaches to dealing with menopause. You may have had strong feelings about whether or not to have natural childbirth, or whether or not to take birth control pills. Similarly, you may have strong feelings about how you want to approach menopause. It's those feelings we're after, because they're the most important factor in your decision. They're sometimes hard to sort out. You're exposed to so many *other* people's feelings, and when those people are health professionals, their feelings are often masked as objective truth. Any consultation with an expert—and that's what a doctor's appointment really is—involves an interaction between your feelings, your values, and those of the expert.

The Doctor's Values

When I was in medical school, we were told to put ourselves in the patient's position. What that really meant was to put the patient in our own, imaginary, position. That is, we were supposed to say, "If I were you, I would..." On the surface this sounds very kind and caring. In fact, it's very arrogant. If there's one thing I've learned in over twenty years as a doctor, it's that I'm not my patients. I don't know what I'd do if I were you, any more than you know what you'd do if you were me. Each of my patients is a unique individual, with her own beliefs, fears, hopes, and life history. When I'm lucky, I can tell her with accuracy what her particular medical situation is; what the available therapies are, if she needs any; and what those therapies can and can't do. In short, I can do, in a very specific way, what I'm trying to do more generally in this book—provide the best information I can so that my patient can make the best decision for herself.

Those of you who have been on hormones a long time may wonder why doctors did not question the widespread use of hormones sooner. There were some suggestive studies showing that hormones were good for women, and doctors jumped on the bandwagon hoping to help women before any definitive studies had been done. After a while hormone replacement therapy became the standard of care, and many doctors did not realize that we lacked proof that it worked.

And in the heyday of HRT, many doctors assumed that they knew best. I was interviewed in Toronto in the 1990s by a television reporter in her sixties, who told me her own story. Her gynecologist had said she needed to be on hormone therapy. She'd rather not, she said; she felt fine. The gynecologist was insistent. He asked her to take hormones for two months, keep a daily chart recording how she felt, and then come back to him. He was sure that she'd feel so much better that she'd never want to stop. Instead, she felt terrible. Her breasts hurt, she had headaches, she was retaining fluid, and she'd started bleeding again. She wanted to stop taking the pills. But he began to pressure her again. Since she was short and thin, he was sure she was at high risk of osteoporosis—she should have her bone density tested. She had the test and found out that her bone density was just fine. He finally gave in and stopped badgering her about hormones. (Ironically, his daily chart might be a good idea—if the doctor approaches it as a real learning tool instead of a propaganda device for hormone therapy. If you've already started taking hormones, keeping such a chart might help you decide whether you want to stop.)

Your Values

There was one big advantage to the idea of the doctor as a god. You didn't have to think for yourself. But even though figuring out what you really want to do and what you really think is best for you can be hard work, it's work worth doing.

Among the values you need to consider is what particular diseases frighten you the most. You may have seen your grandmother trapped for years in bed in a nursing home because of a broken hip. That picture scares you so much that you're willing to do whatever you can to avoid it. On the other hand, you may have lost three friends to breast cancer and be much more scared that this could happen to you. You shouldn't be completely driven by fear, but it certainly is a factor to consider.

Another factor to consider is the issue of animal rights mentioned in Chapter 15. Some women who want to take hormones may decide against taking Premarin because it comes from horse urine and decide instead to take a plant-based hormone such as Cenestin, Ogen, or Estratab. For other women, this may not matter at all.

Another consideration is how you feel about discomfort. Do you find even mild hot flashes so embarrassing that you dread showing up at the office? Are you so uncomfortable with drugs that you'd rather put up with sleepless nights than take a pill you don't absolutely need?

Personally, I decided some time ago not to take hormones unless I found myself having extremely debilitating symptoms—and then only temporarily. The research I've done for this book has strengthened my decision. My research has also made me stock up on herbs, reevaluate my diet, and pursue a regular exercise program. So far, I haven't found hormones necessary.

It's important for you to realize that this isn't necessarily an either/or decision. You can take one route only, or combine more than one route, or do nothing at all.

DECISION 1: SHOULD I START TAKING HORMONES?

In an attempt to help you sort out your own values, I've put together a questionnaire to help you to think about treatments for symptoms. My questionnaire is not scientifically validated. Its purpose is to help you sort out your own thinking and feelings about these topics. Sometimes just doing this will make your decision clear to you. Remember, the questionnaire will not decide for you. Like medicine, like alternative treatments, like exercise and diet, a questionnaire is only a tool—to be used when it's helpful and discarded when it's not.

I've given you a way to score your responses and a way to interpret that score. I'm ambivalent about the scoring because while I want to help you clarify your thinking, I don't want you to get fixated on the score— one point more and you'll do x, one point less and you'll do y. Use your responses as a rough guide, not a mandate. The questionnaire is divided into your symptoms, your values, and your risks and should help you sort through where you stand on these aspects of your decision.

QUESTIONNAIRE PART 1: SYMPTOMS

Perimenopausal Symptoms

Hot Flashes
- Once a day or less, and they're manageable. [1]
- More than once a day, and they occasionally interfere with my life. [2]
- Every fifteen minutes, and they're driving me crazy. [3]
- I could deal with them if I knew they were transient. [2]
- I have to do something to stop them. [3]

Night Sweats, Insomnia
- Occasionally I throw the covers off. [1]
- Most nights I wake up once drenched in sweat. [2]
- Every hour I wake up drenched in sweat and I have trouble falling asleep again. [3]
- I could manage if I didn't have to go to work. [2]
- I don't sleep as well as I used to. [1]
- I can't get back to sleep once I wake up. [2]
- I can't function unless I get a full night's sleep. [3]

Mood Swings
- I am more irritable than I used to be. [1]
- I have uncontrollable rages. [3]
- I have crying jags. [2]
- I just want to be alone. [2]
- I am fine one minute and then suddenly angry or depressed and then fine again. [3]
- I am driving my family crazy. [3]
- I haven't noticed any difference. [0]

Vaginal Dryness
- Intercourse is a little uncomfortable. [1]
- I can't even consider intercourse because of the pain involved. [3]
- I feel raw and sore all of the time. [3]
- I am uncomfortable during intercourse but fine otherwise. [2]
- I haven't noticed any change. [0]
- My partner and I are happy with nonpenetrating sex. [1]

Other Symptoms
- My brain does not work right any more. [2]
- I am not as sharp as I used to be, and my job is beginning to suffer. [3]
- I can't remember names but can always find a way around it. [1]
- I have lost my interest in sex, and that devastates me. [3]
- I am not interested in sex, but I find that a relief. [1]
- I haven't noticed any change in my libido. [0]
- I have migraines that are getting worse. [3]
- I sometimes lose urine when I cough or sneeze. [1]
- I sometimes can't get to the bathroom in time. [1]

SCORING: The higher your score, the more symptomatic you are and the more likely you are to benefit from hormones. If your score is 17 or less, hormones are unlikely to improve the quality of your life.

Risks
- I have gallstones. [3]
- I have had thrombophlebitis (clots in my veins). [3]
- I have had heart disease. [3]
- I have high blood pressure. [3]
- I have high cholesterol. [3]
- I have a family history of heart disease. [3]
- I have a family history of stroke. [3]
- I have had a stroke. [3]
- I have a family history of breast cancer. [3]
- I have had a breast biopsy showing atypical hyperplasia or lobular carcinoma in situ. [3]
- I have had breast cancer. [3]
- I have taken birth control pills for over ten years. [3]

SCORING: Although there is always some risk, the higher your score, taking hormones even for symptom relief is more risky for you.

Values

Lifestyle
- I hate pills and would rather tough it out. [1]
- I don't care what it takes, I just want it to get better, and fast. [3]
- I have always favored natural remedies. [2]
- I don't have time to exercise or change my diet—just give me a pill. [3]

- I have always thought that herbs were useless. [3]
- I go to the doctor because she or he is the expert, so I'll do what the doctor says. [3]
- It's important to me to be actively involved in all my own decisions about health care. [1]
- I am willing to experiment with other ways of seeking health care to get rid of my symptoms. [2]
- I am willing to experiment with different approaches to get rid of my symptoms. [2]
- I don't care what the studies say: women on hormones look younger to me. [3]
- I think menopause almost always includes unpleasant symptoms that need treatment. [3]
- I can't let anyone at work know that I am old enough to be going through menopause. [3]
- I don't have time for menopause. [3]
- I couldn't take anything that came from horse urine. [2]

SCORING: The higher your score (>15), the more you favor hormone therapy. If less than 10, you are unlikely to want to use hormones.

This questionnaire is designed to help you with decision one: should I start taking hormones? When you've answered the questionnaire, you'll know that I'm not trying to trick you. If you have a high score in the section on perimenopausal symptoms, you have the most severe symptoms; and if you also score high in the section on values, you'll most likely want to take hormones. On the other hand, if you have low scores for symptoms and low scores for values, you'll be happy with lifestyle changes or with doing nothing. If you score in the middle for both symptoms and values, you're most likely to want to do something, but that something may not be drugs—you'll probably want at least to consider the alternative route. The score on risks helps you see what the tradeoffs are for you. Even taking hormones for one year has some risks, but they are small. It still may be worth it, but you might want to try an alternative first.

Of course, most of us are mismatches. We have terrible symptoms but hate drugs, or our symptoms aren't that bad but are annoying enough that we like the idea of taking a pill to get rid of them. That's okay. If you have terrible symptoms but hate drugs, you'll be very motivated to try lifestyle changes and alternatives. If after several months they don't work, then you can reconsider drugs. And if you'd rather take a pill than put up with any degree of symptoms, you can do that and think about tapering off in a few years.

If you've had a premature menopause or a surgical menopause, you may want to take estrogen, alone or combined with a progesterone, to tide you over what are usually more abrupt and severe symptoms. This doesn't mean you need to take it forever. Give yourself a year or two and then taper off gradually over another six months to a year. If you had a hysterectomy and ovary removal at a young age, you can consider taking hormones until around the natural age of menopause (about fifty) and then taper off. For those of you in this category, lifestyle changes are even more important to maintain your bones and heart in optimum condition. You might also want to start on some of the alternative regimens as you taper off your hormones.

If you've had breast cancer and are faced with sudden menopausal symptoms, you're in a different situation. One problem is that women who have been on hormone therapy are often diagnosed with breast cancer and then are told to stop their hormones cold turkey. This, needless to say, will cause your symptoms to come back with a vengeance. I suggest tapering off over at least two months if possible. The cancer has been there a long time, and I'm not sure that two months will make a difference. Discuss this with your doctor. If you're a premenopausal woman with breast cancer who has undergone chemotherapy and has been abruptly put into menopause as a result, you can also have a lot of problems. There's a 30 percent chance that your periods will come back and the symptoms will go away. If they don't, the symptoms can be intense. (I think that young women who go through menopause abruptly, either surgically or because of drugs, tend to have more intense symptoms than older women, probably because the hormonal shifts are greater.) You might want to consider looking very seriously at lifestyle changes (most of which are also good for preventing a recurrence of breast cancer) and exploring some of the alternatives: soy, paced respiration, acupuncture, black cohosh (RemiFemin), or low-dose antidepressants for hot flashes, nonestrogenic Chinese herbal formulas, vitamin E, or even Estring for vaginal dryness.

If breast cancer isn't a major concern and you decide to take hormones for symptoms, then you have to decide which ones and how to take them. This may be more complicated than it seems. In spite of their eagerness to have you take hormones, some gynecologists feel that you shouldn't take postmenopausal hormones until after you haven't had a period for a year, and so they suggest other, nonhormonal approaches. Others feel that it's better to start on hormone therapy as soon as you have symptoms. One approach is to take the birth control pill in this situation to "regulate your cycle." (Remember when they did that to many of us in puberty?) This approach makes sense because the dose of hormones in the current third-generation pill is still high enough to suppress your own hormonal flux, but there are no studies about it, and it does raise concerns about breast cancer. Another approach is to use progesterone or progestin to try to balance things out. (This is especially appropriate for heavy bleeding, as we discussed in Chapter 11.) And you always want to take the lowest dosage that will help your symptoms.

It's important to realize that any of these approaches could make you feel better or worse. There are whole menus of types of hormones and routes of administration and you should work with your gynecologist to find one that helps you. If they all make you feel bad then you should stop. Since you're taking these pills to control symptoms, it makes no sense to continue them if you're feeling worse.

Have a discussion with your health care provider, and together you can determine the best approach for you. If you feel that your doctor isn't listening to your concerns or doesn't have enough time for you, shop around. This is your body, and your choice. There is no right answer, and your doctor has to be willing to work with you on finding the best solution for you.

Once you've made your choice and found a clinician who'll work with you, it's a good idea to follow the example of the reporter in Toronto and keep a diary of how you feel on the hormone you're taking. This will clarify your symptoms and their timing and help you assess what you want to do. Sometimes you'll need to try several different approaches before you find what works for you. And by that time, your symptoms may even be gone—they're transient, remember. And remember that this decision may be good only for now: be ready to change when circumstances dictate.

DECISION 2: WHEN AND HOW SHOULD I STOP HORMONES?

Many women are on hormones and have been for many years. Should you stop or leave well enough alone? In fact, the data from the WHI and most of the observational studies would indicate that you should stop if you have been on them for more than five years after fifty. Why five years? Because the risk of breast cancer starts going up after five years and increases the more years you have been taking the hormones. This risk happens even if you have no risk factors for breast cancer. We don't think this applies to women who undergo menopause before fifty since early menopause decreases the risk of breast cancer. But by the time they reach fifty the clock starts.

The first thing to ask yourself is why am I on them? If the answer is symptom relief and it has been over five years, you can probably get off gradually and your symptoms will not return. At the very least you can get down to a lower dose. If it was to prevent cardiac disease or stroke, we have sufficient evidence to suggest that you should get off. Hormones increase heart attacks and strokes. If it is to prevent Alzheimer's disease, we have insufficient data to know whether it works, but the harm from other problems outweighs the potential benefit. If it is to protect your bones and you have osteoporosis, you are probably better off with one of the other drugs that have been proven to prevent fractures (see Chapter 5). Finally, there are the less serious but nonetheless compelling reasons of looking young and staying sexually appealing. In this situation I would still suggest getting off because the risks of chronic diseases outweigh the questionable but certainly evanescent chance of holding on to your youth. Overall there are no proven reasons to continue on hormones long term. The good news is that the risk of breast cancer and gall bladder disease goes away as soon as you stop taking the hormones. We do not yet know how long the cardiac and stroke risk lasts. There are some women who are taking hormones to treat a disease where nothing else seems to work. I have talked to women with severe seizures, or migraines that only respond to hormones. Obviously they need to talk the situation over with their doctors to determine the risks and benefits in their specific cases.

But what about quality of life? Every time I get into an argument about hormone therapy with my colleagues (and, mind you, I get into a lot of these arguments), their parting shot is always: "Women feel so much better on hormones." How do they know? My guess is that they're talking about their own experience, or that of their mothers, wives, or girlfriends, rather than any actual study. Why is it that the vast majority of women who start on hormones stop within two years, if they feel so much better? Some women do indeed feel better, but some, like the reporter in Toronto, don't. In fact, when the women who participated in the HERS study were questioned about the quality of their lives, those who were experiencing hot flashes did find that taking Prempro improved the quality of their lives, while the other women did not.

Stopping Hormones

How do you stop? If you've been on hormones for several years and you decide to get off, be sure to taper off slowly, over six to twelve months, rather than quitting abruptly (see Chapter 15). Remember that if you go off and do nothing additional, your cholesterol will probably go up and your bone density will start to go down. A friend of mine told me that she stopped taking Premarin and was surprised to find that her cholesterol was the same as it had been before she had started. So if you're worried about cholesterol, when you stop hormones you should probably change your diet, or exercise, and if your cholesterol is dangerously high, consider specific cholesterol-lowering drugs. A few women will get their symptoms back even if they taper slowly. It then becomes an issue of deciding on the quality of your life. At the very least, get down to the lowest dose you can tolerate.

DECISION 3: WHAT SHOULD I DO FOR PREVENTION?

As you consider stopping your hormones what should you do for prevention? As always there are choices. Depending on your situation you might need preventive drugs such as those that lower cholesterol or blood pressure or those that increase bone density. Sometimes you can have the same effect by quitting smoking, losing weight, and exercising.

If you're a smoker and you quit, you can add 11.5 percent to your life expectancy. Lower your cholesterol, and you'll move into a group whose mortality rate is 40.5 percent lower. Lower your blood pressure, and you'll move into a group whose mortality rate is 55.1 percent lower. If you can avoid non-insulin-dependent diabetes (by weight control), you'll be in a group whose mortality rate is 70 percent lower.[10]

As you look at this information, you begin to realize how right the physical fitness gurus have been all along. Lifestyle changes can be as effective as drugs, and sometimes even more effective. Exercise is beneficial for fighting osteoporosis, heart disease, and breast cancer. It's a little closer to the "designer drugs" the pharmaceutical companies are looking for, but far less expensive.

While we all know we should change our lifestyle, some of us are more likely to do it than others. Sometimes realizing you are indeed at risk can be the impetus to start. Or it can show you that maybe you need to see your doctor and discuss if there are preventive drugs you can take. The second questionnaire will help you sort out your own feelings, risk factors, values, and habits. As with the first questionnaire this is an attempt to help you figure our your risks and values.

QUESTIONNAIRE PART 2: PREVENTION

Risk Factors for Future Disease

Osteoporosis
- I have had a fracture after age fifty. [3]
- My mother has severe osteoporosis. [3]
- I have lost more than an inch in height. [3]
- I spent most of my life dieting. [2]
- I had anorexia nervosa when I was younger. [2]
- I have been an athlete or ballet dancer and lost my period for a while. [2]
- I have taken cortisone or corticosteroids (such as prednisone) for more than five years. [2]
- I have taken thyroid replacement for most of my life. [2]
- I had a hysterectomy and my ovaries out before age forty. [2]
- I had chemotherapy and stopped menstruating before age forty. [2]
- I smoke cigarettes. [2]
- I take medication for seizures. [2]
- I was an athlete as a child and a teenager. [1]
- I exercise at least three times a week. [1]
- I have big bones. [1]
- I have always eaten a high-calcium diet. [1]
- I am overweight. [1]
- I am African American. [1]
- I am Asian. [1]
- I am Caucasian. [3]

Heart Disease
- My mother had a heart attack before age sixty-five. [1]
- My father had a heart attack before age fifty-five. [1]
- I have had a heart attack. [1]
- I have high blood pressure. [1]

- I have a cholesterol count between 230 and 300. [1]
- I have a cholesterol count over 300. [1]
- I have chest pain (angina). [1]
- I am more than twenty pounds overweight. [2]
- I am a couch potato. [2]
- I have a high-stress job, and it's driving me crazy. [2]
- I have diabetes. [2]
- I smoke cigarettes. [2]
- I eat mostly junk food and am unlikely to stop. [2]
- I went through menopause naturally before age forty. [2]
- I had a surgical menopause before age forty. [2]
- I had menopause caused by chemotherapy before age forty. [2]
- I exercise at least three times a week. [1]
- My cholesterol is less than 200. [1]
- I eat a low-fat diet. [1]
- I drink a cocktail or glass of wine a night. [1]

Breast Cancer
- I have had breast cancer or precancer. [1]
- My mother, sister, or daughter has had breast cancer. [1]
- There is breast cancer on my father's side of the family. [1]
- There is colon cancer in my family. [2]
- There is uterine or ovarian cancer in my family. [2]
- I took DES during a pregnancy. [2]
- My first full-term pregnancy was before age thirty. [3]
- My first full-term pregnancy was after thirty-five. [2]
- I have never had children. [2]
- I took birth control pills for more than ten years. [2]
- I am Caucasian. [2]
- I had radiation treatment for acne, or to shrink my thymus gland, or for Hodgkin's disease. [2]
- I received a lot of X rays as a teenager for TB, scoliosis, or chest problems. [2]
- I drink more than three alcoholic drinks a week. [1]
- I rarely drink alcohol. [2]
- I had my first period before age thirteen. [2]
- I had my menopause after age fifty. [2]
- I had my menopause before age forty-five and did not take hormones. [3]

- I exercised more than three times a week when I was premeno-pausal. [3]
- I was an athlete as a teenager and a young adult. [3]
- I rarely exercised as a child or a young adult. [1]
- I have been exercising for the past five years or more. [2]

Endometrial cancer
- My mother had endometrial cancer. [1]
- I am overweight. [2]
- I have more than three alcoholic drinks a week. [2]
- I almost never drink alcohol. [3]

Values
Fears
- I am particularly afraid of breast cancer. [1]
- I am particularly afraid of endometrial cancer. [1]
- I am particularly afraid of heart disease. [1]
- I am particularly afraid of osteoporosis. [3]
- I am particularly afraid of taking drugs. [1]

Habits
- I love junk food. [3]
- I buy vegetables, but they rot in my refrigerator. [3]
- I have never in my life been able to stick to a diet. [3]
- I have never been able to stick to my New Year's resolutions. [3]
- I hate taking vitamins or supplements. [3]
- I think that herbs are worthless. [3]
- I'm willing to try "health foods" if I can find creative, tasty ways to cook them. [1]
- Once I set my mind to do something, I always succeed. [1]
- My family sabotages me every time I try to change. [3]
- I will never quit smoking. [3]
- I drink a glass or more of wine a night and am not about to change now. [3]
- I rarely drink alcohol. [1]
- I have never been able to keep up an exercise program for more than two weeks. [3]

- My stationary bike is a clothes hanger. [3]
- I have never been able to find a sport I like doing. [3]
- I have no time for lifestyle changes. [3]
- I have lost the same twenty pounds fifty times. [3]
- My weight is stable. [1]
- I have never been on a diet. [1]
- I have never been able to take a pill (even for birth control) every day—I always forget. [1]
- I am extremely reliable and will take any medication exactly as directed. [3]
- I always trust my doctor and think he or she knows best. [3]
- My mother went through menopause without drugs and is fine. [1]

A high score for any one disease means you're at higher risk. Don't take this too seriously, either, because these risk factors don't necessarily add up. As I said in an earlier chapter, some of them are like concurrent life sentences. But generally, the more risk factors you have, the greater your chance of getting the disease in question. In the section on values and habits, the higher your score, the more likely you are to lean toward drugs for prevention. The lower your score, the more likely you are to want to explore lifestyle changes and alternatives.

Once you take hormones out of the mix, the decisions become easier: lifestyle changes, drugs, or both. That's when you need to look at your values. Are you at risk for fractures but unlikely to exercise? Then talk to your doctor about drugs to prevent bone loss. If your cholesterol is high but you hate drugs, get to work on losing weight and exercising. (Remember, there are no guarantees with any of this. You can take Fosamax and still get a hip fracture. You can eat well and exercise and still get all of these diseases, or you can smoke, drink, and eat cheesecake every day and live to ninety. We're looking at odds, not certainties.)

So What Should You Do?

At fifty or at the onset of menopause you should reevaluate your lifestyle and health. Get a mammogram and repeat yearly. Have a screening test for colorectal cancer (sigmoidoscopy or colonoscopy). Have your cholesterol, fasting glucose, and blood pressure checked. Repeat normal levels every five years. Stop smoking. Avoid extreme weight loss (risk for osteoporosis) or gain (heart disease and breast cancer). Make sure that you have a diet adequate in calcium and vitamin D (1500mg of calcium and 600–800IU/day of vitamin D). Reduce your salt and animal fat while increasing your fruits, vegetables (DASH diet), fish, and omega-3 fatty acids. Start an exercise program that includes a half an hour three times a week of moderate-intensity dynamic exercise as well as weight training. Make sure you are also exercising your brain. If you decide to take hormone therapy, it should be with the goal of symptom relief and not for the prevention of heart attacks or fractures. If you are at high risk for heart disease, osteoporosis, or breast cancer, you should consult with specialists regarding the use of appropriate drugs for prevention. At sixty-five years, have a DEXA scan to see where you stand regarding bone density. If you are normal or osteopenic, continue the good work. For women sixty or older who have osteoporosis but are not at high risk for nonspine fracture, raloxifene can be used to decrease the risk of spine fracture. Older women with severe osteoporosis and prior fractures might want to consider alendronate or risedronate for their ability to decrease all types of fractures. When available, parathyroid hormone may also be an option.

If you decide to take hormones for symptom relief, you can take bioidentical hormones, conjugated equine estrogen (Premarin), estradiol (Estrace), estrone (Ogen), or esterified estrogen (Estratab); you can wear a patch or take a pill. You should take the lowest dose of hormone that will address your problem. For example, new data are showing that half the standard dose of esterified estrogen (0.3 milligram or even .15mg) can reduce symptoms in some women and has the same beneficial effects on the bones with fewer side effects and possibly less breast cancer risk. And it eliminates the need for a progestin. If you are on a "standard" dose of estrogen and have a uterus, you will need either progesterone or a progestin.

For women who have had breast cancer, the issue is more complex. Although there's a growing trend toward putting women who have had breast cancer on hormone therapy, it scares me a lot. There really are no data confirming its safety. In addition, even if your first cancer is cured, the possibility of a second tumor in the other breast caused by the hormones overshadows any possible protection they might offer against osteoporosis. If you also have osteoporosis, you might consider raloxifene or Fosamax. And don't forget your calcium and vitamin D. For now I'd stick to lifestyle changes.

So what is the final word on ERT/HRT? Short-term use (three to five years) of hormone therapy for relief of severe symptoms is relatively low risk for most women. But according to our current studies, there is no benefit to long-term use, and there is significant harm.

If you have been on hormones for more than five years and are over fifty, you should taper off gradually over six to nine months. You should evaluate your risk for the diseases of aging and look to your lifestyle as the foundation of prevention, adding specific drugs as needed.

What Do I Tell My Doctor?

A friend of mine, a professor of public health, knowing that I was writing this book, said to me, "Whatever else you talk about, be sure you tell your readers how to tell your doctor or provider if you decide to stop taking hormones." She admitted that, for all of her professional success, she was afraid to tell her gynecologist that she wanted to go off hormones after ten years. With all the new data, this should not be as hard as it would have been in 1997 when I wrote the first edition of this book. Most gynecologists are very receptive to a discussion on this issue. Some, however, feel that the data are not all in and that there still may be some benefit. If you want to have a discussion with them, the best way to do this is to come well prepared.

First, call ahead and let your provider know that you want to have a discussion about menopause and hormones. Trying to have this discussion in the middle of a routine yearly visit can be frustrating to both provider and patient. With advance warning, your provider can make sure there's enough time scheduled. Before you go, marshal all of your questions and arguments. Write down your points. Bring a friend with you to the appointment for moral support if you need to. It's often helpful to bring a tape recorder as well. When you're nervous, it can be hard to hear what the doctor is actually saying. And often providers will be more circumspect about what they say when they're being recorded. If your provider has an opinion, ask why, and what data she or he is basing it on. It's important to feel that your provider is a partner you can work with in order to find the right approach to fit your life and values. If it doesn't feel right, it probably isn't—and you should see someone else. Don't forget other options—an herbalist, a traditional Chinese doctor, a homeopath. Remember: this isn't a disease you're treating; it is a normal part of life.

A FINAL THOUGHT: YOU ARE THE EXPERT

For some of you, taking hormones—short term for symptoms—will be the right decision. For others, it won't. There are lots of options open to you, and there will always be different options you can consider, at any time. Medical science doesn't have the right answer—it has only the best guess at the moment. I've tried to give you as much information as possible, so that you'll have some tools to help you make your decision. But the most important tool is one I can't give you: self-knowledge. In the final analysis, it isn't me, or your doctor, or anyone else, who knows what's best for you. For that knowledge, you and you alone are the expert.

And stay tuned. Pay attention to the new studies and try to evaluate the information based on the foundation I have given you. Medicine is a work in progress—and thank God we are finally making some progress in studying menopause.

APPENDIX I

How to Find a Practitioner

Menopause in General

American College of Obstetrics and Gynecology (ACOG)
409 12th Street S.W.
Washington, DC 20024
202-638-5577
www.acog.org

ACOG can give you a list of board-certified physicians. It also publishes pamphlets and reports. Generally its bias is toward HRT.

North American Menopause Society (NAMS)
PO Box 94527
Cleveland, OH 44101
216-844-8748
www.menopause.org

Although they receive support from the pharmaceutical companies, they have become more open lately to alternative viewpoints.

Alternative Approaches

Naturopathy and Herbs

American Association of Naturopathic Physicians
8201 Greensboro Drive, Suite 300
McLean, VA 22102
877-969-2267
www.naturopathic.org

Can provide referrals to naturopaths; also publishes a quarterly newsletter.

National College of Naturopathic Medicine
049 S.W. Porter Street
Portland, OR 97201
503-499-4343
www.ncnm.edu

This college offers a degree in naturopathic medicine and provides referrals.

Northeastern Herbal Association
PO Box 103
Manchaug, MA 01526-0103
www.northeastherbal.org

A membership organization of practicing herbalists, growers of herbs, and students. It has a journal and directory of herbalists in the Northeast.

Vermont School of Herbal Studies
PO Box 232
Marshfield, VT 05658
802-456-1402

An association of practicing herbalists.

Traditional Chinese

New England School of Acupuncture
40 Belmont Street
Watertown, MA 02472
617-926-1788
www.nesa.edu

This school offers a master's-level training in acupuncture and Chinese medicine. It also offers a three-year herbal medicine program.

American College of Traditional Chinese Medicine
455 Arkansas Street
San Francisco, CA 94107
415-282-7600
www.actcm.edu

This college offers a master of science degree in traditional Chinese medicine. Contact for information and referrals to local professional associations and practitioners.

Acupuncture and Oriental Medicine Alliance
14637 Starr Road S.E.
Olalla, WA 98359
253-851-6896
www.acupuncturealliance.org

Makes referrals.

American Association of Oriental Medicine
433 Front Street
Catasaugua, PA 18032-2506
610-266-1433
www.aaom.org

Makes referrals.

Accreditation Commission for Acupuncture and Oriental Medicine
7501 Greenway Drive, Suite 820
Greenbelt, MD 20770
301-313-0855
www.acaom.org

National accrediting agency for established acupuncture and oriental medicine schools and colleges.

National Commission for the Certification of Acupuncturists
11 Canal Center Plaza, Suite 300
Alexandria, VA 22314
703-548-9004
www.nccaom.org

Ensures minimal entry-level professional competence.

In states where acupuncture is licensed and state regulated, you can find the names of local practitioners in the Yellow Pages or by contacting the Department of Health, Board of Medical Examiners, or Department of Licensing. In states without licensing, seek out practitioners who are nationally board certified and have "Dipl. Ac." (for Diplomate of Acupuncture) after their names.

No license is required to practice Chinese herbal medicine. Ask practitioners what their training was and where they went to school. Ask for references from previous patients. Make sure that you can communicate with them. A professional practitioner of Chinese medicine should be able and willing to give a written traditional Chinese diagnosis of the case. Practitioners should also belong to local and national Chinese medicine-acupuncture professional associations.

Homeopathy
North American Society of Homeopaths
1122 East Pike Street, Suite 1122
Seattle, WA 98122
206-720-7000
www.homeopathy.org

Membership organization with certification program and directory of practitioners.

National Center for Homeopathy
801 North Fairfax Street, Suite 306
Alexandria, VA 22314
703-548-7790
www.homeopathic.org

Maintains a directory of homeopaths with a wide range of training and education.

Homeopathic Academy of Naturopathic Physicians
12132 S.E. Foster Place
Portland, OR 97266
503-761-3298
www.healthy.net/HANP

Specialty society affiliated with the American Association of Naturopathic Physicians.

Other: Biofeedback
Association for Applied Psychophysiology and Biofeedback
10200 West 44 Avenue, Suite 304
Wheat Ridge, CO 80033
303-422-8436
www.aapb.org

Its affiliate trains and certifies biofeedback practitioners.

Other: Massage
American Massage Therapy Association
820 Davis Street, Suite 100
Evanston, IL 60201
847-864-0123 and 847-864-1178
www.amtamassage.org

Members must pass a certification exam or graduate from a massage therapy program approved or accredited by an AMTA commission on massage training.

Lifestyle Changes

Support
American Psychological Association
750 First Street N.E.
Washington, DC 20002-4242
202-336-5500
www.apa.org

Published a short book called *Women and Depression: Risk Factors and Treatment.* Also issues a pamphlet, "Choosing a Psychotherapist."

American Association for Marital and Family Therapists
112 S. Alfred Street
Alexandria, VA 22314
703-838-9808
www.aamft.org

Will provide you with a list of certified marital or family therapists in your area.

National Mental Health Association
Information Center
1021 Prince Street
Alexandria, VA 22314-2971
703-684-7722 or 800-969-6642
www.nmha.org

Will give referrals, support, and information.

Meditation and Hypnosis
Maharishi Vedic Schools
888-LearnTM
www.tm.org

Can provide information about local teachers of Transcendental Meditation.

Guided Imagery
Academy for Guided Imagery
PO Box 2070
Mill Valley, CA 94942
800-726-2070
www.interactiveimagery.com

Has a 150-hour training program for health care professionals and publishes a directory of trained imagery practitioners.

Hypnosis

National Guild of Hypnotists
PO Box 308
Merrimack, NH 03054
603-429-9438
www.ngh.net

Offers training and certification programs.

American Institute of Hypnotherapy
2002 E. McFadden, Suite 100
Santa Ana, CA 92705
800-872-9996
www.hypnosis.com

Offers a doctoral program in hypnotherapy.

American Society of Clinical Hypnosis
140 N. Bloomingdale Road
Bloomingdale, IL 60108
630-980-4740
www.asch.net

Will provide a list of medical doctors and dentists who also do hypnosis.

APPENDIX 2

BOOKS, VIDEOS, PAMPHLETS, AND THE INTERNET

Menopause in General

Janine O'Leary Cobb. *Understanding Menopause: Answers and Advice for Women in the Prime of Life.* New York: Penguin, 1993. *A very good and friendly book by the founder of the newsletter "A Friend Indeed."*

Paula Brown Doress, Diana Laskin Siegal (and the Midlife and Older Women Book Project). *Ourselves Growing Older: Women Aging with Knowledge and Power.* New York: Simon and Schuster, 1996. *Very good overview of the second half of life.*

Carol Landau, Ph.D., Michele G. Cyr, M.D., and Anne W. Moulton, M.D. *The Complete Book of Menopause.* New York: Perigee Books, 1995. *Written by two gynecologists and a psychologist, this book is a good overall guide to menopause in all of its aspects. It sticks to traditional medicine and lifestyle issues and doesn't discuss alternative approaches.*

Susan Perry and Katherine A. O'Hanlan, M.D. *Natural Menopause: The Complete Guide to a Woman's Most Misunderstood Passage.* Mass.: Perseus Press, 1996. *A good guide to all of the aspects of menopause from a friendly balanced approach (does not include alternatives).*

Ann M. Voda, R.N., Ph.D. *Menopause, Me, and You: The Sound of Women Pausing.* Binghamton, N.Y.: Haworth Press, 1997. *A wonderful book filled with women's experiences. It is especially strong in describing women's experiences of bleeding.*

ON THE INTERNET

Power Surge: A Virtual Community for Women in the Pause
www.power-surge.com. *This is a wonderful website chock-full of information; has chats with experts in women's health at midlife.*

Menopause with a Slant Toward Drugs

Lila Nachtigall, M.D., and Joan Rattner Heilman. *Estrogen: A Complete Guide to Reversing the Effects of Menopause Using Hormone Replacement Therapy.* New York: HarperCollins, 2000. *Listed in the interest of fair play; this book is very pro-hormone therapy.*

Morris Notelovitz, M.D., and Diana Tonnessen. *Estrogen: Yes or No.* New York: St. Martin's Press, 1993.

————. *Menopause & Midlife Health.* New York: St. Martin's Press, 1993. *A good overall look at midlife, with hints for lifestyle change.*

Menopause with a Slant Toward Natural Approaches

Ellen Brown and Lynne Walker. *Menopause and Estrogen: Natural Alternatives to Hormone Replacement Therapy.* Berkeley, Calif.: Frog, 1996. *An alternative book about menopause.*

Sadja Greenwood, M.D. *Menopause, Naturally: Preparing for the Second Half of Life.* Volcano, Calif.: Volcano, 1996. *A wonderful overview of all the aspects of menopause. To order, call 800-879-9636.*

Dee Ito. *Without Estrogen: Natural Remedies for Menopause and Beyond.* New York: Random House, 1994. *A wonderful tour of the alternative approaches to menopause, complete with examples of how women incorporate them into their lives.*

Susan M. Lark, M.D. *The Estrogen Decision.* Los Altos, Calif.: Westchester, 1994. *Covers hormone therapy and its alternatives. Especially good chapters on yoga and acupressure for menopause.*

Christiane Northrup, M.D. *The Wisdom of Menopause: Creating Physical and Emotional Healing During the Change.* New York: Bantam Doubleday, 2001. *Women's health with a strong holistic philosophy.*

Linda Ojeda, Ph.D. *Menopause Without Medicine.* Alameda, Calif.: Hunter House, 2000. *A good overall book on alternatives to hormones.*

ON THE INTERNET

www.menopause.org
Good site sponsored by North American Menopause Society.

Menopause Textbooks

Karen J. Carlson, M.D., Stephanie A. Eisenstat, M.D., Fredric Frigoletto, Jr., M.D., and Isaac Schiff, M.D. *Primary Care of Women.* St. Louis: Harcourt, 2002. *A multiauthor textbook from Harvard about primary care of women's health.*

Phyllis L. Carr, M.D., Karen M. Freund, M.D., and Sujata Somani, M.D. *The Medical Care of Women.* Philadelphia: Saunders, 1995. *A textbook on all of women's health issues.*

Rogerio A. Lobo, M.D. *Treatment of the Postmenopausal Woman: Basic and Clinical Aspects.* Philadelphia: Lippincott Williams & Wilkins, 1999. *A textbook for physicians. One of the more balanced ones regarding hormone therapy.*

Menopause Culture and Stories

Germaine Greer. *The Change: Women, Aging and the Menopause.* New York: Ballantine, 1993. *A classic.*

Gail Sheehy. *The Silent Passage: Menopause.* New York: Random House, 1992. *The book that started women talking.*

Dena Taylor and Amber Coverdale Sumrall, eds. *Women of the 14th Moon: Writings on Menopause.* Capitola, Calif.: Crossing, 1991. *An anthology of women's experiences.*

Robert A. Wilson. *Feminine Forever.* New York: Evans, 1966. *This is the original and worth a read if you can find it tucked away in the library. He is truly an evangelist for estrogen.*

Menopause Cross-culturally

Y. Beyene. *From Menarche to Menopause: Reproductive Lives of Peasant Women in Two Cultures.* Albany: State University of New York Press, 1989. *An anthropological comparison of menopause among the Mayans in southern Mexico and rural Greek islanders.*

Margaret Lock. *Encounters with Aging: Mythologies of Menopause in Japan and North America.* Berkeley, Calif.: University of California Press, 1995. *Results of twenty years of study of menopause in Japan and North America.*

The Business of Menopause

Sandra Coney. *The Menopause Industry: How the Medical Establishment Exploits Women.* Alameda, Calif.: Hunter House, 1994. *One of the first books to look at the business side of menopause. The pictures of the old ads for hormones alone are worth the price of the book.*

Barbara Seaman and Gideon Seaman. *Women and the Crisis in Sex Hormones.* New York: Rawson, 1977. *One of the first books to look at the widespread use of sex hormones in normal women.*

Heart Disease

Dean Ornish, M.D. *Dr. Dean Ornish's Program for Reversing Heart Disease.* New York: Ivy Books, 1996. *The lifestyle approach to preventing and reversing heart disease. It works.*

American Heart Association. *Women and Heart Disease: The Silent Epidemic* (videotape and brochure). To order, write 7320 Greenville Avenue, Dallas TX 75231, call 800–AHA–USA1, or log on to www.americanheart.org for listing of brochures.

Breast Cancer

Susan Love, M.D. *Dr. Susan Love's Breast Book.* Cambridge, Mass.: Perseus Publishing, 2000. *Everything you want or need to know about benign and malignant breast disease. Women tell me it's the bible.*

Susun S. Weed. *Breast Cancer? Breast Health: The Wise Woman Way.* Woodstock, N.Y.: Ash Tree, 2001. *The herbal approach to breast problems.*

Incontinence

Kathryn L. Burgio. *Staying Dry: A Practical Guide to Bladder Control.* Baltimore and London: Johns Hopkins University Press, 1990. *A best-selling book explaining incontinence; gives an action plan that helps 90 percent of the people who try it.*

Rebecca Chalker and Kristene E. Whitmore, M.D. *Overcoming Bladder Disorders.* New York: Harper and Row, 1991. *An excellent book by a woman urologist.*

Lifestyle Changes

NUTRITION

Mark Messina. *The Simple Soybean and Your Health.* Wayne, N.J.: Avery, 1994. *An authoritative book by one of the world's experts.*

Earl Mindell. *Earl Mindell's Soy Miracle.* New York: Simon and Schuster, 1998. *Good source of information and recipes.*

Elaine Moquette-Magee. *Eat Well for a Healthy Menopause.* New York: Wiley, 1997. *A good healthy approach to nutrition.*

Dean Ornish. *Everyday Cooking.* New York: HarperCollins, 1997.

Harriet Roth. *Deliciously Simple.* New York: Penguin, 1998.

Nina Shandler. *Estrogen: The Natural Way—Over 250 Easy and Delicious Recipes for Menopause.* New York: Villard, 1998.

Walter Willett, P. J. Skerrett, and E. L. Giovannucci. *Eat, Drink and Be Healthy: The Harvard Medical School Guide to Healthy Eating.* New York: Simon and Schuster, 2001.

Marcia S. Williams. *The No Salt, No Sugar, No Apologies Cookbook.* Freedom, Calif.: Crossing, 1986.

———. *More Healthy Cooking.* Freedom, Calif.: Crossing, 1991.

STRETCHING, MUSCLE BUILDING, AND AEROBIC EXERCISES

Bob Anderson, Ed Burke, and Bill Pearl. *Getting in Shape.* Bolinas, Calif.: Shelter Publications, 1995.

Collage Video. *The Complete Guide to Exercise Videos.* Catalog of more than three hundred exercise workout tapes. To order, write 5390 Main St. N.E., Dept. 1, Minneapolis, MN 55421 or call 800-433-6769.

Bob Greene and Oprah Winfrey. *Make the Connection.* New York: Hyperion, 1996.

Lisa Hoffman. *Better Than Ever: The Four-Week Workout Program for Women over Forty.* Chicago: McGraw-Hill, 1997. *A great way to get started.*

Judy Mahle Lutter, Lynn Jaffee, and Staff and Researchers of Melpomene Institute for Women's Health Research. *The Bodywise Woman.* Champaign, Ill.: Human Kinetics, 1996. *Reliable information about physical activity and health.*

Casey Meyers. *Walking: A Complete Guide to the Complete Exercise.* New York: Random House, 1992.

Leora Myers. *Menopause and Beyond: A Fitness Plan for Life.* San Francisco, Calif.: Adelaide, 1996. *Guides you in fitness: stretching, weight training, aerobics, and more.*

Miriam E. Nelson, Ph.D. *Strong Women Stay Young.* New York: Bantam Double-day, 2000. *Especially good on weight training.*

MEDITATION
Herbert Benson. *The Relaxation Response.* New York: Avon, 1975 (reissue 1990). *Classic book about this deceptively simple technique.*

Joan Borysenko. *Minding the Body, Mending the Mind.* New York: Bantam, 1993. *Best-selling book discussing mind-body healing techniques.*

Lawrence LeShan. *How to Meditate.* New York: Bantam, 1974. *Classic book on meditation.*

SUPPORT
Lonnie Barbach. *For Each Other: Sharing Sexual Intimacy.* New York: Signet, 2001.

―――. *The Pause: Positive Approaches to Perimenopause and Menopause.* New York: Plume, 2000.

Karen Johnson, M.D. *Trusting Ourselves: The Complete Guide to Emotional Well-Being for Women.* New York: Atlantic Monthly, 1991. *This book addresses stress, anxiety, depression, and relaxation.*

QUITTING SMOKING
T. Ferguson. *The Smoker's Book of Health.* New York: Putnam, 1987. *How to quit when you are ready and decrease the consequences until you are.*

Alternative Approaches
Craig Clayton and Virginia McCullough. *A Consumer's Guide to Alternative Health Care.* Holbrook, Mass.: Adams, 1995. *A survey of all the alternatives out there.*

Michael Lerner. *Choices in Healing: Integrating the Best of Conventional and Complementary Approaches to Cancer.* Boston: MIT Press, 1994. *A wonderful book on ways to integrate alternative approaches and traditional medicine.*

ON THE INTERNET
Rosenthal Center
www.rosenthal.hs.columbia.edu

Herbs

German Commission E Monograph. Translated and made available by the American Botanical Council ($149), PO Box 201660, Austin, TX 78720. *This is the German government's analysis of indication and safety of commonly used herbs.*

Michael T. Murray, M.D. *The Healing Power of Herbs: The Enlightened Person's Guide to the Wonders of Medicinal Plants.* Rocklin, Calif.: Prima, 1995. *Careful look at selected herbs. Can be ordered by calling 916-632-4400.*

Varro E. Tyler. *The Honest Herbal: A Sensible Guide to the Use of Herbs and Related Remedies.* Binghamton, N.Y.: Haworth, 1993.

Susun Weed. *New Menopausal Years: The Wise Woman Way.* Woodstock, N.Y.: Ash Tree, 2001. *A description of a natural approach to menopause. Includes how to identify and prepare herbs.*

Michael A. Weiner, Ph.D., and Janet Weiner. *Herbs That Heal.* Mill Valley, Calif.: Quantum, 1994. *A good compendium of herbs in general with reviews of the most recent articles.*

On the Internet
American Botanical Council/HerbalGram
www.herbalgram.org

Herb Research Foundation
www.herbs.org

Traditional Chinese Approaches

John Boik. *Cancer and Natural Medicine: A Textbook of Basic Science and Clinical Research.* Princeton, Minn.: Oregon Medical Press, 1996. *This is a wonderfully researched medical book on herbs and how they relate to cancer treatment. It leans toward traditional Chinese herbs.*

Bob Flaws. *Imperial Secrets of Health and Longevity.* Boulder, Colo.: Blue Poppy, 1999. *Introduction to the theories and practices that support longevity and health according to traditional Chinese medicine.*

Ted Kaptchuk. *The Web That Has No Weaver,* 2d edition. New York: McGraw-Hill, 2000. *Said to be the best introduction for anyone interested in exploring Chinese medicine and its theories.*

Honora Lee Wolfe. *Menopause: A Second Spring.* Boulder, Colo.: Blue Poppy Press, 1998. *A good overview of traditional Chinese medicine and how it views menopause.*

Honora Wolfe and Bob Flaws. *Managing Menopause Naturally with Chinese Medicine.* Boulder, Colo.: Blue Poppy Press, 1998.

Mind-Body

Deepak Chopra, M.D. *Perfect Health: The Complete Mind/Body Guide.* New York: Three Rivers Press, 2001. *Nearly everything you need to know to adopt an Ayurvedic lifestyle.*

Alice D. Domar, Ph.D., and Henry Dreher. *Healing Mind, Healthy Woman: Using the Mind-Body Connection to Manage Stress and Take Control of Your Health.* New York: Delta, 1997. *A book applying the principles of the mind-body connection to women's lives.*

Martin Rossman. *Healing Yourself: A Step-by-Step Program for Better Health Through Imagery.* New York: Pocket Books, 1989.

HOMEOPATHY
Trevor Smith. *Homeopathy for the Menopause.* Worthing, England: Insight, 1994.

SUPPLEMENTS
Sherry W. Sultenfuss and Thomas Sultenfuss. *A Woman's Guide to Vitamins and Minerals.* New York: McGraw-Hill, 1999.

Drugs

John Lee and Virginia Hopkins. *What Your Doctor May Not Tell You About Menopause: The Breakthrough Book on Natural Progesterone.* New York: Warner, 1996. *A critical evaluation of the current use of estrogen. Lee is an evangelist for "natural progesterone," however. As I mention in this book, some of the data are provocative, but we aren't quite there yet.*

Susan Rako, M.D. *The Hormone of Desire: The Truth About Sexuality, Menopause, and Testosterone.* New York: Three Rivers Press, 1999. *Provocative look at some women's apparent need for testosterone. More conjecture than science at this point.*

Surgery

Winifred Berg Cutler. *Hysterectomy: Before and After.* New York: HarperCollins, 1990. *A comprehensive book on this often unnecessary surgery.*

William Parker. *A Gynecologist's Second Opinion.* New York: Plume, 1996. *Good descriptions of alternative procedures to hysterectomy.*

Decision Making

Harvard Health Publications Special Report: "Managing Menopause." To order, write to Harvard Health Publications, PO Box 421073, Palm Coast, FL 32142-1073 (or www.health.harvard.edu). *A very good overview of the issues ($16.00).*

National Women's Health Network. "The Truth About Hormone Replacement Therapy," Roseville Calif.: Prima Publishing, 2002. To order, write to National Women's Health Network, 514 10th Street N.W., Suite 400; Washington, DC 20004. *www.womenshealthnetwork.org.*

APPENDIX 3

NEWSLETTERS AND JOURNALS

Menopause in General
A Friend Indeed
Box 260
Pembina, ND 58271
204-989-8028
www.afriendindeed.ca

This newsletter was founded by Janine O'Leary Cobb and is published six times a year. It is chock-full of good information and provides a forum for women to exchange their experiences. $30 a year.

Harvard Women's Health Watch
PO Box 424448
Palm Coast, FL 32142-0448
800-829-5379
www.health.harvard.edu

A very open-minded and balanced view of women's health. $24 a year.

Lifestyle Changes—Nutrition
Nutrition Action Healthletter
Center for Science in the Public Interest, Suite 300
1875 Connecticut Avenue N.W.
Washington, DC 20009-5728
202-332-9110
www.cspinet.org/nah
$15 a year (10 issues).

Soy Connection Newsletter
PO Box 237
Jefferson City, MO 65102
888-772-8445
www.talksoy.com
Free.

Tufts University Health and Nutrition Letter
PO Box 420912
Palm Coast, FL 32142
800-274-7581
www.healthletter.tufts.edu

Published monthly by Tufts University; $28 a year.

Alternative Approaches—Herbs

HerbalGram
American Botanical Council
PO Box 144345
Austin, TX 78714
800-373-7105
www.herbalgram.org

A source of information about herbs; $35 a year, published quarterly.

ON THE INTERNET

www.remifemin.com

Website maintained by Glaxo SmithKline, makers of RemiFemin Menopause. This black cohosh preparation is an herbal preparation that has been extensively studied.

APPENDIX 4

ORGANIZATIONS

Menopause in General
National Women's Health Network
514 10th Street N.W., Suite 400
Washington, DC 20004
202-347-1140
www.womenshealthnetwork.org

This is a national public-interest organization dedicated to women's health issues. It has a booklet on menopause and a newsletter, "The Network News."

National Black Woman's Health Project
600 Pennsylvania Ave S.E., Suite 310
Washington, DC 20003
202-543-9311
202-543-9743 fax
www.nbwhp.org

An advocacy and support group.

The North American Menopause Society (NAMS)
PO Box 94527
Cleveland, OH 44101
440-442-7550
440-442-2660 fax
www.menopause.org

The preeminent professional menopause association in the United States holds a yearly meeting and publishes a journal. It has some ties with the pharmaceutical industry but is becoming more open to alternatives.

International Menopause Society
Av. des Cattleyas, 3, Box 1
1150 Brussels, Belgium
(011) 32.2.772.2183

Primarily a group of gynecologists promoting the study of medical intervention in menopause. Publishes the journal *Climacteric.*

Older Women's League
666 11th Street N.W., Suite 700
Washington, DC 20001
202-783-6686
www.owl-national.org

An advocacy organization that focuses on issues of concern to middle-aged and older women.

Society for Menstrual Cycle Research
c/o Mary Anna Friederich, M.D.
10559 N. 104 Place
Scottsdale, AZ 85258
maryannafriederich@msn.com

Membership is $20 a year and includes a quarterly newsletter.

Boston Women's Health Book Collective
PO Box 192
Somerville, MA 02144
617-414-1230
617-414-1233 fax
www.ourbodiesourselves.org

In addition to publishing *The New Our Bodies, Ourselves* and *The New Ourselves, Growing Older,* the collective maintains a public information center.

Osteoporosis
National Osteoporosis Foundation
2100 M Street N.W., Suite 602
Washington, DC 20037
800-223-9994
www.nof.org

Heart Disease
American Heart Association
7272 Greenville Avenue
Dallas, TX 75231
800-242-8721
www.americanheart.org

Breast Cancer
National Breast Cancer Coalition
1707 L Street N.W., Suite 1060
Washington, DC 20036
202-296-7477
www.natlbcc.or

Advocates for more breast cancer research money and monitors how it is spent.

Susan Love MD Breast Cancer Foundation
427 East Carrillo Street
Santa Barbara, CA 93101
805-963-2877
805-963-2877 fax
www.susanlovemdfoundation.org

Funds research into the intraductal approach and maintains the SusanLoveMD.org website.

Y-ME National Breast Cancer Organization
212 West Van Buren Street
312-986-8338
800-221-2141
www.y-me.org

Runs support groups and maintains a hotline in English and Spanish.

Cancer in General
Commonweal Cancer Help Program
PO Box 316
Bolinas, CA 94924
415-868-0970
www.commonweal.org

Holds retreats for individuals with cancer.

National Coalition for Cancer Survivorship
1010 Wayne Avenue, Suite 770
Silver Spring, MD 20910
301-650-9127
301-565-9670 fax
www.canceradvocacy.org

Wellness Community—National
35 East 7th Street, Suite 412
Cincinnati, OH 45202
888-793-WELL
513-421-7119 fax
www.wellness-community.org

Free support groups; many local chapters.

Wellness Community (L.A.)
2716 Ocean Park Boulevard
Santa Monica, CA 90405
310-314-2571
310-314-7586 fax
www.la.wellnesscommunity.org

Other: Lupus

Lupus Foundation of America, Inc.
1300 Piccard Drive, Suite 200
Rockville, MD 20850-4303
301-670-9292
301-670-9486 fax
www.lupus.org

Other: Incontinence

National Association for Continence
PO Box 8310
Spartanburg, SC 29305-8310
800-BLADDER
864 579-7902 fax
www.nafc.org

$15 membership fee; free quarterly newsletter and a *Resource Guide of Continence Aids and Services* ($10).

Lifestyle Changes

Exercise
Melpomene Institute for Women's Health Research
1010 University Avenue
St. Paul, MN 55104
612-642-1951
www.melpomene.org

This group has been studying the relationship between women's health and physical activity since 1981. It publishes the *Melpomene Journal* three times a year.

Prevention Walking Club
Rodale Press/Prevention Magazine
33 E. Minor Street
Emmaus, PA 18098-0099
610-967-5171
610-967-8963 fax
www.prevention.com/cda/center

Free monthly email newsletter and folks to motivate you.

Runner's World
Rodale Press
800-666-2828
www.runnersworld.com

Popular running-related website and magazine.

Support
Self-Help Clearinghouse
St. Clares–Riverside Medical Center
25 Pocono Road
Denville, NJ 07834
www.mentalhelp.net/selfhelp/

This group has information about support groups for various illnesses.

National Mental Health Consumers' Self-Help Clearinghouse
1211 Chestnut Street, Suite 1207
Philadelphia, PA 19107
800-553-4539
215-636-6312 fax
www.mhselfhelp.org

This group provides technical assistance to mental health support groups.

Quitting Smoking
American Lung Association
1740 Broadway
New York, NY 10019-4374
212-315-8700
www.lungusa.org

Information about quitting smoking.

Alternative Approaches

Herbs
Herb Research Foundation
1007 Pearl Street, Suite 200
Boulder, CO 80302
303-449-2265
303-449-7849
www.herbs.org

HRF is a clearinghouse for information about herbalism, and especially new research. It is a membership-based organization.

California School of Herbal Studies
PO Box 39
Forestville, CA 95436
707-887-7457
www.cshs.com

A school offering a nine-month program in Western herbalism.

Mind-Body
Mind/Body Medical Institute
Beth Israel—Deaconess Hospital
110 Francis Street
Boston, MA 02215
617-632-9530
www.mbmi.org

A good source of relaxation tapes.

Mind-Body Health Sciences, Inc.
393 Dixon Road
Boulder, CO 80302
303-440-8460
303-440-7580 fax
www.joanborysenko.com

Drugs
American College of Obstetricians and Gynecologists Resource Center
409 12th Street S.W.
PO Box 96920
Washington, DC 20090-6920
202-638-3577
www.acog.org

Surgery
Hysterectomy Educational Resources and Services (HERS Foundation)
422 Bryn Mawr Avenue
Bala Cynwyd, PA 19004
610-667-7757
888-750HERS
www.hersfoundation.com

APPENDIX 5

THE DASH DIET

This eating plan is from the "Dietary Approaches to Stop Hypertension" (DASH) clinical study. The research was funded by the National Heart, Lung, and Blood Institute (NHLBI), with additional support by the National Center for Research Resources and the Office of Research on Minority Health, all units of the National Institutes of Health. DASH's final results appear in the April 17, 1997, issue of *The New England Journal of Medicine*. The results show that the DASH "combination diet" lowered blood pressure and, so, may help prevent and control high blood pressure.

The "combination diet" is rich in fruits, vegetables, and low-fat dairy foods, and low in saturated and total fat. It also is low in cholesterol, high in dietary fiber, potassium, calcium, and magnesium, and moderately high in protein.

The DASH eating plan shown below is based on two thousand calories a day. The number of daily servings in a food group may vary from those listed depending on your caloric needs. The DASH eating diet was not designed to promote weight loss but it is rich in lower-calorie foods such as fruits and vegetables. You can make it lower in calories by replacing higher-calorie foods with more fruits and vegetables or decreasing portion size.

The DASH Diet and accompanying twenty pages of information (NIH Publication NO. 01-4082) may be found on the web at www.nhlbi.nih.gov/health/public/heart/hbp/dash or ordered from NHLBI Information Center, PO 30105, Bethesda MD 20824. Single copies are free of charge.

THE DASH DIET

FOOD GROUP	DAILY SERVING SIZES (EXCEPT AS NOTED)	SERVING OF EACH FOOD GROUP TO THE DASH EATING PLAN	EXAMPLES OF SIGNIFICANCE; NOTES
Grains and grain products	7–8	1 slice bread 1 oz dry cereal* ½ cup cooked rice, pasta or cereal	whole wheat bread, English muffin, pita bread, bagel, cereals, grits, oatmeal, crackers, unsalted pretzels and popcorn; major sources of energy and fiber
Vegetables	4–5	1 cup raw leafy vegetable ½ cup cooked vegetable 6 oz vegetable juice	tomatoes, potatoes, carrots, peas, squash, broccoli, turnip greens, collards, kale, spinach, artichokes, green beans, lima beans, sweet potatoes; rich sources of potassium, magnesium, and fiber
Fruits	4–5	6 oz fruit juice 1 medium fruit ¼ cup dried fruit ½ cup fresh, frozen, or canned fruit	apricots, bananas, dates, grapes, oranges, orange or grapefruit juice, mangoes, melons, peaches, prunes, pineapples, raisins, figs, strawberries, tangerines; important sources of potassium, magnesium, and fiber
Low-fat or fat-free dairy foods	2–3	8 oz milk 1 cup yogurt 1½ oz cheese	fat-free (skim) or low-fat (1%) milk or buttermilk, fat-free or low-fat regular or frozen yogurt, low-fat and fat-free cheeses; major sources of calcium and protein

* Equals ½–1¼ cup, depending on cereal type. Check the product's nutrition label.

THE DASH DIET

FOOD GROUP	DAILY SERVING SIZES (EXCEPT AS NOTED)	SERVING OF EACH FOOD GROUP TO THE DASH EATING PLAN	EXAMPLES OF SIGNIFICANCE; NOTES
Meats, poultry, and fish	2 or less	3 oz cooked meats, poultry, or fish	select only lean; trim away visible fats; broil, roast, or boil, instead of frying; remove skin from poultry; rich sources of protein and magnesium
Nuts, seeds, and dry beans	4–5 per week	$\frac{1}{3}$ cup or 1$\frac{1}{2}$ oz nuts 2 tbsp or $\frac{1}{2}$ oz seeds $\frac{1}{2}$ cup cooked dry beans	almonds, filberts, mixed nuts, peanuts, walnuts, sunflower seeds, kidney beans, lentils; rich sources of energy, magnesium, potassium, protein, and fiber
Fats and oils**	2–3	1 tsp soft margarine 1 tbsp low-fat mayonnaise 2 tbsp light salad dressing 1 tsp vegetable oil	soft margarine, low-fat mayonnaise, light salad dressing, vegetable oil (such as olive, canola, or safflower); DASH has 27 percent of calories as fat, including that in or added to foods
Sweets	5 per week	1 tbsp sugar 1 tbsp jelly or jam $\frac{1}{2}$ oz jelly beans 8 oz lemonade	maple syrup, sugar, jelly; sweets should be jam, fruit-flavored gelatin, low in fat beans, hard candy, fruit punch sorbets, ices

** Fat content changes serving counts for fats and oils: For example, 1 tablespoon of regular salad dressing equals 1 serving; 1 tablespoon of a low-fat dressing equals $\frac{1}{2}$ serving; 1 tablespoon of a fat-free dressing equals 0 servings.

NOTES

Introduction

1. Yoffe, Emily. "Hormonal imbalances: Why were all those women taking hormones in the first place?" http://slate.msn.com, July 11, 2002, at 3:14 P.M. PT.

Chapter 1. What Is Menopause?

1. Neugarten, B. L., and Kraines, R. J. "Menopausal symptoms in women of various ages." *Psychosomatic Medicine* 1965; 27: 266–273.

2. Sherman, B. M., and Korenman, S. G. "Hormonal characteristics of the human menstrual cycle throughout reproductive life." *Journal of Clinical Investigation* 1975; 55: 699–706.

3. Shideler, S. E., DeVane, G. W., Kalra, P. S., Benirschke, K., and Lasley, B. I. "Ovarian-pituitary hormone interactions during the perimenopause." *Maturitas* 1989; 11(4): 331–339.

4. Santorro, N., Brown, Jr., Asa, T., and Skjrnick, J. H. "Characterization of reproductive hormonal dynamics in the perimenopause." *Journal of Clinical Endocrinology and Metabolism* 1996; 81: 1495–1501.

5. Burger, H. G. "The menopause: When it is all over or is it?" *Australian New Zealand Journal Obstetrics and Gynaecology* 1994; 34(3): 293–295.

6. New England Research, Inc. *Women and Their Health in Massachusetts: Final Report 1991*. Watertown, Mass.: New England Research Institute, 1991.

7. Sluijmer, A. V., Heineman, M. J., De Jong, F. H., and Evers, J. L. "Endocrine activity of the postmenopausal ovary: The effects of pituitary down-regulation and oophorectomy." *Journal of Clinical Endocrinology and Metabolism* 1995; 80: 2163–2167.

Ushiroyama, T., and Sugimoto, O. "Endocrine function of the peri- and postmenopausal ovary." *Hormone Research* 1995; 44: 64–68.

8. Hreshchyshyn, M. M., Hopkins, A., Zylstra, S., and Anbar, M. "Effects of natural menopause, hysterectomy, and oophorectomy on lumbar spine and femoral neck bone densities." *Obstetrics and Gynecology* 1988; 72: 631.

9. Cauley, J. A., Gutal, J. P., Kuller, L. H., LeDonne, D., and Powell, J. G. "The epidemiology of serum sex hormones in postmenopausal women." *American Journal of Epidemiology* 1989; 129(6): 1120–1131.

10. Yen, S. C., and Jaffe, R. B. *Reproductive Endocrinology.* Philadelphia: Saunders, 1991, p. 585.

11. Petrakis, N. L. "Oestrogens and other biochemical and cytological componenets in nipple aspirates of breast fluid: Relationship to risk factors for breast disease." *Proceedings of the Royal Society of Edinburgh* 1989; 95B: 169–181.

12. Hreshchyshyn, op. cit.

13. Stone, L. *The Family, Sex, and Marriage.* New York: Harper and Row, 1979, p. 67.

14. Hale, J. R. *Renaissance Europe.* Berkeley: University of California Press, 1971, p. 15.

15. Fraser, A. *The Weaker Vessel.* New York: Vintage, 1984, p. 101.

16. Utian, W. "Overview on menopause." *American Journal of Obstetrics and Gynecology* 1987; 156(5): 1280–1283.

17. Lock, M. "Menopause: Lessons from anthropology." Presentation at annual meeting, North American Menopause Society, San Francisco, Sept. 21–23, 1995.

18. Diamond, J. "Why women change." *Discover* July 1996: 131–137.

19. Weed, S. *The Menopausal Years: The Wise Woman Way.* Woodstock, N.Y.: Ash Tree, 1992.

20. Quoted in Gray, F. D. "The third age." *The New Yorker* (Special Women's Issue), Feb. 26/March 4, 1996: 191.

21. Quoted ibid.

Chapter 2. The Medicalization of Menopause

1. Coney, S. *The Menopause Industry.* Alameda, Calif.: Hunter House, 1994, p. 67.

2. Utian, W. H. "Overview on menopause." *American Journal of Obstetrics and Gynecology* 1987; 156: 1280–1283.

3. Ibid., p. 1280.

4. Wilson, R. *Feminine Forever.* New York: Evans, 1966.

5. Rhoades, F. P. "Minimizing the menopause." *Journal of the American Geriatric Society* 1967; 15(4): 346–354.

6. Utian, op. cit., p. 1281.

7. Ibid., p. 1283.

8. Barrett-Connor, E., and Miller, V. "Estrogens, lipids, and heart disease." *Clinics in Geriatric Medicine* 1993(9): 57–67.

9. McCullough, M. "Hope or hype?" *Philadelphia Inquirer,* May 13, 1996.

10. Pike, M. C., Pike, A., Rude, R., Shoupe, D., and Richardson, J. "Pilot trial of a gonadotropin hormone agonist with replacement hormones as a prototype contraceptive to prevent breast cancer." *Contraception* 1993; 47(5): 427–444.

11. van Keep, P. A. "The history and rationale of hormone replacement therapy." *Maturitas* 1990; 12: 163–170.

12. Ibid., p. 167.

13. Leiblum, S. R., and Swartzman, L. C. "Women's attitudes toward the menopause: An update." *Maturitas* 1986; 8(1): 47–56.

14. Lock, M., Kaufert, P., and Gilbert, P. "Cultural construction of the menopausal syndrome: The Japanese case." *Maturitas* 1988; 10: 317–332.

15. Lock, M. "Menopause in cultural context." *Experimental Gerontology* 1994; 29(3/4): 307–317.

16. Ibid., p. 313.

17. Flint, M., and Samil, R. S. "Cultural and subcultural meanings of the menopause." In *Multidisciplinary Perspectives on Menopause,* Flint, M.,

Kronenberg, F., and Utian, W. (eds.). *Annals of New York Academy of Sciences,* 1990, pp. 134–148, discussion 185–192.

18. Martin, M. C., Block, J. E., Sanchez, S. D., Arnaud, C. D., and Beyene, Y. "Menopause without symptoms: The endocrinology of menopause among rural Mayan Indians." *American Journal of Obstetrics and Gynecology* 1993; 168(6): 1839–1845.

19. Flint, M., and Samil, R. S. op. cit.

20. Beyene, Y. "Cultural significance and physiological manifestation of menopause: A biocultural analysis." *Culture, Medicine, and Psychiatry* 1986; 10: 47–71.

21. Chirawitkul, T., and Manderson, L. "Perception of menopause in Northeast Thailand: Contested meaning and practice." *Social Science Medicine* 1994; 39(11): 1545–1554.

22. Ibid., p. 1546.

23. Cooper, W. *No Change: A Biological Revolution for Women.* London: Arrow, 1983.

24. Hunt, K. "Perceived value of treatment among a group of long-term users of hormone replacement therapy." *Journal of the Royal College of General Practitioners* 1988; 38: 398–401.

25. Ibid., pp. 399–400.

26. Hunter, M. S., and Liao, K. L. "Intentions to use hormone replacement therapy in a community sample of 45 year old women." *Maturitas* 1994; 20: 13–23.

27. Doress-Worters, P. B. Preface to Coney, op. cit., p. 9.

28. Wilson, op. cit., pp. 18ff.

29. Cyran, W. "Estrogen replacement therapy and publicity." In *Aging and Estrogens. Frontiers of Hormone Research,* Vol. 2, Lauritzen, C., and van Keep, P. A. (eds.). Basel: Karger, 1973, p. 152.

30. Lee, J. R. *What Your Doctor May Not Tell You About Menopause.* New York: Warner, 1996.

31. Seaman, B., and Seaman, G. *Women and the Crisis in Sex Hormones.* New York: Bantam, 1977.

32. Wilson, op. cit., p. 97.

33. Hemminki, E., and Sihvo, S. "A review of postmenopausal hormone therapy recommendations: Potential for selection bias." *Obstetrics and Gynecology* 1993; 82(6): 1021–1028.

34. Coronary Drug Project Research Group. "The Coronary Drug Project: Initial findings leading to modifications of its research protocol." *Journal of the American Medical Association* 1970; 214: 1303–1313.

35. Ziel, H. K., and Finkle, W. D. "Increased risk of endometrial carcinoma among users of conjugated estrogens." *New England Journal of Medicine* 1970; 293: 1167–1170.

36. *Wall Street Journal,* June 15, 1995: 5.

37. Hemminki and Sihvo, op. cit.

38. Meyers, J. H. *The U.S. Retail Prescription Market Year in Review.* Boca Raton, Fla. CPSNET, 1966.

39. Bowman, M. A., and Pearle, D. L. "Changes in drug prescribing patterns related to commercial company funding of continuing medical education." *Journal of Continuing Education of the Health Professions* 1988; 8(1): 13–20.

40. Tanouye, E. "Estrogen study shifts ground for women and for drug firms." *Wall Street Journal,* June 15, 1995: A5.

41. Utian, W. "Nonhormonal medication." In *Modern Approach to the Menopausal Years,* Greenblatt, Robert (ed.). Berlin, N.Y.: DeGruyter, 1986, pp. 117–125.

42. Prior, J. "One voice on menopause." *Journal of the American Women's Association* Jan.–Feb. 1994; 49(1): 27–29.

43. Seaman and Seaman, op. cit., pp. 6–7.

44. Fletcher, S., and Colditz, G. A. "Failure of estrogen plus progestin therapy for prevention." *Journal of the American Medical Association* 2000; 288(3).

45. Kreling, D., Mott, D., Wiederholt, J., et al. "Prescription drug trends: A chartbook update." Menlo Park, Cal.: Kaiser Family Foundation, November 2001.

46. *Osteoporosis Report* 1995; 11(3): 7.

Chapter 3. "What Does It Feel Like?"

1. Cobb, J. O. *Understanding Menopause*. New York: Plume, 1993.

2. New England Research Institute, Inc. *Women and Their Health in Massachusetts: Final Report*. Watertown, Mass.: NERI, 1991.

3. Bungay, G. T., Vessey, M. P., and McPherson, C. K. "Study of symptoms in middle life with special reference to the menopause." *British Medical Journal* 1980; 281(6234): 181–183.

4. Gambone, J., Meldrum, D. R., Laufer, L., Chang, R. J., Lu, J. K. H., and Judd, H. L. "Further delineation of hypothalamic dysfunction responsible for menopausal hot flashes." *Journal of Clinical Endocrinology Metabolism* 1984; 59: 1097.

5. New England Research Institute, op. cit.

6. Judd, H. L. "The pathophysiology of menopausal hot flushes." In *Neuroendocrinology of Aging*, Meites, J. (ed.). New York: Plenum, 1983, pp. 173–202.

7. Voda, A. "Climacteric hot flashes." *Maturitas* 1981; 3: 73–90.

8. Weed, S. *The Menopausal Years: The Wise Woman Way*. Woodstock, N.Y.: Ash Tree, 1992.

9. Greenwood, S. *Menopause Naturally*. Volcano, Calif.: Volcano, 1996, p. 32.

10. Holte, A. "Influences of natural menopause on health complaints: A prospective study of healthy Norwegian women." *Maturitas* 1992; 14: 127–141.
    Kaufert, P. A., Gilbert, P., and Tate, R. "The Manitoba Project: A reexamination of the link between menopause and depression." *Maturitas* 1992; 14: 143–155.
    New England Research Institute, op. cit.

11. Greene, J. G., and Cooke, D. J. "Life stress and symptoms at the climacterium." *British Journal of Psychiatry* 1980; 136: 486–491.

12. New England Research Institute, op. cit.

13. Yesavage, J. A., and Sheikh, J. I. "Nonpharmacologic treatment of age-associated memory impairment." *Comprehensive Therapy* 1988; 14(6): 44–46.

14. Sherwin, B. B. "Estrogenic effects on memory in women." *Annals of New York Academy of Sciences* 1994; 14(743): 213–230.

15. Sherwin, B. B. "Estrogen and/or androgen replacement therapy and cognitive functioning in surgically menopausal women." *Psychoneuroendocrinology* 1988; 10: 325–335.

16. Barrett-Connor, E., and Kritz-Silverstein, D. "Estrogen replacement therapy and cognitive function in older women." *Journal of the American Medical Association* 1993; 260: 2637–2641.

17. Robinson, D., Friedman, L., Marcus, R., Tinklenberg, J., and Yesavage, J. "Estrogen replacement therapy and memory in older women." *Journal of the American Geriatric Society* 1994; 42(9): 919–922.

18. Voytko, M. L. "Estrogen effects on cognition in brain biology." Presentation at IBC Menopause Conference, Philadelphia, Penn., May 9–10, 1996.

19. New England Research Institute, op. cit.

20. Hunter, M., Battersby, R., and Whitehead, M. "Relationships between psychological symptoms, somatic complaints, and menopausal status." *Maturitas* 1986 (8): 217–228.

21. Ibid.

22. Castelo-Branco, C., Duran, M., and Gonzalez-Merlo, J. "Skin collagen changes related to age and hormone replacement therapy." *Maturitas* 1992; 15: 113–119.

23. Savas, M., Bishop, J., Laurent, G., Watson, N., and Studd, J. "Type III collagen content in the skin of postmenopausal women receiving oestradiol and testosterone implants." *British Journal of Obstetrics and Gynaecology* 1993; 100(2): 154–156.

24. Holland, E. F., Studd, J. W., Mansell, J. P., Leather, A. T., and Bailey, A. J. "Changes in collagen composition and cross-links in bone and skin of osteoporotic postmenopausal women treated with percutaneous estradiol implants." *Obstetrics and Gynecology* 1994; 83(2): 180–183.

25. Dunn, L. B., Damesyn, M., Moore, A. A., Reuben, D. B., and Greendale, G. A. "Does estrogen prevent skin aging? Results from the First National Health and Nutrition Examination Survey (NHANES 1)." *Archives of Dermatology* 1997; 133(3): 339–342.

26. Brown, J. S., Sawaya, G., Thom, D. H., and Grady, D. "Hysterectomy and urinary incontinence: A systematic review." *Lancet* 2000; 356(9229): 535–539.

27. Hulley, S., Grady, D., Bush, T. et al. Randomized trial of estrogen plus progestin for secondary prevention of coronary heart disease in postmenopausal women. Heart and Estrogen/progestin Replacement Study (HERS) Research Group. *Journal of the American Medical Association* 1998; 28050–280513.

28. Raz, R., and Stamm, W. E. "A controlled trial of intravaginal estriol in postmenopausal women with recurrent urinary tract infections." *New England Journal of Medicine* 1993; 329(11): 753–756.

29. Pfeiffer, E., and Davis, G. C. "Determinants of sexual behavior in middle and old age." *Journal of the American Geriatric Society* 1972; 20(4): 151–158.

30. Sarrel, P. M., and Whitehead, M. I. "Sex and menopause: Defining the issues." *Maturitas* 1985; 7(3): 217–224.

31. McCoy, N., and Davidson, J. M. "A longitudinal study of the effects of menopause on sexuality." *Maturitas* 1985; 7(3): 203–210.

32. Chirawitkul, T., and Manderson, L. "Perception of menopause in Northeast Thailand: Contested meaning and practice." *Social Science Medicine* 1994; 39(11): 1545–1554.

33. Michael, R. P., and Keverne, E. B. "A male sex-attractant on rhesus monkey vaginal secretions." *Journal of Endocrinology* 1970; 46(2): xx–xxi.

34. Sherwin, B. B. "Changes in sexual behavior as a function of plasma sex steroid levels in post-menopausal women." *Maturitas* 1985; 7: 225–233.

35. Rako, S. *The Hormone of Desire.* New York: Harmony Books, 1996.

36. Cauley, J. A., Lucas, F. L., Kuller, L. H., et al. "Elevated serum estradiol and testosterone concentrations are associated with a high risk for breast cancer. Study of Osteoporotic Fractures Research Group." *Annals of Internal Medicine* 1999; 130(4 Pt 1): 270–277.

Chapter 4. Prevention and Risk: Understanding Research

1. Writing Group for the Women's Health Initiative Investigators. "Risks and benefits of estrogen plus progestin in healthy postmenopausal women: Principal results from the Women's Health Initiative randomized controlled trial." *Journal of the American Medical Association* 2002; 288 (3): 321–333.

2. Stampfer, M. J., Colditz, G. A., Willett, W. C., Manson, J. E., Rosner, B., Speizer, F. E., and Hennekens, C. H. "Postmenopausal estrogen therapy and

cardiovascular disease: Ten-year follow up from the Nurses' Health Study." *New England Journal of Medicine* 1991; 325: 756–762.

3. Writing Group for the Women's Health Initiative Investigators, op. cit.

4. Coronary Drug Project Research Group. "The Coronary Drug Project: Initial findings leading to modifications of its research protocol." *Journal of the American Medical Association* 1970; 214: 1303–1313.

5. Matthews, K. A., Kuller, L. H., Wing, R. R., Meilahn, E. N., and Plantinga, P. "Health prior to use of estrogen replacement therapy: Are users healthier than nonusers?" *American Journal of Epidemiology* 1996; 143: 971–978.

6. Matthews, K. A., Kuller, L. H., Wing, R. R., Meilahn, E. N., and Platinga, P. "Health prior to hormone use: Matthews et al. reply to Grodstein." *American Journal of Epidemiology* 1996; 143: 983–984.

7. Petitti, D. B. "Coronary heart disease and estrogen replacement therapy: Can compliance bias explain the results of observational studies?" *Annals of Epidemiology* 1994; 4: 115–118.

8. Matthews et al., ". . . Reply to Grodstein."

9. Colditz, G. A., Hankinson, S. E., Hunter, D. J., Willett, W. C., Manson, J. E., Stampfer, M. J., Hennekens, C., Rosner, B., and Speizer, F. E. "The use of estrogens and progestins and the risk of breast cancer in postmenopausal women." *New England Journal of Medicine* 1995; 332: 1589–1593.

10. Stanford, J. L., Weiss, N. S., Voight, L. F., Daling, J. R., Habel, L. A., and Rosing, M. "Combined estrogen and progestin hormone replacement therapy in relation to risk of breast cancer." *Journal of the American Medical Association* 1995; 274: 37–142.

11. Adami, H. O., and Persson, I. "Hormone replacement and breast cancer: A remaining controversy?" *Journal of the American Medical Association* 1995; 274: 178–179.

Chapter 5. Osteoporosis: Are We All Going to Crumble?

1. Tenenhouse, A. "Epidemiology of osteoporosis." *First McGill International Symposium on Recent Advances in Infertility and Reproductive Endocrinology Pre IX World Congress on Human Reproduction Symposium,* May 28, 1996.

2. Kanis, J. A. "Are oestrogen deficiency and hormone replacement a distraction to the field of osteoporosis?" *Osteoporosis International* 1998 Suppl. 1: S51–S56.

3. Pocock, N. A., Eisman, J. A., Hopper, J. L., Yeates, M. G., Sambrook, P. N., and Eberl, S. "Genetic determinants of bone mass in adults: A twin study." *Journal of Clinical Investigations* 1987; 80: 706–710.

4. Hughes, B. D., Harris, S. S., Krall, E. A., and Dallal, G. E. "Effect of calcium and vitamin D supplementation on bone density in men and women sixty-five years of age or older." *New England Journal of Medicine* 1997; 337: 670–676.

5. Conference Report Consensus Development Conference. "Prophylaxis and treatment of osteoporosis." *American Journal of Medicine* 1991; 90: 107–110.

6. McClung, M. R. "Clinical utility of bone density testing." *Menopause Management* 2000; July/Aug.: 6–10.

7. Ettinger, B. "Guidelines for established osteoporosis treatment." *Menopause Management* 1997; Sept./Oct.: 7–9.

8. Kanis, J. A., Melton, J., Christiansen, C., Johnston, C. C., and Khaltaev, N. "The diagnosis of osteoporosis." *Journal of Bone and Mineral Research* 1994; 9: 1137–1141.

9. Ibid., p. 1138.

10. Melton L. J., Chrischilles, E. A., Cooper, C., Lane, A. W., and Riggs, B. L. "How many women have osteoporosis?" *Journal of Bone and Mineral Research* 1992; 9: 1005–1009.

11. Tobias, J. H., Cook, D. G., Chambers, T. J., and Dalsell, N. "A comparison of bone mineral density between Caucasian, Asian and Afro-Caribbean women." *Clinical Science* 1994; 87: 587–591.

12. Kanis, J. A., Johnell, O., et al. "Risk of hip fracture according to the World Health Organization criteria for osteopenia and osteoporosis." *Bone* 2000; 27: 585–590.

13. "Understanding osteoporosis and osteopenia," available at www.susanlovemd.org. Accessed September 2, 2002.

14. Ibid.

15. Kanis et al., 2000, op cit.

16. Prior, J. C., Vigna, Y. M., Barr, S. I., Kennedy, S., Schulzer, M., and Li, D. K. B. "Ovulatory premenopausal women lose cancellous spinal bone: A five-year prospective study." *Bone* 1996; 18: 261–267.

17. Riis, B. J. "The role of bone loss." *American Journal of Medicine* 1995; 98(Supp. 12A): 2A/29S–2A/32S.

18. Clements, D., Compston, J. E., Evans, C., and Evans, W. D. "Bone loss in normal British women: A 5-year follow up." *British Journal of Radiology* 1993; 66; 1134–1137.

19. Kanis, J. A., and Adami, S. "Bone loss in the elderly." *Osteoporosis International* 1994; Supp. 1: S59–65.

20. Pansini, F., Bagni, B., Bonaccorsi, G., Albertazzi, P., Zanotti, L., Farina, A., Campobasso, C., Orlandi, R., and Mollica, G. "Oophorectomy and spine bone density: Evidence of a higher rate of bone loss in surgical compared with spontaneous menopause." *Menopause: Journal of the North American Menopause Society* 1995; 2(2): 109–115.

21. Bruns, M. E., Overpeck, J. G., Smith, G. C., Hirsch, G. N., Mills, S. F., and Bruns, D. E. "Vitamin D dependent calcium binding protein in rat uterus: Differential effects of estrogen, tamoxifen, progesterones, and pregnancy on accumulation and cellular localization." *Endocrinology* 1988; 122(6): 2371–2378.

22. Martin, M. C., Block, J. E., Sanchez, S. D., Arnaud, C. D., and Beyene, Y. "Menopause without symptoms: The endocrinology of menopause among rural Mayan Indians." *American Journal of Obstetrics and Gynecology* 1993; 168(6): 1839–1845.

23. Siddle, N., Sarrel, P., and Whitehead, M. "The effect of hysterectomy on the age at ovarian failure: Identification of a subgroup of women with premature loss of ovarian function and literature reviews." *Fertility and Sterility* 1987; 47(1): 94–100.

24. Pike, M. C., Pike, A., Rude, R., Shoupe, D., and Richardson, J. "Pilot trial of a gonadotropin hormone agonist with replacement hormones as a prototype contraceptive to prevent breast cancer." *Contraception* 1993; 47(5): 427–444.

25. Seeman, E., Hopper, J. L., Bach, L. A., Cooper, M. E., Parkinson, E., McKay, J., and Jerums, G. "Reduced bone mass in daughters of women with osteoporosis." *New England Journal of Medicine* 1989; 20(9): 554–558.

26. Cummings, S. R., Nevitt, M. C., Browner, W. S., Stone, K., Fox, K. M., Ensrud, K. E., Cauley, J., Black, D., and Vogt, T. M. "Risk factors for hip fracture in white women." *New England Journal of Medicine* 1995; 332: 767–773.

27. Sarkar, S., Mitlak, B. H., et al. "Relationships between bone mineral density and incident vertebral fracture risk with raloxifene therapy." *Journal of Bone and Mineral Research* 2002; 17: 1–10.

28. Kanis et al., 1994, op. cit.

29. Chrischilles, E. A., Butler, D., Cavis, C. S., and Wallace, R. B. "A model of lifetime osteoporosis impact." *Archives of Internal Medicine* 1991; 151: 2026–2032.

30. Owen, R. A., Melton, L. J., Johnson, K. A., Ilstrup, D. M., and Riggs, B, L. "Incidence of Colles' fracture in a North American community." *American Journal of Public Health* 1982; 72: 605–607.

31. Jensen, G. F., Christiansen, C., Boesen, J., Hegedus, V., and Transbol, I. "Relationship between bone and mineral content and frequency of postmenopausal fractures." *Acta Medica Scandinavia* 1983; 213: 61–63.

32. Melton, L. J. "Epidemiology of fractures." In *Osteoporosis: Etiology, Diagnosis, and Management,* Riggs, B. L., and Melton, L. J. (eds.). New York: Raven, 1988, pp. 133–154.

33. Jensen et al., op. cit.

34. Chrischilles et al., op. cit.

35. Ibid.

36. Clements et al., op. cit.

37. Melton, L. J., Eddy, D. M., and Johnston, C. C. "Screening for osteoporosis." *Annals of Internal Medicine* 1990; 112(7): 516–528.

38. Cummings, S. R., Palerno, L., Browner, W., et al. "Monitoring osteoporosis therapy with bone densitometry: Misleading changes and regression to the mean." *Journal of the American Medical Association* 2000; 283: 1318–1321.

39. Kanis, J. A., 1998, op. cit.

40. Ettinger, B., Genant, H. K., and Cann, C. E. "Long-term estrogen replacement therapy prevents bone loss and fractures." *Annals of Internal Medicine* 1985; 102: 319–324.

41. Lee, J. R. *Natural Progesterone.* Sebastopol, Calif.: BLL, 1993.

42. Leonetti, H. B., Longo, S., and Anasti, J. N. "Transdermal progesterone cream for vasomotor symptoms and postmenopausal bone loss." *Obstetrics and Gynecology* 1999; 94(2): 225–228.

43. Lufkin, E. G., Wahner, H. W., O'Fallon, W. M., et al. "Treatment of postmenopausal osteoporosis with transdermal estrogen." *Annals of Internal Medicine* 1992; 117: 1–9.

44. The Writing Group for the PEPI Trial. "Effects of hormone therapy on bone mineral density: Results from the Postmenopausal Estrogen/Progestin Intervention (PEPI) Trial." *Journal of the American Medical Association* 1996; 276: 1389–1396.

45. Cauley, J. A., Black, D. M., Barrett-Connor, E., et al. "Effects of hormone replacement therapy on clinical fractures and height loss: The Heart and Estrogen/Progestin Replacement Study (HERS)." *American Journal of Medicine* 2001; 110: 442–450.

46. Torgerson, D. J., and Bell-Syer, S. E. M. "Hormone replacement therapy and prevention of nonvertebral fractures: A meta-analysis of randomized trials." *Journal of the American Medical Association* 2001; 285: 2891–2897.

47. Writing Group for the Women's Health Initiative Investigators. "Risks and benefits of estrogen plus progestin in healthy postmenopausal women: Principal results from the Women's Health Initiative randomized controlled trial." *Journal of the American Medical Association* 2002; 288(3): 321–333.

48. Ettinger, B., and Grady, D. "The waning effect of postmenopausal estrogen on osteoporosis." *New England Journal of Medicine* 1993; 329: 1192–1193.

49. Sowers, M., Clark, M., Hollis, B., Wallace, R., and Jannausch, M. "Radial bone mineral density in pre- and perimenopausal women: A prospective study of rates and risk factors." *Journal of Bone and Mineral Research* 1992; 7: 647–657.
    Pouilles, J. M., Tremollieres, F., and Ribbot, C. "The effects of menopause on longitudinal bone loss from the spine." *Calcified Tissue International* 1993; 52: 340–343.

50. Ensrud, K. E., Palermo, L., Black, D. M., et al. "Hip bone loss increases with advancing age: Longitudinal results from the study of osteoporotic fractures." In *Sixteenth Annual Meeting of the American Society for Bone and Mineral Research,* Raisz, L. G. (ed.). Kansas City, Mo.: Liebert, 1994, S153.

51. Black, D. "Alendronate prevents hip and other fractures in some osteoporosis patients." Presentation at 1996 World Conference on Osteoporosis. Amsterdam, Netherlands, May 1996.

52. Black D. M. "Why elderly women should be screened and treated to prevent osteoporosis." *American Journal of Medicine* 1995; 98(Supp. 12A): 2A/67S–2A/75S.

53. "Understanding osteoporosis and osteopenia," op. cit.

54. Ibid.

Chapter 6.   Heart Disease: What's Your Real Risk?

1. Lawlor, D. A., and Smith, G. D. "Sex matters: secular and geographical trends in sex differences in coronary heart disease mortality." *British Medical Journal* 2001 (323): 541–545.

2. Bush, T. L. "The epidemiology of cardiovascular disease in postmenopausal women." *Annals of New York Academy of Sciences* 1990; 592: 263–271; (discussion) 334–345.

3. Berliner, J. A., Navab, M., Fogelman, A. M., Frank, J. S., Demer, L. L., Edwards, P. A., Watson, A. D., and Lusis, A. J. "Atherosclerosis: Basic mechanisms. Oxidation, inflammation, and genetics." *Circulation* 1995; 91(9): 2488–2496.

4. Verhoef, P., Kok, F. J., Kruyssen, D. A., Schouten, E. G., Witteman, J. C., Grobbee, D. E., Ueland, P. M., and Refsum, H. "Plasma total homocysteine, B vitamins, and risk of coronary atherosclerosis." *Arteriosclerosis, Thrombosis and Vascular Biology* 1997; 17(5): 989–995.

5. Schwartz, S. M., Siscovick, D. S., Malinow, M. R., Rosendaal, F. R., Beverly, R. K., Hess, D. L., Psaty, B. M., Longstreth, W. T., Koepsell, T. D., Raghunathan, T. E., and Reitsma, P. H., "Myocardial infarction in young women in relation to plasma total homocysteine, folate, and a common variant in the methylene-tetrahydrofolate reductase gene." *Circulation* 1997; 96(2): 412–417.

6. Rimm, E. B., Willett, W. C., Hu, F. B., et al. "Folate and vitamin B_6 from diet and supplements in relation to risk of coronary heart disease among women." *Journal of the American Medical Association* 1998; 279: 359–364.

7. Ridker, P. M., Rifai, N., Rose, L., et al. "Comparison of C-reactive protein and low-density lipoprotein cholesterol levels in the prediction of first cardiovascular events." *New England Journal of Medicine* 2002; 347(20): 1557–1565.

8. Williams, R. *The Trusting Heart.* New York: Washington Square, 1985.

9. Scherwitz, L., McKelvain, R., Laman, C., et al. "Type A behavior, self-involvement, and coronary atherosclerosis." *Psychosomatic Medicine* 1983; 45(1): 45–57.

10. Clarkson, T. B., Adams, M. R., Kaplan, J. R., Shively, C. A., and Koritnik, D. R. "From menarche to menopause: Coronary artery atherosclerosis and protection in cynomolgus monkeys." *American Journal of Obstetrics and Gynecology* 1989; 160(5): 1280–1285.

11. Haertel, U., Heiss, G., Filipiak, B., and Doering, A. "Cross-sectional and longitudinal associations between high-density lipoprotein cholesterol and women's employment." *American Journal of Epidemiology* 1992; 135: 68–78.

12. Haynes, S. G., and Feinleib, M. "Women, work and coronary heart disease: Prospective findings from the Framingham heart study." *American Journal of Public Health* 1980; 70(2): 133–141.

13. Bush, T. L., "The epidemiology of cardiovascular disease in postmenopausal women." *Annals of New York Academy of Sciences* 1990; 592: 263–271.

14. Grady, D., Rubin, S. M., Petitti, D. B., et al. "Hormone therapy to prevent disease and prolong life in postmenopausal women." *Annals of Internal Medicine* 1992; 117: 1016–1037.

15. Greenland, P., Reicher-Reiss, H., Goldbourt, U., et al. "In hospital and 1 year mortality in 1524 women after myocardial infarction." *Circulation* 1991; 83: 484.

16. Oliver, M., and Boyd, G. "Effect of bilateral ovariectomy on coronary artery disease and serum-lipid levels." *Lancet* 1959; 31: 690–694.

17. Barrett-Connor, E., and Goodman-Gruen, D. "Prospective study of endogenous sex hormones and fatal cardiovascular disease in postmenopausal women." *British Medical Journal* 1995; 311: 1193–1196.

18. Coronary Drug Project Research Group. "The Coronary Drug Project: Findings leading to discontinuation of the 2.5 mg/day estrogen arm." *Journal of the American Medical Association* 1973; 226: 652–657.

19. Bush, T. L., Barrett-Connor, E., Cowan, L. D., Criqui, M. H., Wallace, R. B., Suchindran, C. M., Tyroler, H. A., and Rifkind, B. M. "Cardiovascular mortality and noncontraceptive use of estrogen in women: Results from the Lipid Research Clinics Program Follow-up Study." *Circulation* 1987; 75: 1102–1109.

20. Stampfer, M. J., and Colditz, G. A. "Estrogen replacement therapy and coronary heart disease: A quantitative assessment of the epidemiologic evidence." *Preventive Medicine* 1991; 20: 47–63.

21. Grodstein, F., Stampfer, M. J., Manson, J. E., Colditz, G. A., Willett, W. C., Rosner, B., Speizer, F. E., and Hennekens, C. H. "Postmenopausal estrogen and

progestin use: The risk of cardiovascular disease." *New England Journal of Medicine* 1996; 335.

22. Barrett-Connor, E. "Postmenopausal estrogen and prevention bias." *Annals of Internal Medicine* 1991; 115: 455–456.

23. Matthews, K. A., Kuller, L. H., Wing, R. R., Meilahn, E. N., and Plantinga, P. "Prior to use of estrogen replacement therapy, are users healthier than nonusers?" *American Journal of Epidemiology* 1996; 143: 971–978.

24. Petitti, D. B. "Coronary heart disease and estrogen replacement therapy: Can compliance bias explain the results of observational studies?" *Annals of Epidemiology* 1994; 4: 115–118.

25. LaCroix, A. Z. "Psychosocial factors and risk of coronary heart disease in women: An epidemiologic perspective." *Fertility and Sterility* 1994; 62: 133S–139S.

26. Correspondence between Barbara Kriegsmann (executive director of marketing, Wyeth-Ayerst) and Robyn Lipner (professional staff member, Committee on Labor and Human Resources, United States Senate), April 16, 1991.

27. Writing Group for the PEPI Trial. "Effects of estrogen or estrogen/progestin regimens on heart disease risk factors in postmenopausal women: The postmenopausal estrogen/progestin interventions (PEPI) trial." *Journal of the American Medical Association* 1995; 272(3): 199–208.

28. Ibid.

29. Hulley, S., Grady, D., Bush, T., et al. "Randomized trial of estrogen plus progestin for secondary prevention of coronary heart disease in postmenopausal women." Heart and Estrogen/progestin Replacement Study (HERS) Research Group. *Journal of the American Medical Association* 1998; 28/280(7): 605–613.

30. Herrington, D., Reboussin, D. M., Brosnihan, K. B., et al. "Effects of estrogen replacement on the progression of coronary artery atherosclerosis." *New England Journal of Medicine* 2000; 343(8): 522–529.

31. Grady, D., Herrington, D., Bittner, V., et al. "Cardiovascular disease outcomes during 6.8 years of hormone therapy: Heart and Estrogen/progestin Replacement Study follow-up (HERS II)." *Journal of the American Medical Association* 2002; 288: 49–57.

32. Writing Group for the Women's Health Initiative Investigators. "Risks and benefits of estrogen plus progestin in healthy postmenopausal women: Principal

results from the Women's Health Initiative randomized controlled trial." *Journal of the American Medical Association* 2002; 288(3): 321–333.

33. Humphrey, L. L., Chan, B. K. S., Sox, H. C. "Postmenopausal hormone replacement therapy and the primary prevention of cardiovascular disease." *Annals of Internal Medicine* 2002; 137: 273–284.

Nelson, H. D., Humphrey, L. L., Nygren, P., Teutsch, S. M., and Allan, J. D. "Postmenopausal hormone replacement therapy: Scientific review." *Journal of the American Medical Association* 2002; 288: 872–881.

34. Sherwin, B. B., Gelfand, M. M., Schucher, R., and Gabor, J. "Postmenopausal estrogen and androgen replacement and lipoprotein lipid concentrations." *American Journal of Obstetrics and Gynecology* 1987; 156: 414–419.

35. Mosca, L., Collins, P., Herrington, D., et al. "Hormone replacement therapy and cardiovascular disease: A statement for healthcare professionals from the American Heart Association." *Circulation* 2001; 104: 499–503.

Chapter 7. Breast Cancer: Every Woman's Fear?

1. Writing Group for the Women's Health Initiative Investigators. "Risks and benefits of estrogen plus progestin in healthy postmenopausal women: Principal results from the Women's Health Initiative randomized controlled trial." *Journal of the American Medical Association* 2002; 288(3): 321–333.

2. Horwitz, K. B., Sartorius, C. A., Hovland, A. R., Jackson, T. A., Groshong, S. D., Tung, L., and Takimoto, G. S. "Surprises with antiprogestins: Novel mechanisms of progesterone receptor action." *CIBA Foundation Symposium* 1995; 191: 235–249; (discussion) 250–253.

3. Pike, M., Spicer, D. V., Dahmoush, L., and Press, M. F. "Estrogens, progestogens, normal breast cell proliferation, and breast cancer risk." *Epidemiologic Reviews* 1993; 15(1): 17–35.

4. Kuiper, G. G., Enmark, E., Pelto-Huikko, M., Nilsson, S., and Gustafsson, J. A. "Cloning of a novel receptor expressed in rat prostate and ovary." *Proceedings of National Academy of Sciences U.S.A.* 93(12): 5925–5930, June 11, 1996.

5. Feinleib, M. "Breast cancer and artificial menopause: A cohort study." *Journal of the National Cancer Institute* 1968; 41: 315–329.

6. Zhang, Y., Kiel, D., Kreger, B., et al. "Bone mass and the risk of breast cancer among postmenopausal women." *New England Journal of Medicine* 1997; 336: 611–617.

Verbeek, A. L. M., Hendricks, J. H. C. L., Peeters, P. H. M., and Sturmans, F. "Mammographic breast pattern and the risk of breast cancer." *Lancet,* 1: 591–593, 1984.

7. Hoffman, D. A., Lonstein, J. E., Morin, M. M., et al. "Breast cancer in women with scoliosis exposed to multiple diagnostic X rays." *Journal of the National Cancer Institute* 1989; 81: 1307.

8. Bernstein, L., Hanisch, R., Sullivan-Halley, J., and Ross, R. K. "Treatment with human chorionic gonadotropin and risk of breast cancer." *Cancer Epidemiology Biomarkers and Prevention* 1995; 4: 437–440.

9. Wolff, M. S., Toniolo, P. G., Lee, E. W., Rivera, M., and Dubin, N. "Blood levels of organochlorine residues and risk of breast cancer." *Journal of the National Cancer Institute* 1993; 85: 648.

10. Hunter, D. J., Hankinson, S. E., Laden, F., et al. "Plasma organochlorine levels and the risk of breast cancer." *New England Journal of Medicine* 1997; 337: 1253–1258.

11. Barnes, S., Peterson, T. G., and Coward, L. "Rationale for the use of genistein–containing soy matrices in chemoprevention trials for breast and prostate cancer." *Journal of Cellular Biochemistry* 1995; Supp. 22: 181–187.

12. Berrino, F., Muti, P., Micheli, A., Bolelli, G., Krogh, V., Sciajno, R., Pisani, P., Panico, S., and Secreto, G. "Serum sex hormone levels after menopause and subsequent breast cancer." *Journal of the National Cancer Institute* 1996; 88(5): 291–296.

13. Elia, M., Handpour, S., Terranova, P., Anderson, J., Klemp, J. R., and Fabian, C. J. "Marked variation in nipple aspirate fluid (NAF) estrogen concentration and NAF/serum ratios between ducts in high risk women." *Proceedings Annual Meeting of American Association of Cancer Research* 2002; abstract #4072.

14. Greenberg, E. R., Barnes, A. B., Resseguie, L., et al. "Breast cancer in mothers given diethylstilbesterol in pregnancy." *New England Journal of Medicine* 1984; 311: 1393.

15. Rookus, M. A., and van Leeuwen, F. E. "Oral contraceptives and risk of breast cancer in women aged 20–54 years." *Lancet* 1994; 344: 844–851.

16. Writing Group for the Women's Health Initiative Investigators, op. cit.

17. Schairer, C., Byrne, C., Keyl, P. M., Brinton, L. A., Sturgeon, S. R., and Hoover, R. N. "Menopausal estrogen and estrogen-progestin replacement therapy

and risk of breast cancer (United States)." *Cancer Causes and Control* 1994; 5(6): 491–500.

18. Ross, R. K., Paganini-Hill, A., Wan, P. C., and Pike, M. C. "Effect of hormone replacement therapy on breast cancer risk: Estrogen versus estrogen plus progestin." *Journal of the National Cancer Institute* 2000; 92: 328–332.

19. Colditz, G. A., Hankinson, S. E., Hunter, D. J., Willett, W. C., Manson, J. E., Stampfer, M. J., Hennekens, C., Rosner, B., and Speizer, F. E. "The use of estrogens and progestins and the risk of breast cancer in postmenopausal women." *New England Journal of Medicine* 1995; 332: 1589–1593.

20. Ettinger, B., Quesenberry, C., Schroeder, D. A., and Friedman, G. "Long-term postmenopausal estrogen therapy may be associated with increased risk of breast cancer: A cohort study." *Menopause* 1997; 4(3): 125–129.

21. Greendale, G. A., Reboussin, B. A., Sie, A., et al. "Effects of estrogen and estrogen-progestin on mammographic parenchymal density." *Annals of Internal Medicine* 1999; 130: 262–269.

22. Persson, I., Thurfjell, E., Bergstrom, R., and Holmberg, L. "Hormone replacement therapy and the risk of breast cancer. Nested case-control study in a cohort of Swedish women attending mammography screening." *International Journal of Cancer* 1977; 72(5): 758–761.

23. Collaborative Group on Hormonal Factors in Breast Cancer. "Breast cancer and hormone replacement therapy: Collaborative reanalysis of data from fifty-one epidemiological studies of 52,050 women with breast cancer and 108,411 women without breast cancer." *Lancet* 1997; 350: 1047–1059.

24. Grodstein, F., Stampfer, M. J., Colditz, G. A., et al. "Postmenopausal hormone therapy and mortality." *New England Journal of Medicine* 1997; 336: 1769–1775.

25. Bergkvist, L., Adami, H. O., Persson, I., Bergstrom, R., and Krusemo, U. B. "Prognosis after breast cancer diagnosis in women exposed to estrogen and estrogen-progestin replacement therapy." *American Journal of Epidemiology* 1989; 130(2): 221–227.

26. Chen, C. L., Weiss, N. S., Newcomb, P., Barlow, W., and White, E. "Hormone replacement therapy in relation to breast cancer." *Journal of the American Medical Association* 2002; 287: 734–741.
    Newcomer, L. M., Newcomb, P. A., Daling, J. R., et al. "Postmenopausal hormone use and risk of breast cancer by histologic type." *American Journal of Epidemiology* 1999; 149: S79.

Li, C. I., Weiss, N. S., Stanford, J. L., and Daling, J. R. "Hormone replacement therapy in relation to risk of lobular and ductal breast carcinoma in middle-aged women." *Cancer* 2000; 88: 2570–2577.

Newcomb, P. A., Titus-Ernstoff, L., Egan, K. M., et al. "Postmenopausal estrogen and progestin use in relation to breast cancer risk." *Cancer Epidemiology, Biomarkers and Prevention* 2002; 11: 593–600.

27. Colditz et al., op. cit.

28. Writing Group for the Women's Health Initiative Investigators, op. cit.

29. Stomper, P. C., Van Voorhis, B. J., Ravnikar, V. A., and Meyer, J. E. "Mammographic changes associated with postmenopausal hormone replacement therapy: A longitudinal study." *Radiology* 1990; 174: 487–490.

30. Laya, M. B., Larson, E. B., Taplin, S. H., and White, E. "Effect of estrogen replacement therapy on the specificity and sensitivity of screening mammography." *Journal of the National Cancer Institute* 1996; 88(10): 643–649.

31. Byrne, C., Schairer, C., Wolfe, J., Parekh, N., Salane, M., Brinton, L., Hoover, R., and Haile, R. "Mammographic features and breast cancer risk: Effects with time, age, and menopause status." *Journal of the National Cancer Institute* 1995; 87: 1622–1629.

32. Grady, D., Rubin, S. M., Petitti, D. B., et al. "Hormone therapy to prevent disease and prolong life in postmenopausal women." *Annals of Internal Medicine* 1992; 117: 1016–1037.

33. DiSaia, P. J., Grosen, E. Q., Odicino, F., Cowan, B., Pecorelli, S., Wile, A., and Creasman, W. T. "Replacement therapy for breast cancer survivors: A pilot study." *Cancer* 1995; 76: 2075–2078.

Eden, J. A., Bush, T., Nand, S., and Wren, B. G. "A case-control study of combined continuous estrogen-progestin replacement therapy among women with a personal history of breast cancer." *Menopause* 1995; 2(2): 67–72.

34. Dhodapkar, M. V., Ingle, J. N., and Ahmann, D. L. "Estrogen replacement therapy withdrawal and regression of metastatic breast cancer." *Cancer* 1995; 75: 43–46.

35. Spicer, D., Pike, M. C., and Henderson, B. E. "The questions of estrogen replacement therapy in patients with a prior diagnosis of breast cancer." *Oncology* 1990; 4(12): 49–62.

36. Couzi, R. J., Helzsouer, K. J., and Fetting, J. H. "Prevalence of menopausal symptoms among women with a history of breast cancer and attitudes toward

estrogen replacement therapy." *Journal of Clinical Oncology* 1995; 13: 2737–2744.

Chapter 8. Endometrial Cancer: The First Problem with Estrogen

1. Kurman, R., Kaminski, P. F., and Norris, H. J. "The behavior of endometrial hyperplasia: A long-term study on 'untreated' hyperplasia in 170 patients." *Cancer* 1985; 56: 403–412.

2. Grady, D., Gebretsadik, T., Kerlikowske, K., Ernster, V., and Petitti, D. "Hormone replacement therapy and endometrial cancer risk: A meta-analysis." *Obstetrics and Gynecology* 1995; 85(2): 304–313.

3. Grady, D., Rubin, S. M., Petitti, D. B., Fox, C. S., Black, D., Ettinger, B., Ernster, V. L., and Cummings, S. R. "Hormone therapy to prevent disease and prolong life in postmenopausal women." *Annals of Internal Medicine* 1992; 117(12): 1016–1037.

4. Greendale, G. A., and Judd, H. L. "Hormone therapy in the menopause." In *The Medical Care of Women,* Carr, P. T., Freund, K. M., and Somani, S. (eds.). New York: Saunders, 1995, pp. 635–642.

5. Writing Group for the PEPI Trial. "Effects of estrogen or estrogen/progestin regimens on heart disease risk factors in postmenopausal women." *Journal of the American Medical Association* 1994; 273(3): 199–208.

6. Ettinger, B., Pressman, A., and Van Gessel, A. "Low-dosage esterified estrogens opposed by progestin at 6-month intervals." *Obstetrics and Gynecology* 2001; 98: 205–211.

Chapter 9. For Better or Worse: Hormone Therapy and Other Diseases

1. Hebert, L. E., Scherr, P. A., Beckett, L. A., Albert, M. S., Pilgrim, D. M., Chown, M. J., Funkenstein, H. H., and Evans, D. A. "Age-specific incidence of Alzheimer's disease in a community population." *Journal of the American Medical Association* 1995; 273(17): 1354–1359.

2. Barrett-Connor, E. "Rethinking estrogen and the brain." *Journal of the American Geriatric Society* 1998; 46: 918–920.

3. Mulnard, R. A., Cotman, C. W., Kawas, C., et al. "Estrogen replacement therapy for treatment of mild to moderate Alzheimer's disease: A randomized controlled trial." *Journal of the American Medical Association* 2000; 283: 1007–1015.

4. Henderson, V. W. "Alzheimer's disease in women: Is there a role for estrogen replacement therapy?" *Menopause Management* 1995; 4(6): 10–14.

5. Yaffe, K., Grady, D., Pressman, A., and Cummings, S. "Serum estrogen levels, cognitive performance, and risk of cognitive decline in older community women." *Journal of the American Geriatric Society* 1998; 46: 816–821.

6. McEwen, B. S., Alves, S. E., Bulloch, K., and Weiland, N. G. "Ovarian steroids and the brain: Implications for cognition and aging." *Neurology* 1997; 48(5 Suppl 7): S8–15.

7. LeBlanc, E. S., Janowsky, J., Chan, B. K., and Nelson, H. D. "Hormone replacement therapy and cognition: Systematic review and meta-analysis." *Journal of the American Medical Association* 2001; 285: 1489–1499.

8. Yaffe, K., Krueger, K., Srkar, S., Grady, D., Barrett-Connor, E., Cox, D. A., Nickelsen. "Cognitive function in postmenopausal women treated with raloxifene." *New England Journal of Medicine* 2001; 344(16): 1207–1213.

9. Calle E. E., Miracle-McMahill, H. L., Thun, M. J., and Heath, C. W., Jr. "Estrogen replacement therapy and risk of fatal colon cancer in a prospective cohort of postmenopausal women." *Journal of the National Cancer Institute* 1995; 87(7): 517–523.

10. Giovannucci, E., Egan, K. M., Hunter, D. J., Stampfer, M. J., Colditz, G. A., Willett, W. C., and Speizer, F. E. "Aspirin and the risk of colorectal cancer in women." *New England Journal of Medicine* 1995; 333(10): 609–614.

11. Schoen, R. E., Weissfeld, J. L., and Kuller, L. H. "Are women with breast, endometrial, or ovarian cancer at increased risk for colorectal cancer?" *American Journal of Gastroenterology* 1994; 89(6): 835–842.

12. Broeders, M. J., Lambe, M., Baron, J. A., and Leon, D. A. "History of child-bearing and colorectal cancer risk in women aged less than 60: An analysis of Swedish routine registry data 1960–1984." *International Journal of Cancer* 1996; 66(2): 170–175.
    Chute, C. G., Willett, W. C., Colditz, G. A., Stampfer, M. J., Rosner, B., and Speiz, F. E. "A prospective study of reproductive history and exogenous estrogens on the risk of colorectal cancer in women." *Epidemiology* 1991; 2(3): 201–207.

13. Wu, A. H., Paganini-Hill, A., Ross, R. K., et al. "Alcohol, physical activity, and other risk factors for colorectal cancer: A prospective study." *British Journal of Cancer* 1987; 55: 687–694.

14. Newcomb, P. A., and Storer, B. E. "Postmenopausal hormone use and risk of large-bowel cancer." *Journal of the National Cancer Institute* 1995; 87(18): 1416.

15. Writing Group for the Women's Health Initiative Investigators. "Risks and benefits of estrogen plus progestin in healthy postmenopausal women: Principal results from the Women's Health Initiative randomized controlled trial." *Journal of the American Medical Association* 2002; 288(3): 321–333.

16. Nevitt, M. C., Cummings, S. R., Lane, N. E., Hochberg, M. C., Scott, J. C., Pressman, A. R., Genant, H. K., and Cauley, J. A., for the Study of Osteoporotic Fractures Research Group. "Association of estrogen replacement therapy with the risk of osteoarthritis of the hip in elderly white women." *Archives of Internal Medicine* 1996; 156: 2073–2080.

17. Paganini-Hill, A., Ross, R. K., and Henderson, B. E. "Postmenopausal oestrogen treatment and stroke: A prospective study." *British Medical Journal* 1988; 297(20–27): 519–522.
    Thompson, S. G., Meade, T. W., and Greenberg G. "The use of hormonal replacement therapy and the risk of stroke and myocardial infarction in women." *Journal of Epidemiology and Community Health* 1989; 43(2): 173–178.

18. Paganini-Hill, A. "Estrogen replacement therapy and stroke." *Progress in Cardiovascular Diseases* 1995; 38(3): 223–242.

19. Pedersen, A. T., Lidegaard, O., Kreiner, S., and Ottesen, B. "Hormone replacement therapy and risk of non-fatal stroke." *Lancet* 1997; 350: 1277–1283.

20. Simmon, J. A., Hsia, J., Cauley, J. A., et al. "Postmenopausal hormone therapy and the risk of stroke: The heart and estrogen-progestin replacement study." *Circulation* 2001; 103: 638–642.

21. Viscoli, C. M., Brass, L. M., Kernan, W. N., Sarrel, P. M., Suissa, S., and Horwitz, R. I. "A clinical trial of estrogen-replacement therapy after ischemic stroke." *New England Journal of Medicine* 2001; 345(17): 1243–1249.

22. Writing Group for the Women's Health Initiative Investigators, op. cit.

23. Kerlikowske, K., Brown, J. S., and Grady, D. G. "Should women with familial ovarian cancer undergo prophylactic oophorectomy?" *Obstetrics and Gynecology* 1992; 80(4): 700–707.

24. Kaufman, S. C., Spiritas, R., Alexander, N. J. "Do fertility drugs cause ovarian tumors?" *Journal of Women's Health* 1995; 4(3): 241–259.

25. Hartge, P., Hoover, R., McGowan, L., Lesher, L., and Norris, H. J. "Menopause and ovarian cancer." *American Journal of Epidemiology* 1988; 127: 990–998.

26. Rodriguez, C., Calle, E. E., Coates, R. J., Miracle-McMahill, H. L., Thun, M. J., and Heath, C. W., Jr. "Estrogen replacement therapy and fatal ovarian cancer." *American Journal of Epidemiology* 1995; 141(9): 828–835.

27. Garg, P. P., Kerlikowske, K., Subak, L., and Grady, D. "Hormone replacement therapy and the risk of epithelial ovarian carcinoma: A meta-analysis." *Obstetrics and Gynecology* 1998; 92: 472–479.

28. Lacey, J. V., Mink, P. J., Lubin, J. H., et al. "Menopausal hormone replacement therapy and risk of ovarian cancer." *Journal of the American Medical Association* 2002; 2888: 334–341.

29. Rodriguez, C., Patel, A. V., Calle, E. E., Jacob, E. J., and Thun, M. J. "Estrogen replacement therapy and ovarian cancer mortality in a large prospective study of US women." *Journal of the American Medical Association* 2001; 285: 1460–1465.

30. Grodstein, F., Colditz, G. A., and Stampfer, M. J. "Postmenopausal hormone use and colecystectomy in a large prospective study." *Obstetrics and Gynecology* 1994; 83(1): 5–11.

31. Simon, J. A., Hunninghake, D. B., Agarwal, S. K., Lin, F., et al. "Effect of estrogen plus progestin on risk for biliary tract surgery in postmenopausal women with coronary artery disease." *Annals of Internal Medicine* 2001; 135: 493–501.

32. Craft, P., and Hannaford, P. C. "Risk factors for acute myocardial infarction in women: Evidence from the Royal College of General Practitioners' oral contraception study." *British Medical Journal* 1989; 298: 165–168.

33. Report from the Boston Collaborative Drug Surveillance Program, Boston University Medical Center. "Surgically confirmed gallbladder disease, venous thromboembolism, and breast tumors in relation to postmenopausal estrogen therapy." *New England Journal of Medicine* 1974; 290(1): 15–19.

34. Daly, E., Vessey, M. P., Hawkins, M. M., Carson, J. L., Gough, P., and Marsh, S. "Risk of venous thromboembolism in users of hormone replacement therapy." *Lancet* 1996; 348: 977–980.
   Jick, H., Derby, L. E., Myers, M. W., Vasilakis, C., and Newton, K. M. "Risk of hospital admission for idiopathic venous thromboembolism among users of postmenopausal oestrogens." *Lancet* 1996; 348: 981–983.
   Grodstein, F., Stampfer, M. J., Goldhaber, S. Z., Manson, J. E., Colditz, G. A., Speizer, F. E., Willett, W. C., and Hennekens, C. H. "Prospective study of

exogenous hormones and risk of pulmonary embolism in women." *Lancet* 1996; 348: 983–987.

35. Price, D. T., and Ridker, P. M. "Factor V Leiden mutation and the risks for thromboembolic disease: A clinical perspective." *Annals of Internal Medicine* 1997; 127(10): 895–903.

36. Grady, D., Wenger, N. K., Herrington, D., Khan, S., Furberg, C., Hunninghake, D., et al. "Postmenopausal hormone therapy increases risk for venous thromboembolic disease. The Heart and Estrogen/progestin Replacement Study." *Annals of Internal Medicine* 2000; 132(9); 689–696.

37. Writing Group for the Women's Health Initiative Investigators, op. cit.

38. Akkad, A. A., Habiba, M. A., Ismail, N., Abrams, K., and al-Azzawi, F. "Abnormal uterine bleeding on hormone replacement: The importance of intrauterine structural abnormalities." *Obstetrics and Gynecology* 1995; 86(3): 330–334.

39. Sener, A. B., Seckin, N. C., Ozmen, S., Gokmen, O., Dogu, N., and Ekici, E. "The effects of hormone replacement therapy on uterine fibroids in postmenopausal women." *Fertility and Sterility* 1996; 65(2): 354–357.

40. Namnoum, A. B., Hickman, T. N., Goodman, S. B., Gehlbach, D. L., and Rock, J. A. "Incidence of symptoms' recurrence after hysterectomy for endometriosis." *Fertility and Sterility* 1995; 64(5): 898–902.
    Goh, J. T., and Hall, B. A. "Postmenopausal endometrioma and hormonal replacement therapy." *Australia New Zealand Journal of Obstetrics and Gynaecology* 1992; 32(4): 384–385.

41. Sanchez-Guerrero, J., Liang, M. H., Karlson, E. W., Hunter, D. J., and Colditz, G. A. "Postmenopausal estrogen therapy and the risk for developing systemic lupus erythematosus." *Annals of Internal Medicine* 1995; 122(6): 430–433.

42. Petris, M. "Exogenous estrogen in systemic lupus eythematosus: Oral contraceptives and hormone replacement therapy." *Lupus* 2001; 10(3): 222–226.

43. Troisi, R. J., Speizer, F. E., Willett, W. C., Trichopoulos, D., and Rosner, B. "Menopause, postmenopausal estrogen preparations, and the risk of adult-onset asthma. A prospective cohort study." *American Journal of Respiratory and Critical Care Medicine* 1995; 152(Part 1): 1183–1188.

44. Adami, H. O., Persson, I., Hoover, R., Schairer, C., and Bergkvist, L. "Risk of cancer in women receiving hormone replacement therapy." *International Journal of Cancer* 1989; 44(5): 833–839.

45. Zang, E. A., and Wynder, E. L. "Differences in lung cancer risk between men and women: Examination of the evidence." *Journal of the National Cancer Institute* 1996; 88(3/4): 183–192.

46. Writing Group for the Women's Health Initiative Investigators, op. cit.

Chapter 10. What Are My Options for Feeling Better Right Now?

1. Anonymous. "Complementing mainstream medicine." *Nature Medicine* 1996; 2(6): 619.

2. Kaufert, P., Boggs, P. P., Ettinger, B., et al. "Woman and menopause: Beliefs, attitudes, and behaviors. The North American Menopause Society 1997 Menopause Survey." *Menopause* 1998; 5: 197–202.

3. Kam, I. W., Dennehy, C. E., et al. "Dietary supplement use among menopausal women attending a San Francisco health conference." *Menopause* 2002; 9: 72–78.

4. Dickstein, E. S., and Kunkel, F. W. "Foxglove tea poisoning." *American Journal of Medicine* 1980; 9(1): 167–169.

5. Weed, S. *Wise Woman Herbal Healing.* Woodstock, N.Y.: Ash Tree, 1989.

6. Cargill, Marie. Personal conversation, November 1995.

7. Elghamry, M. I., and Shihata, I. M. "Biological activity of phytoestrogens." *Planta Medica* 1965; 13: 352–357.

8. Cargill, op. cit.

Chapter 11. From Flashes to Fuzzy Thinking: What You Can Do Right Now

1. Kronenberg, F., and Barnard, R. M. "Modulation of menopausal hot flashes by ambient temperature." *Journal of Thermal Biology* 1992; 17: 43–49.

2. Kronenberg, F. "Hot flashes: Epidemiology and physiology." *Annals of the New York Academy of Sciences* 1990; 592: 52–86.

3. Hammar, M., Berg, G., and Lindgren, R. "Does physical exercise influence the frequency of postmenopausal hot flushes?" *Acta Obstetrica et Gynecologica Scandinavica* 1990; 69: 409–412.

4. Notelovitz, M., and Tonnessen, D. *Menopause and Midlife Health.* New York: St. Martin's Press, 1993, p. 244.

5. Upmalis D. H., Lobo, R., et al. "Vasomotor symptom relief by soy isoflavone extract tablets in postmenopausal women: A multicenter, double-blind randomized placebo-controlled study." *Menopause* 2000; 7: 236–242.

6. Messina, M. J., and Loprinzi, C. L. "Soy for breast cancer survivors: A critical review of the literature." *Journal of Nutrition* 2001; 131: 3095S–3108S.

7. Freedman, R. R., and Woodard, S. "Behavioral treatment of menopausal hot flushes: Evaluation by ambulatory monitoring." *American Journal of Obstetrics and Gynecology* 1992; 167: 436–439.

8. Irvin, J. H., Domar, A., Clark, C., Zuttermeister, P. C., and Friedman, R. "The effects of relaxation response training on menopausal symptoms." Paper presented at the Annual Meeting of the Society of Behavioral Medicine. Boston: April 13–16, 1994.

9. Wyon, Y., Lingrem, T., Lundeberg, T., and Hammar, M. "Effects of acupuncture on climacteric vasomotor symptoms, quality of life, and urinary excretion of neuropeptides among postmenopausal women." *Menopause: Journal of the NAMS* 1995; 2(1): 3–12.

10. Blatt, M. H. G., Wiesbader, H., and Kupperman, H. S. "Vitamin E and climacteric syndrome." *Archives of Internal Medicine* 1953; 91: 792–796.

11. Barton, D. L., Loprinzi, C. L., Quella, S. K., et al. "Prospective evaluation of vitamin E for hot flashes in breast cancer survivors." *Journal of Clinical Oncology* 1998: 16(2): 495–500.

12. Kronenberg, F. "Hot flashes: Phenomenology, quality of life, and search for treatment options." *Experimental Gerontology* 1994; 29(3/4): 319–336.

13. Kushi, L. H., Fee, R. M., Sellers, T. A., Zheng, W., and Folsom, A. R. "Intake of vitamins A, C, and E and postmenopausal breast cancer: The Iowa Women's Health Study." *American Journal of Epidemiology* 1996; 144(2): 165–174.

14. Verhoeven, D. T., Assen, N., Goldbohm, R. A., Dorant, E., van't Veer, P., Sturmans, F., Hermus, R. J., and van den Brandt, P. A. "Vitamins C and E, retinol, beta-carotene, and dietary fibre in relation to breast cancer risk: A prospective cohort study." *British Journal of Cancer* 1997; 75(1): 149–155.

15. Hunter, D. J., Manson, J. E., Colditz, G. A., Stampfer, M. J., Rosner, B., Hennekens, C. H., Speizer, F. E., and Willet, W. C. "A prospective study of the intake of vitamins C, E, and A and the risk of breast cancer." *New England Journal of Medicine* 1993; 329(4): 234–240.

van't Veer, P., Strain, J. J., Fernandez-Crehuet, J., Martin, B. C., Thamm, M., Kardinaal, A. F., Kohlmeier, L., Huttunen, J. K., Martin-Moreno, J. M., and Kok, F. J. "Tissue antioxidants and postmenopausal breast cancer: The European Community Multicentre Study on Antioxidants, Myocardial Infarction, and Cancer of the Breast (EURAMIC)." *Cancer Epidemiology Biomarkers and Prevention* 1996; 5(6): 441–447.

Rohan, T. E., Howe, G. R., Friedenreich, C. M., Jain, M., and Miller, A. B. "Dietary fiber, vitamins A, C, and E, and risk of breast cancer: A cohort study." *Cancer Causes and Control* 1993; 4(1): 29–37.

16. London, S. J., Stein, E. A., Henderson, I. C., Stampfer, M. J., Wood, W. C., Remine, S., Dmochowski, J. R., Robert, N. J., and Willet, W. C. "Carotenoids, retinol, and vitamin E and risk of proliferative benign breast cancer." *Cancer Causes and Control* 1992; 3(6): 503–512.

17. Gerber, M., Cavallo, F., Marubini, E., Richardson, S., Barbieri, A., Capitelli, E., Costa, A., Crastes de Paulet, A., Crastes de Paulet, P., Decarlki, A., et al. "Liposoluble vitamins and lipid parameters in breast cancer: A joint study in northern Italy and southern France." *International Journal of Cancer* 1988; 42(4): 489–494.

Gerber, M., Richardson, S., Cavallo, F., Marubini, E., Crastes de Paulet, P., Crastes de Paulet, A., and Pujol, H. "The role of diet history and biologic essays in the study of 'diet and breast cancer.'" *Tumori* 1990; 76(4): 321–330.

Gerber, M., Richardson, S., Salkeld, R., and Chappuis, P. "Antioxidants in female breast cancer patients." *Cancer Investigations* 1991; 9(4): 421–428.

18. Waald, N. J., Boreham, J., Hayward, J. L., and Bulbrook, R. D. "Plasma retinol, beta carotene, and vitamin E levels in relation to the future risk of breast cancer." *British Journal of Cancer* 1984; 49: 321–324.

Torun, M., Akgul, S., and Sargin, H. "Serum vitamin E level in patients with breast cancer." *Journal of Clinical Pharmacology and Therapeutics* 1995; 20(3): 173–178.

19. Chajes, V., Lhuillery, C., Sattler, W., Kostner, G. M., and Bougnoux, P. "Alpha tocopherol and hydroperoxide content in breast and adipose tissue from patients with breast tumors." *International Journal of Cancer* 1996; 67(2): 170–175.

20. Schwartz, J., and Shklar, G. "The selective cytoxic effect of carotenoids and alpha-tocopherol on human cancer cell lines in vitro." *Journal of Oral and Maxillofacial Surgery* 1992; 50(4): 367–373.

21. Saintot, M., Astre, C., Pujol, H., and Gerber, M. "Tumor progression and oxidant-antioxidant status." *Carcinogenesis* 1996; 17(6): 1267–1271.

22. Weed, Susun. Personal communication, July 1996.

23. Stoll, W. "Phytotherapeutic influences atrophic vaginal epithelium. Double-blind study on Cimicifuga versus an estrogen preparation." *Therapeutikon* 1987; 1: 23–31.

24. Lehmann-Willenbrock, E., and Riedal, H. H. "Clinical and endocrinologic studies of the treatment of ovarian insufficiency manifestations following hysterectomy with intact adnexa." *Zentralbl Gynakol* (Germany, East) 1988; 110(10): 611–618.

25. Jacobson, J. S., Troxel, A. B., Evans, J., et al. "Randomized trial of black cohosh for the treatment of hot flashes among women with a history of breast cancer." *Journal of Clinical Oncology* 2001; 19(10): 2739–2745.

26. Liske, E., et al. "Physiological investigation of a unique extract of black cohosh (*Cimicifugae racemosae* rhizome): A 6-month clinical study demonstrates no systemic estrogenic effect." *Journal of Women's Health and Gender-Based Medicine* 2002; 11(2): 163–174.

27. Baber, R. J., et al. "Randomized placebo-controlled trial of an isoflavone supplement and menopausal symptoms in women." *Climacteric* 1999; 2: 85–92.
   Knight, D. C., et al. "The effect of Promensil, an isoflavone extract, on menopausal symptoms." *Climacteric* 1999; 2: 79–84.

28. Ota, H., Fukushima, M., and Maki, M. "Stimulatory action of shakuyaku on aromatase activity in cultured rat follicles." *Nippon Sanka Fujinka Gakkai Zasshi* 1989; 41(5): 525–529.
   Kato, T., and Okamoto, R. "Effect of shakuyaku-kanzo-to on serum estrogen levels and adrenal gland cells in ovariectomized rats." *Nippon Sanka Fujinka Gakkai Zasshi* 1992; 44(4): 433–439.

29. Epstein, M. T., Espiner, E. A., Donald, R. A., Hughes, H., Cowles, R. J., and Lun, S. "Licorice raises urinary cortisol in man." *Journal of Clinical Endocrinology Metabolism* 1978; 47(2): 397–400.

30. Walker, B. R., and Edwards, C. R. "Licorice-induced hypertension and syndromes of apparent mineralocorticoid excess." *Endocrinology Metabolism Clinics of North America* 1994; 23(2): 359–377.

31. Bernardi, M., D'Intino, P. E., Trevisani, F., Cantelli-Forti, G., Raggi, M. A., Turchetto, E., and Gasbarrini, G. "Effects of prolonged ingestion of graded doses of licorice by healthy volunteers." *Life Science* 1994; 55(11): 863–872.

32. Zhang, J. P., and Zhou, D. J. "Changes in leucocytic estrogen receptor levels in patients with climacteric syndrome and therapeutic effect of liu wei di huang pills." *Chung Hsi I Chieh Ho Tsa Chih* 1991; 11(9): 521–523, 515.

Zhang, G. L. "Treatment of breast proliferation disease with modified xiao yao san and er chen decoction." *Chung Hsi I Chieh Ho Tsa Chih* 1991; 11(7): 400–402, 388.

33. Coope, J., Thomson, J. M., and Poller, L. "Effects of 'natural oestrogen' replacement therapy on menopausal symptoms and blood clotting." *British Medical Journal* 1975; 4: 139–143.

34. Lebherz, T. B., and French, L. "Nonhormonal treatment of the menopausal syndrome." *Obstetrics and Gynecology* 1969; 33: 795–799.

35. Clayden, J. R., and his group (Clayden, J. R., Bell, J. W., and Pollard, P.). "Menopausal flushing: Double-blind trial of a nonhormonal medication." *British Medical Journal* 1974; 1: 409–412.

36. Tulandi, T., Lal, S., and Kinch, R. A. "Effect of intravenous clonidine on menopausal flushing and luteinizing hormone secretion." *British Journal of Obstetrics and Gynaecology* 1983; 90: 854–857.

37. Jones, K. P., Ravnikar, V., and Schiff, I. "A preliminary evaluation of the effect of lofexidene on vasomotor flushes in postmenopausal women." *Maturitas* 1985; 7: 135–139.

38. Loprinzi, C. L., Kugler, J. W., Sloan, J. A., et al. "Venlaflaxine in management of hot flashes in survivors of breast cancer: A randomized controlled trial." *Lancet* 2000; 356(9247): 2059–2063.
    Quella, S. K., Loprinzi, C. L., Sloan, J., et al. "Pilot evaluation of venlafaxine for the treatment of hot flashes in men undergoing androgen ablation for prostate cancer." *Journal of Urology* 1999; 162 (1): 98–102.

39. Cottershio, M., Kreiger, N., Darlington, G., Steingart, A. "Antidepressant medication use and breast cancer risk." *American Journal of Epidemiology* 2000; 151(10): 951–957.

40. Kelly, J. P., Rosenberg, L., Palme, J. R., et al. "Risk of breast cancer according to use of antidepressants, phenothiazines, and antihistamines." *American Journal of Epidemiology* 1999; 150(8): 861–868.
    Wang, P. S., Walker, A. M., Tsuang, M. T., et al. "Antidepressant use and the risk of breast cancer; A non association." *Journal of Clinical Epidemiology* 2001; 54(7): 728–734.

41. Loprinzi, C. L., Michalak, J. C., Quella, S. K., O'Fallon, J. R., Hatfield, A. K., Nelimark, R. A., Dose, A. M., Fischer, T., Johnson, C., Klatt, N. E., et al. "Megestrol acetate for the prevention of hot flashes." *New England Journal of Medicine* 1994; 331(6): 347–352.

42. Rookus, M. A., and van Leeuwen, F. E. "Oral contraceptives and risk of breast cancer in women aged 20–54 years." *Lancet* 1994; 344(8926): 844–851.

43. Pethö, A. Ärztl. *Praxis* 1987; 47: 1551–1553.

44. Milewicz, A., Gejdel, E., Sworen, H., Sienkiewicz, K., Jedrzejak, J., Teucher, T., and Schmitz, H. "Vitex agnus castus-Extrakt zur Behandlung von Regeltempoanomalien infolge latenter Hyperprolaktinamie. Ergebnisse einer randomisierten Plazebo-kontrollierten Doppelblindstudie." *Arzneimittelforschung* 1993; 43(7): 752–756.

45. Sliutz, G., Speiser-Schultz, A. M., Spona, J., and Zeillinger, R. "Agnus castus extracts inhibit prolactin secretion of rat pituitary cells." *Hormone Metabolism Research* 1993; 25(5): 253–255.

46. Nilsson, L., and Rybo, G. "Treatment of menorrhagia." *American Journal of Obstetrics and Gynecology* 1971; 110: 713–720.

47. Archer, D. F., Viniegra-Sibal, A., Hsiu, J.-G., et al. "Endometrial histology, uterine bleeding, and metabolic changes in postmenopausal women using progesterone-releasing intrauterine device and oral conjugated estrogens for hormone replacement therapy." *Menopause* 1994; 1: 109–116.

48. Makarainen, L., and Yikorkala, O. "Primary and myoma associated menorrhagia: Role of prostaglandin and effects of ibuprofen." *British Journal of Obstetrics and Gynaecology* 1986; 93: 974–978.

49. O'Connor, H., and Magos, A. "Endometrial resection for the treatment of menorrhagia." *New England Journal of Medicine* 1996; 335: 151–156.

50. Carlson, K. J., Miller, B. A., and Fowler, F. J. "The Maine Women's Health Study: I. Outcomes of hysterectomy." *Obstetrics and Gynecology* 1994; 83: 556–565.

51. Tobachman, J. K., Tucker, M. A., Kase, R., et al. "Intra-abdominal carcinomatosis after prophylactic oophorectomy in ovarian cancer prone families." *Lancet* 1982; 11: 795–797.

52. Wilcox, G. "Oestrogenic effects of plant foods on postmenopausal women." *British Medical Journal* 1991; 301: 905–906.

53. Nachtigall, L. E. "Comparative study: Replens versus local estrogen in menopausal women." *Fertility and Sterility* 1994; 61(1): 178–180.

54. Punnonen, R., and Lukola, A. "Oestrogen-like effect of ginseng." *British Medical Journal* 1980; 281: 1110.

55. DiRaimondo, C. V., Roach, A. C., and Meador, C. K. "Gynecosmastia from exposure to vaginal estrogen cream." *New England Journal of Medicine* 1980; 302(9): 1089–1090.

56. Zhdanova, I. V., Wurtman, R. J., Lynch, H. J., Ives, J. R., Dollins, A. B., Morabito, C., Matheson, J. K., and Schomer, D. L. "Sleep inducing effects of low doses of melatonin ingested in the evening." *Clinical Pharmacology and Therapeutics* 1995; 57(5): 552–558.
    Garfinkel, D., Laudon, M., Nof, D., and Zisapel, N. "Improvement of sleep quality in elderly people by controlled-release melatonin." *Lancet* 1995; 346(8974): 541–544.

57. Brown, E., and Walker, L. *Breezing Through the Change*. Berkeley, Calif.: Frog, p. 107.
    Also Ito, D. *Natural Remedies for Menopause and Beyond*. New York: Random House, p. 143.

58. Baulieu, E. E., et al. "Dehydroepiandrosterone (DHEA), DHEA sulfate and aging: Contribution of the DHEAge Study to a sociobiomedical issue." *Proceedings of the National Academy of Science* 2000; 97: 4279–4284.

59. Barrett-Connor, E., and Khaw, K. T. "Absence of an inverse relationship of dehydroepiandrostenedione sulfate with cardiovascular disease mortality in postmenopausal women." *New England Journal of Medicine* 1987; 317: 711.
    Morris, K. T., Toth-Fejel, S., Schmidt, J., et al. "High dehydroepiandrosterone-sulfate predicts breast cancer progression during new aromatase inhibitor therapy and stimulates breast cancer cell growth in tissue culture: A renewed role for adrenalectomy." *Surgery* 2001; 130 (6): 947–953.

60. Ito, T. Y., et al. "A double-blind placebo-controlled study of ArginMax, a nutritional supplement for enhancement of female sexual function." *Journal of Sex and Marital Therapy* 2001; 27: 541–549.

61. Weed, op. cit.

62. Petkov, V. D., Kehayov, R., Belcheva, S., Konstantinova, E., Petkov, V. V., Getova, D., and Markovska, V. "Memory effects of standardized extracts of Panax ginseng (G115), Gingko balboa (GK501), and their combination Gincosan (PHL-00701)." *Planta Medica* 1993; 59(2): 106–114.

63. Liberti, L. E., and Marderosian, A. D. "Evaluation of commercial ginseng products." *Journal of Pharmacology Science* 1978; 67: 1487–1489.

64. Murray, M. *The Healing Power of Herbs: The Enlightened Person's Guide to the Wonders of Medicinal Plants*. Rocklin, Calif.: *Prima*, 1995.

65. Semlitsch, H. V., Anderer, P., Saletu, B., Binder, G. A., and Decker, K. A. "Cognitive psychophysiology in nootropic drug research: Effects of Ginkgo biloba on event-related potentials (P300) in age-associated memory impairment." *Pharmacopsychiatry* 1995; 28(4): 134–142.

66. Solomon, P. R., Adams, F., Silver, A., Zimmer, J., De Veaux, R. "Ginkgo for memory enhancement: A randomized controlled trial." *Journal of the American Medical Association* 2002; 288: 835–840.

67. LeBars, P. L., Katz, M. M., Erman, N., et al. "A placebo-controlled, double-blind randomized trial of an extract of ginkgo biloba for dementia." *Journal of the American Medical Association* 1997; 278: 1327–1332.

68. Brown, J. S., Seeley, D. G., Fing, J., et al. "Urinary incontinence in older women: Who is at risk? Study of Osteoporotic Fractures Research Group." *Obstetrics and Gynecology* 1996; 87 (5 Pt 1): 715–721.

69. Nygaard, I. "Prevention of exercise incontinence with mechanical devices." *Journal of Reproductive Medicine* 1995; 40(2): 89–94.

70. Dunn, M., Brandt, D., and Nygaard, I. *Physician and Sportsmedicine* January 2002.

71. Thom, D. H., and Brown, J. S. "Reproductive and hormonal risk factors for urinary incontinence in later life: A review of the clinical and epidemiologic literature." *Journal of the American Geriatric Society* 1998; 46(11): 1411–1417.

72. Grady, D., Brown, J. S., Vittinghoff, E., et al. "Postmenopausal hormones and incontinence: The Heart and Estrogen/progestin Replacement Study." *Obstetrics and Gynecology* 2001; 97: 116–120.

73. Brown and Walker, op. cit.

Chapter 12. For Prevention: First, Look to Your Lifestyle!

1. Mulrow, C. "Sound clinical advice for hypertensive patients." *Annals of Internal Medicine* 2001; 135(12): 1084–1086.

2. Vollmer, W. M., Sacks, F. M., et al. "Effects of diet and sodium intake on blood pressure: Subgroup analysis of the DASH-Sodium Trial." *Annals of Internal Medicine* 2001; 135: 1019–1028.

3. Sacks, F. M., Svetkey, L. P., Vollmer, W. M., et al. "Effects on blood pressure of reduced dietary sodium and the Dietary Approaches to Stop Hypertension (DASH) diet." DASH-Sodium Collaborative Research Group. *New England Journal of Medicine* 2001; 344: 3–10.

Appel, L. J., Moore, T. J., Obarzanek, E., et al. "A clinical trial of the effects of dietary patterns on blood pressure." *New England Journal of Medicine* 1997; 336: 1117–1124.

4. Vasan, R., Larson, M., Liep, E. P., et al. "Impact of high-normal blood pressure on the risk of cardiovascular disease." *New England Journal of Medicine* 2001; 345: 1291–1297.

5. Willet, W. C., and Ascherio, A. "Trans fatty acids: Are the effects only marginal?" *American Journal of Public Health* 1994; 84: 722–724.

6. Oomen, C. M., Ocke, M. C., Feskens, E. J. M., et al. "Association between trans fatty acid intake and 10 year risk of coronary heart disease in the Zutphen Elderly Study: A prospective population-based study." *Lancet* 2001; 357: 746–751.

7. Rose, D. P., Connolly, J. M., Rayburn, J., and Coleman, M. "Influence of diet containing eicosapentaenoic or docosahexaenoic acid on growth and metastasis of breast cancer cells in nude mice." *Journal of the National Cancer Institute* 1995; 87: 587–592.

8. Ornish, D. *Dr. Dean Ornish's Program for Reversing Heart Disease.* New York: Random House, 1990.

9. Heaney, R. P., "Protein intake and bone health: The influence of belief systems on the conduct of nutritional science." *American Journal of Clinical Nutrition* 2001; 75: 5–6.

10. Bennetts, H. W., Underwood, E. J., and Shier, F. L. "A specific breeding problem of sheep on subterranean clover pastures in Western Australia." *Australian Veterinarian Journal* 1946; 22: 2–129.

11. Findlay, J. K., Buckmaster, J. M., Chamley, W. A., Cummings, I. A., Hearnshaw, H., and Goding, J. R. "Release of luteinizing hormone by oestradiol 17 beta and gonadotrophin-releasing hormone in ewes affected with clover disease." *Neuroendocrinology* 1973; 11: 57–66.

12. Hughes, C. L. "Phytochemical mimicry of reproductive hormones and modulation of herbivore fertility by phytoestrogens." *Environmental Health Perspectives* 1988; 78: 171–175.

13. Anderson, J. W., Johnstone, B. M., and Cook-Newell, M. E. "Meta-analysis of the effects of soy protein intake on serum lipids." *New England Journal of Medicine* 1995; 333: 276–282.

14. Barnes, S. Presentation at Menopause Conference: Advances in Hormone Replacement and Alternative Therapeutic Strategies. Philadelphia, Penn., May 9–10, 1996.

15. Erdman, J. W., Jr. "Soy protein and cardiovascular disease: A statement for healthcare professionals from the nutrition committee of the AHA." *Circulation* 2000; 102: 2555–2559.

16. Messina, M., Grugger, E. T., Alekel, D. L. "Soy protein, soy bean isoflavones and bone health: A review of the animal and human data." In *Handbook of Nutraceuticals and Functional Goos,* Wildman, R. (ed.). Boca Raton: CRC Press, 2001, pp. 77–98.

17. Naomi, O., Syuichi, A., Katumi, M., and Ikuko, E. "Evaluation of the effect of soybean milk and soybean milk peptide on bone metabolism in the rat model with ovariectomized osteoporosis." *Journal of Nutritional Sciences and Vitaminol* 1994; 40, 201–211.

18. Wang, C., and Kurzer, M. S. "Effects of isoflavones flavinoids and lignans on proliferation of estrogen–dependent and independent human breast cancer cells." *Proceedings of the American Association for Cancer Research* 1996; 37: 277.

19. Messina, M. J., and Loprinzi, C. L. "Soy for breast cancer survivors: A critical review of the Literature." *Journal of Nutrition* 2001; 131: 3095S–3108S.

20. Seraino, S. "The effect of flaxseed supplementation on the initiation and promotional stages of mammary tumorgenesis." *Nutrition and Cancer* 1992; 17(2): 153–159.

21. Bierenbaum, M. L. "Reducing atherogenic risk in hyperlipemic humans with flaxseed supplementation: A preliminary report." *Journal of the American College of Nutrition* 1993; 12(5): 501–504.

22. Cumnane, S. C. "Nutritional attributes of traditional flaxseed in healthy young adults." *American Journal of Clinical Nutrition* 1993; 69(2): 443–453.

23. Shandler, N. *Estrogen: The Natural Way: Over 250 Easy and Delicious Recipes for Menopause.* New York: Villard, 1997.

24. Guillemant, J., Le, H., Accarie, et al. "Mineral water as a source of dietary calcium: Acute effects on parathyroid function and bone resorption in young men." *American Journal of Clinical Nutrition* 2000; 71: 999–1002.

25. Zheng, W., Doyle, T. J., Hong, C. P., Kushi, L. H., Sellers, T. A., and Folsom, A. R. "Tea consumption and cancer incidence in a prospective cohort study of

postmenopausal women." *Proceedings of the Annual Meeting of the American Association for Cancer Research* 1995; 36: A1654 (meeting abstract).

26. Reid, I. R., Ames, R. W., Evans, M. C., Gamble, G. D., and Sharpe, S. J. "Effect of calcium supplementation on bone loss in postmenopausal women." *New England Journal of Medicine* 1993; 328(7): 460–464.
    Prince, R. "The calcium controversy revisited: Implications of new data." *Medical Journal of Australia* 1993; 159: 404–407.

27. Manson, J. E., Willett, W. C., Stampfer, M. J., Colditz, G. A., Hunter, D. J., Hankinson, S. E., Hennekens, C. H., and Speizer, F. E. "Body weight and mortality among women." *New England Journal of Medicine* 1995; 333(11): 677–685.

28. Nishizawa, T., Akaoka, I., Nishida, Y., Kawaguchi, Y., and Hayashi, E. "Some factors related to obesity in the Japanese sumo wrestler." *American Journal of Clinical Nutrition* 1976; 29(10): 1167–1174.

29. Notelovitz, M., and Tonnessen, D. *Menopause and Midlife Health.* New York: St. Martin's Press, 1993.

30. Weed, S. *Menopausal Years: The Wise Woman Way.* Woodstock, N.Y.: Ash Tree, 1992.

31. Freudenheim, J. L., Marshall, J. R., Vena, J. E., Laughlin, R., Brasure, J. R., Swanson, M. K., Nemoto, T., and Graham, S. "Premenopausal breast cancer risk and intake of vegetables, fruits, and related nutrients." *Journal of the National Cancer Institute* 1966; 88(6): 340–348.

32. Hennekens, C. H., Buring, J. E., Manson, J. E., Stampfer, M., Rosner, B., Cook, N. R., Belanger, C., LaMotte, F., Gaziano, J. M., Ridker, P. M., Willett, W., and Peto, R. "Lack of effect of long-term supplementation with beta carotene on the incidence of malignant neoplasms and cardiovascular disease." *New England Journal of Medicine* 1996; 334(18): 1145–1149.

33. Hu, F. B., et al. "Frequent nut consumption and risk of coronary heart disease in women: Prospective cohort study." *British Medical Journal* 1998; 317: 1341–1345.

34. Ginsberg, E. S., Mello, N. K., Mendelson, J. H., et al. "Effects of alcohol ingestion on estrogens in postmenopausal women." *Journal of the American Medical Association* 1996; 76(2): 1747–1751.

35. Manson et al., op. cit.

36. Bernstein, L., Henderson, B. E., Hanisch, R., Sullivan-Halley, J., and Ross, R. K. "Physical exercise and reduced risk of breast cancer in young women." *Journal of the National Cancer Institute* 1994; 86(18): 1403–1408.

37. Thune, I., Brenn, T., Lund, E., and Gaard, M. "Physical activity and the risk of breast cancer." *New England Journal of Medicine* 1997; 336(18): 1269–1275.

38. Notelovitz and Tonnessen, op. cit., p. 98.

39. Bravo, G. "Physical exercise benefits postmenopausal women." *Journal of the American Geriatric Society* 1996; 44: 756–762.

40. Blair, S. N., Kohl, H. W., Paffenbarger, R. S., Clark, D. G., Cooper, K. H., and Gibbons, L. W. "Physical fitness and all cause mortality: A prospective study of healthy men and women." *Journal of the American Medical Association* 1989; 262: 2395–2401.

41. Notelovitz and Tonnessen, op. cit.

42. Weed, op. cit.

43. Cousins, N. *Anatomy of an Illness.* New York: Bantam, 1979.

44. Benson, H. *Beyond the Relaxation Response.* New York: Berkeley, 1985.

45. Stolbach, Leo. Quoted in Love, S. *Dr. Susan Love's Breast Book.* Reading, Mass.: Addison-Wesley, 1995, pp. 438–439.

46. Benson, op. cit.

47. Jarte, J. L., Eifert, G. H., and Smith, R. "The effects of running and meditation on beta endorphin, corticotropin releasing hormone and cortisol in plasma and on mood." *Biological Psychology* 1995; 40(3): 251–265.

48. Smith, W. P., Compton, W. C., and West, W. B. "Meditation as an adjunct to a happiness enhancement program." *Journal of Clinical Psychology* 1995; 51(2): 269–273.

49. Fiore, N. *The Road Back to Health.* New York: Bantam, 1984.

50. Cousins, op. cit.

51. LeShan, L. *How to Meditate.* New York: Bantam, 1974, pp. 33, 39, 40.

52. Spiegel, D., Bloom, J. R., Kraemer, H. C., and Gottheil, E. "Effect of psychosocial treatment on survival of patients with metastatic breast cancer." *Lancet* 1989; 2(8668): 888.

Chapter 13. Alternatives: From Acupuncture to Herbs

1. Omenn, G. S., Goodman, G. E., Thornquist, M. D., Balmes, J., Cullen, M. R., Glass, A., Keogh, J. P., Meyskens, F. L., Valanis, B., Williams, J. H., Barnhart, S., and Hammar, S. "Effects of a combination of beta carotene and vitamin A on lung cancer and cardiovascular disease." *New England Journal of Medicine* 1966; 334(18): 1150–1155.

2. Pennington, J. A. T. "Mineral content of foods and total diets: The selected minerals in foods survey." *Journal of the American Dietetic Association* 1986; 86(7): 876–891.

3. Sempos, C. T., et al. "A two-year dietary survey of middle-aged women: Repeated dietary records as a measure of usual intake." *Journal of the American Dietetic Association* 1984; 1008–1013.

4. Cumming, R. G. "Calcium intake and bone mass: A quantitative review of the evidence." *Calcified Tissue International* 1990; 47: 194–201.

5. Garland, C., Barrett-Connor, E., Rossof, A. H., Shekelle, R. B., Criqui, M. H., and Paul, O. "Dietary vitamin D and calcium and risk of colorectal cancer: A 19-year prospective study in men." *Lancet* 1985; February: 307–325.

6. Sowers, M. R., Wallace, R. B., and Lemke, J. H. "The association of intakes of vitamin D and calcium with blood pressure among women." *American Journal of Clinical Nutrition* 1985; 42: 135–142.

7. Weed, S. *The Menopausal Years: The Wise Woman Way.* Woodstock, N.Y.: Ash Tree, 1992.

8. Sojka, J. E., and Weaver, C. M. "Magnesium supplementation and osteoporosis." *Nutrition Reviews* 1995; 53(3): 71–80.

9. Abraham, G. E., and Grewal, H. "A total dietary program emphasizing magnesium instead of calcium." *Journal of Reproductive Medicine* 1990; 35: 503–507.

10. Koskinen, T., Pyykko, K., Kudo, R., Jokela, H., and Punnonen, R. "Serum selenium, vitamin A, vitamin E and cholesterol concentrations in Finnish and Japanese postmenopausal women." *International Journal for Vitamin and Nutrition Research* 1987; 57: 111–114.

11. Free-Graves, J., et al. "Manganese status of osteoporotics and age matched, healthy women." *FASEB Journal* 1990; 4: A777.

12. National Research Council. *Recommended Dietary Allowances.* Washington, D.C.: National Academy, 1989, p. 186.

13. Notelovitz, M., and Tonnessen, D. *Menopause and Midlife Health.* New York: St. Martin's Press, 1993, p. 86.

14. Krall, E. A., et al. "Effect of vitamin D intake on seasonal variations in parathyroid hormone secretion in postmenopausal women." *New England Journal of Medicine* 1989; 321: 1777–1783.

15. Willett, W. C., and Stampfer, M. J. "What vitamin should I be taking, doctor?" *New England Journal of Medicine* 2001; 345(25): 1819–1824.

16. Sultenfuss, S. W., and Sultenfuss, T. J. *A Woman's Guide to Vitamins and Minerals.* Chicago: Contemporary, 1995.

17. Cargill, M. *Acupuncture: A Viable Medical Alternative.* Westport, Conn.: Praeger, 1994, p. 26.

18. Wolfe, H. L. *Menopause: A Second Spring.* Boulder, Colo.: Blue Poppy, 1995.

19. Dickens, P., Tai, Y. T., But, P. P., Tomlinson, B., Ng, H. K., and Yan, K. W. "Fatal accident aconitine poisoning following ingestion of Chinese herbal medicine: A report of two cases." *Forensic Science International* 1994; 67(1): 55–58.

20. Gertner, E., Marshall, P. S., Filandrinos, D., Potek, A. S., and Smith, T. M. "Complications resulting from the use of Chinese herbal medications containing undeclared prescription drugs." *Arthritis Rheumatism* 1995; 38(5): 614–617.

21. Chan, T. Y., Chan, A. Y., and Critchley, J. A. "Hospital admissions due to adverse reactions to Chinese herbal medicines." *Journal of Tropical Medicine Hygiene* 1992; 95(4): 296–298.

22. Yamamoto, M., Uemura, T., Nakama, S., Uemiya, M., and Kumagai, A. "Serum HDL-cholesterol-increasing and fatty liver improving actions of Panax ginseng in high-cholesterol-diet fed rats with clinical effect on hyperlipidemia in man." *American Journal of Chinese Medicine* 1983; 11(1–4): 96–101.

23. Bai, Y. R., and Wang, S. Z. "Hemodynamic study on nitroglycerin compared with salvia miltiorrhiza chung kuo." *Chung Hsi I Chieh Ho Tsa Chih* 1994; 14(1): 24–25.

24. Jiu, L. J., Morikawa, N., Omi, N., and Ezawa, I. "The effect of tochu bark on bone metabolism in the rat model with ovariectomized osteoporosis." *Nutrition Science Vitaminology* 1994; 40(3): 261–273.

25. Chopra, D. *Perfect Health.* New York: Harmony, 1991.

26. Ibid.

27. Thakur, C. P., Thakur, B., Singh, S., Sinha, P. K., and Sinha, S. K. "The ayurvedic medicines haritaki, amala, and bahira reduce cholesterol-induced atherosclerosis in rabbits." *International Journal of Cardiology* 1988; 21(2): 167–175.

28. Shaila, H. P., Udupa, A. L., and Udupa, S. L. "Preventative actions of *Terminalia belerica* in experimentally induced atherosclerosis." *Journal of Cardiology* 1995; 49(2): 101–106.
    Sharma, H. M., Hanna, A. N., Kauffman, E. M., and Newman, H. A. "Inhibition of human low-density lipoprotein oxidation in vitro by Maharishi Ayur-Veda herbal mixtures." *Pharmacology, Biochemistry, and Behavior* 1992; 43(4): 1175–1182.
    Shanmugasundaram, E. R., Sundaram, P., Srinivas, K., Shanmugasundaram, K. R., and Shankara, J. R. "Double-blind crossover study of modified Anna Pavala Sindhooram in patients with hyperlipidemia or ischemic heart disease." *Ethnopharmacology* 1991; 31(1): 85–99.

29. Zamarra, J. W., Schneider, R. H., Besseghini, I., Robinson, D. K., and Salerno, J. W. "Usefulness of the transcendental meditation program in the treatment of patients with coronary heart disease." *American Journal of Cardiology* 1996; 77(10): 867–870.

30. Schneider, R. H., Staggers, F., Alexander, C. N., Sheppard, W., Rainforth, M., Kondwani, K., Smith, S., and King, C. G. "A randomized controlled trial of stress reduction for hypertension in older African Americans." *Hypertension* 1995; 26(5): 820–827.

31. Collinge, W. *The American Holistic Health Association Complete Guide to Alternative Medicine.* New York: Warner, 1996.

Chapter 14. Drugs: Other Means of Prevention

1. Landman, J. O., Hamdy, N. A., Pauwels, E. K., and Papapoulos, S. E. "Skeletal metabolism in patients with osteoporosis after discontinuation of long-term treatment with oral pamidronate." *Journal of Clinical Endocrinology Metabolism* 1995; 8 (12): 3465–3468.

2. Black, D. M., Cummings, S. R., Karpf, D. B., et al. "Randomized trial of effect of alendronate on risk of fracture in women with existing vertebral fractures." *Lancet* 1996; 348: 1535–1541.

3. Cummings, S. R., Black, D. M., Thompson, D. E., et al. "Effect of alendronate on risk of fracture in women with low bone density but without vertebral

fractures: Results from the Fracture Intervention Trial." *Journal of the American Medical Association* 1998; 280: 2077–2082.

4. McClung, M. R., Geusens, P., Miller, P. D., et al. "Effect of risedronate on the risk of hip fracture in elderly women." *New England Journal of Medicine* 2001; 344: 333–340.

5. Anonymous. "Warning about oesophagitis with Fosamax." *Lancet* 1996; 347: 959.

6. Reginster, J. Y., Deroisy, R., Lecart, M. P., Sarlet, N., Zegels, B., Jupsin, I., de Longueville, M., and Franchimont, P. "A double-blind, placebo-controlled, dose-finding trial of intermittent nasal salmon calcitonin for prevention of postmenopausal lumbar spine bone loss." *American Journal of Medicine* 1995; 98: 452–458.

7. Rico, H., Revilla, M., Hernandez, E. R., Villa, L. F., and Alvarez de Buergo, M. "Total and regional bone mineral content and fracture rate in postmenopausal osteoporosis treated with salmon calcitonin: A prospective study." *Calcified Tissue International* 1995; 56: 181–185.

8. Downs, R. W., Bell, N. H., Ettinger, M. P., et al. "Comparison of alendronate and intranasal calcitonin for treatment of osteoporosis in postmenopausal women." *Journal of Clinical Endocrinology and Metabolism* 2000; 85: 1783–1788.

9. Lyritis, G. P., Tsakalakos, N., Magiasis, B., Karachalios, T., Yiatzides, A., and Tsekoura, M. "Analgesic effect of salmon calcitonin in osteoporotic vertebral fractures: A double-blind placebo-controlled clinical study." *Calcified Tissue International* 1991; 49: 369–372.

10. Neer, R. M., Arnaud, C. D., Zanchetta, J. R., et al. "Effect of parathyroid hormone (1-34) on fracture and bone mineral density in postmenopausal women with osteoporosis." *New England Journal of Medicine* 2001; 344: 1434–1441.

11. Brandi, M. L. "New treatment strategies: Ipriflavone, strontium, vitamin D metabolites and analogs." *American Journal of Medicine* 1993; 95: 5A69S–5A74S.

12. Alexandersen, P., Toussaint, A., Christiansen, C., et al. "Ipriflavone in the treatment of postmenopausal osteoporosis: A randomized controlled trial." *Journal of the American Medical Association* 2001; 285: 1482–1488.

13. Early Breast Cancer Trialists' Collaborative Group. "Tamoxifen for early breast cancer: An overview of the randomised trials." *Lancet* 1998; 351(9114): 1451–1467.

14. Ettinger, B., Black, D. M., Mitlak, B. H., et al. "Reduction of vertebral fracture risk in postmenopausal women with osteoporosis treated with raloxifene: Results from a 3-year randomized clinical trial." *Journal of the American Medical Association* 1999; 282: 637–645.

15. Kloosterboer, H. "Intracrinology: The secret of the tissue-specificity of tibolone." *Journal of British Menopause Society* 2000; 6 (Suppl): 23–27.

16. Valdivia, I., and Ortega, D. "Mammographic density in postmenopausal women treated with tibolone, etriol or conventional hormone replacement therapy." *Clinical Drug Investigations* 2000; 20: 101–107.
    Gompel, A., Kandouz, M., Siromachkova, M., et al. "The effects of tibolone on proliferation, differentiation and apoptosis in human breast cells." *Gynecology and Endocrinology* 1997: 11 (Suppl 1): 77–79.

17. Tax, L., Goorstein, E., Kicovic, P. "Clinical profile of Org OD 14." *Maturitas* 1987; (Suppl 1): 3–13.

18. Moore, R. A. "Livial: A review of clinical studies." *British Journal of Obstetrics and Gynaecology* 1999; 106 (Suppl 19): 1–21.

19. Gotto, A. M., Jr. "Primary and secondary prevention of coronary artery disease." *Current Opinion Cardiology* 1992; 7: 553.

20. Bradford, R. H., Downtown, M., Chremos, A. N., et al. "Efficacy and tolerability of lovastatin in 3390 women with moderate hypercholesterolemia." *Annals of Internal Medicine* 1993; 118: 50.

21. "The Scandinavian Simvastatin Survival Study Group randomized trial of cholesterol lowering in 4444 patients with coronary heart disease. The Scandinavian Simvastatin Survival Study (4S)." *Lancet* 1994; 344: 1383.

22. Manson, J. E., Stampfer, M. J., Colditz, G. A., Willet, W. C., Rosner, B., Speizer, F. E., and Hennekens, C. H. "A prospective study of aspirin use and primary prevention of cardiovascular disease in women." *Journal of the American Medical Association* 1991; 266: 521–527.

23. SHEP Cooperative Research Group. "Prevention of stroke by antihypertensive drug treatment in older persons with isolated systolic hypertension: Final results of the Systolic Hypertensions in the Elderly Program (SHEP)." *Journal of the American Medical Association* 1991; 265: 3255–3264.
    Staessen, J. A., Fagard, R., Thijis, L., et al. "Randomized double blind comparison of placebo and active treatment for older patients with isolated systolic hypertension. The Systolic Hypertension in Europe (Syst-Eur) Trial Investigators." *Lancet* 1997; 350: 757–764.

24. Yusuf, S., Sleight, P., et al. "Effects of an angiotensin-converting-enzyme inhibitor, rampiril, on cardiovascular events in high-risk patients. The Heart Outcomes Prevention Evaluation Study Investigators." *New England Journal of Medicine* 2000; 342: 145–153.

Chapter 15. Hormones: The Menu of Options

1. Spicer, D., Pike, M. C., and Henderson, B. E. "The question of estrogen replacement therapy in patients with a prior diagnosis of breast cancer." *Oncology* 1990; 4(12): 49–59.

2. McDonnell, D. P., Clemm, D. L., Hermann, T., Goldman, M. E., and Pike, J. W. "Analysis of estrogen receptor function in vitro reveals three distinct classes of antiestrogens." *Molecular Endocrinology* 1995; 9: 659–669.

3. McDonnell, D. P., Clevenger, B., Dana, S. L., Santiso-Mere, D., Tzukerman, T., and Gleeson, M. A. "The mechanism of action of steroid hormones: A new twist to an old tale." *Journal of Clinical Pharmacology* 1993; 33: 1165–1172.

4. Shang, Y., and Brown, M. "Molecular determinants for the tissue specificity of SERMs." *Science* 2002; 295 (29): 2465–2468.

5. Clark, J. H., Paszko, Z., and Peck, E. J., Jr. "Nuclear binding and retention of the receptor estrogen complex: Relation to the agonistic and antagonistic properties of estriol." *Endocrinology* 1977; 100(1): 91–96.

6. Whittaker, P. G., Morgan, M. R., Dean, P. D., Cameron, E. H., and Lind, T. "Serum equilin, oestrone, and oestradiol levels in postmenopausal women receiving conjugated equine oestrogens ('Premarin')." *Lancet* 1980; 1(8158): 14–16.

7. Barrett-Connor, Elizabeth. Personal communication, 1996.

8. Ettinger, B., Pressman, A., and Van Gessel A. "Low-dosage esterified estrogens opposed by progestin at 6-month intervals." *Obstetrics and Gynecology* 2001; 98: 205–211.

9. Ettinger, B., Golditch, I. M., and Friedman, G. "Gynecologic consequences of long-term unopposed estrogen replacement therapy." *Maturitas* 1988; 10: 271–282.

10. Grady, D. "Clinical crossroads: 60-year-old woman trying to discontinue Hormone Replacement Therapy." *Journal of the American Medical Association* 2002; 287(16): 2130–2137.

11. Lemon, H. M. "Antimammary carcinogenic activity of 17–alpha-ethinyl estiol." *Cancer* 1987; 60(12): 2873–2881.

12. Adlercreutz, H., Gorbach, S. L., Goldin, B. R., Woods, M. N., Dwyer, J. T., and Hamalainen, E. "Estrogen metabolism and excretion in Oriental and Caucasian women." *Journal of the National Cancer Institute* 1994; 86(14): 1076–1082.

13. Going, J. J., Anderson, T. J., Battersby, S., et al. "Proliferative and secretory activity in human breast during natural and artificial menstrual cycles." *American Journal of Pathology* 1988; 130: 193–204.

14. Chang, K. J., Fournier, S., Lee, T. T., de Lignieres, B., and Linares-Cruz, G. "Influences of percutaneous administration of estradiol and progesterone on human breast epithelial cell cycle in vivo." *Fertility and Sterility* 1995; 63(4): 785–791.

15. Groshong, S. D., Owen, G. I., et al. "Biphasic regulation of breast cancer cell growth by progesterone: Role of the cyclin-dependent kinase inhibitors, p21 and p27." *Molecular Endocrinology* 1997; 11: 1593–1607.

16. Ewertz, M. "Influence of non-contraceptive exogenous and endogenous sex hormones on breast cancer risk in Denmark." *International Journal of Cancer* 1988; 42: 832–838.
    Bergkvist, L. et al. "The risk of breast cancer after estrogen and estrogen-progestin replacement." *New England Journal of Medicine* 1989; 321: 293–297.
    Hunt, K., et al. "Long-term surveillance of mortality and cancer incidence in women receiving hormone replacement therapy." *British Journal of Obstetrics and Gynecology* 1987; 94: 620–635.
    Magnusson, C., et al. "Breast cancer risk following long-term oestrogen- and oestrogen-progestin-replacement therapy." *International Journal of Cancer* 1999; 81: 339–344.

17. Writing Group for the PEPI Trial. "Effects of estrogen or estrogen/progestin regimens on heart disease risk factors in postmenopausal women." *Journal of the American Medical Association* 1994; 273(3): 199–208.

18. Prior, J. C. "Progesterone as a bone-trophic hormone." *Endocrine Reviews* 1990; 11(2): 386–398.

19. Greendale, G. A., Reboussin, B. A., et al. "Effects of estrogen and estrogen-progestin on mammographic parenchymal density. Postmenopausal Estrogen/Progestin Interventions (PEPI) Investigators." *Annals of Internal Medicine* 1999; 130 (Feb 16, 4 pt 1): 262–269.

20. Greendale, G. A., Reboussin, B. A., et al. "Symptom relief and side effects of postmenopausal hormones: Results from the Postmenopausal Estrogen/Progestin Interventions Trial." *Obstetrics and Gynecology* 1998; 92(6): 982–988.

21. Groshong, S. D., op. cit.

22. Plu-Bureau, Le M. G., et al. "Progestogen use and decreased risk of breast cancer in a cohort study of premenopausal women with benign breast disease." *British Journal of Cancer* 1994; 70: 270–277.

23. Leonetti, H. B., Longo, S., and Anasti, J. N. "Transdermal progesterone cream for vasomotor symptoms and postmenopausal bone loss." *Obstetrics and Gynecology* 1999; 94: 225–228.

24. Lee, J. R. "Osteoporosis reversal with transdermal progesterone." *Lancet* 1990; 336: 1327.
   Riis, B. J., et al. "The effect of percutaneous estraciol and natural progesterone on postmenopausal bone loss." *American Journal of Obstetrics and Gynecology* 1987; 156: 61–65.

25. Writing Group for the PEPI Trial, op. cit.

26. Marslew, U., Riis, B. J., and Christiansen, C. "Bleeding patterns during continuous combined estrogen-progestogen therapy." *American Journal of Obstetrics and Gynecology* 1991; 164: 1163–1168.

27. Hickok, L. R., Toomey, C., and Speroff, L. "A comparison of esterified estrogens with and without Methyltestosterone: Effects on endometrial histology and serum lipoproteins in postmenopausal women." *Obstetrics and Gynecology* 1993; 82: 919–924.

28. Colditz, G. A., Hankinson, S. E., Hunter, D. J., Willet, W. C., Manson, J. E., Stampfer, M. J., Hennekens, C., Roser, B., and Speizer, F. E. "The use of estrogens and progestins and the risk of breast cancer in postmenopausal women." *New England Journal of Medicine* 1995; 332: 1589–1593.

29. Rako, S. *The Hormone of Desire.* New York: Harmony Books, 1996.

Chapter 16. Decisions: What Should I Do?

1. Grady, D., Herrrington, D., Bittner, V., et al. "Cardiovascular disease outcomes during 6.8 years of hormone therapy: Heart and estrogen/progestin replacement study follow-up (HERS II). *Journal of the American Medical Association* 2002; 288: 49–57.
   Writing Group for the Women's Health Initiative Investigators. "Risks and benefits of estrogen plus progestin in healthy postmenopausal women: Principal results from the Women's Health Initiative randomized controlled trial." *Journal of the American Medical Association* 2002; 288 (3): 321–333.

2. Foundation for Informed Medical Decision Making. *Hormone Replacement Therapy. A Shared Decision Making Program Videotape*, Boston MA: Foundation for Informed Decision Making, 1995.

3. Grady, D., Rubin, S. M., Petitti, D. B., et al. "Hormone therapy to prevent disease and prolong life in postmenopausal women." *Annals of Internal Medicine* 1992; 117(12): 1016.

4. Greendale, G. A., Espeland, M., Slone, S., Marcus, R., Barrett-Connor, E. "Bone mass response to discontinuation of long-term hormone replacement therapy: Results from the Postmenopausal Estrogen/Progestin Interventions (PEPI) safety follow-up study." *Archives of Internal Medicine* 2002; 162 (6): 665–72.

5. Nelson, H. D., Humphrey, L. L., Nygren, P., Teutch, S. M., Allan, J. D. "Postmenopausal hormone replacement therapy: Scientific review." *Journal of the American Medical Association* 2002; 288: 872–881.

6. Writing Group for the Women's Health Initiative Investigators, op. cit.

7. Grady, D. "Postmenopausal hormone therapy: Balancing the risks and benefits," Presentation at the NIH Scientific Workshop on Menopausal Hormone Therapy, Bethesda, MD, October 23, 2002.

8. Ibid.

9. Ibid.

10. Blair, S. N., Kohl, H. W., Paffenbarger, R. S., Clark, D. G., Cooper, K. H., and Gibbons, L. W. "Physical fitness and all-cause mortality: A prospective study of healthy men and women." *Journal of the American Medical Association* 1989; 262: 2395–2401.

INDEX

About the Author

SUSAN M. LOVE, M.D., is an author, teacher, surgeon, researcher, and activist. She has written many books and articles, including *Atlas of Techniques in Breast Surgery* and *Dr. Susan Love's Breast Book*, which has been called the bible for women with breast cancer. In 1996, after twenty years of direct patient care, Dr. Love left clinical practice to devote more time to her basic research as an adjunct professor of clinical surgery at UCLA and president of the Susan Love, M.D., Breast Cancer Foundation, a nonprofit organization dedicated to the eradication of breast cancer. She lives in Southern California with her life partner, Helen Cooksey; their daughter, Katie; Brownie and Maggie, the dogs; and Cream and Pickle, the cats.

If you are interested in supporting her work, you can reach her at Susan Love, M.D., Breast Cancer Foundation, P.O. Box 846, Pacific Palisades, CA 90272, or at www.SusanLoveMD.org.

KAREN LINDSEY is the coauthor of *Dr. Susan Love's Breast Book*. She is the author of *Friends as Family* and *Divorced, Beheaded, Survived: A Feminist Reinterpretation of the Wives of Henry VIII*. She teaches writing at Emerson College and women's studies at the University of Massachusetts in Boston.